Probiotics
A Clinical Guide

Probiotics
A CLINICAL GUIDE

Martin H. Floch, MD, MACG, FACP, AGAF
Chief of Ambulatory Gastroenterology
Yale New Haven Hospital
Clinical Professor
Yale Medical Group, Digestive Disease Section
New Haven, CT

Adam S. Kim, MD
Minnesota Gastroenterology, PA
Minneapolis, MN

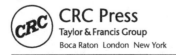
CRC Press
Taylor & Francis Group
Boca Raton London New York

CRC Press is an imprint of the
Taylor & Francis Group, an **informa** business

First published 2010 by SLACK Incorporated

Published 2024 by CRC Press
2385 NW Executive Center Drive, Suite 320, Boca Raton FL 33431

and by CRC Press
4 Park Square, Milton Park, Abingdon, Oxon, OX14 4RN

CRC Press is an imprint of Taylor & Francis Group, LLC

Library of Congress Cataloging-in-Publication Data

Probiotics : a clinical guide / [edited by] Martin H. Floch, Adam S. Kim.
   p. ; cm.
  Includes bibliographical references.
  ISBN 978-1-55642-909-5
 1. Probiotics--Therapeutic use. I. Floch, Martin H. II. Kim, Adam S.
 [DNLM: 1. Probiotics--therapeutic use. QU 145.5 P9213 2010]
 RM666.P835P76 2010
 615'.329--dc22

                              2010004022

ISBN: 9781556429095 (pbk)
ISBN: 9781003525967 (ebk)

DOI: 10.1201/9781003525967

DEDICATION

To our wives, Gladys Floch and Stephanie Kim.

CONTENTS

SECTION I: BASIC PHYSIOLOGY

ABOUT THE EDITORS

Martin H. Floch, MD, MACG, FACP, AGAF is a graduate of New York University, has a master's degree from the University of New Hampshire in Durham, and received his MD from New York Medical College, Valhalla, NY. He completed his residency at Beth Israel Hospital, New York and gastroenterology training at the former Seton Hall College of Medicine, South Orange, NJ.

He is a Master of the American College of Gastroenterology, and a Fellow of the American College of Physicians, as well as the American Gastroenterology Association. Dr. Floch has had numerous NIH grants at Yale University, New Haven and Norwalk Hospital, Norwalk, CT. He was Chairman of Internal Medicine at Norwalk Hospital from 1970 to 1994, and founding Chief of Gastroenterology and Nutrition at Norwalk Hospital, which he assumed after founding the Norwalk Medical Group.

Presently Dr. Floch is Chief of Ambulatory Gastroenterology at Yale New Haven Hospital and sees patients as well as teaches at the Yale Medical Group, Digestive Disease Section. In addition to his clinical responsibilities, Dr. Floch is conducting research on irritable bowel syndrome (IBS), diverticulitis, and probiotics. A registry for IBS patients has been formed and there will be several trials of the effects of probiotics on IBS patients. Dr. Floch is renowned for his work in probiotics, and has lectured on the subject at numerous universities and medical centers in this country and internationally.

Adam S. Kim, MD was raised in the suburbs of Minneapolis, Minnesota and is currently a gastroenterologist working in the Twin Cities area with Minnesota Gastroenterology, PA.

He received his bachelor's degree at Colorado College in Colorado Springs. He then attended medical school at the University of Minnesota, where he studied the intestinal flora and its role in disease and health. Dr. Kim completed his Internal Medicine Internship and Residency at Hennepin County Medical Center in Minneapolis, Minnesota. He then went on to complete his Gastroenterology Fellowship at Yale University School of Medicine in New Haven, Connecticut.

During his time at Yale University, Dr. Kim became increasingly interested in the use of probiotics and started collaborating with Dr. Martin Floch on how best to use probiotics in clinical medicine.

CONTRIBUTING AUTHORS

Katie L. Blackett, BSc, PhD (Chapter 7)
Research Scientist
University of Dundee
Centre for Oncology and Molecular
Medicine
Ninewells Hospital Medical School
Dundee, UK

Ian M. Carroll, PhD (Chapter 5)
Assistant Professor of Medicine
Division of Gastroenterology
and Hepatology
University of North Carolina
Chapel Hill, NC

Erika C. Claud, MD (Chapter 12)
Assistant Professor
Departments of Pediatrics and Medicine
Sections of Neonatology and
Gastroenterology
University of Chicago
Chicago, IL

Anne M. Dattilo, PhD, RD, CDE (Chapter 11)
Nutrition Research and Practice Service
Lemont, PA

Levinus A. Dieleman, MD, PhD (Chapter 17)
Associate Professor of Medicine
Division of Gastroenterology
University of Alberta
Edmonton, AB, Canada

Shira Doron, MD (Chapter 16)
Assistant Professor of Medicine
Tufts University School of Medicine
Attending Physician
Division of Geographic Medicine and
Infectious Diseases
Tufts Medical Center
Boston, MA

Sylvia H. Duncan, BSc, PhD (Chapter 6)
Research Scientist
Gut Health Division
Microbial Ecology Group
Rowett Institute of Nutrition and Health
University of Aberdeen
Aberdeen, UK

Giuseppe Famularo, MD, PhD (Chapter 21)
Department of Internal Medicine
San Camillo Hospital
Rome, Italy

Richard N. Fedorak, MD, FRCP(C) (Chapter 18)
Division of Gastroenterology
University of Alberta
Edmonton, AB, Canada

Harry J. Flint, BSc, PhD (Chapter 6)
Head of the Gut Health Division
Leader of the Microbial
Ecology Group
Rowett Institute of Nutrition and Health
University of Aberdeen
Aberdeen, UK

Miguel Freitas, PhD (Chapter 10)
Health Affairs Director
The Dannon Company Inc.
White Plains, NY

Pramod Gopal, PhD (Chapter 9)
Principal Research Scientist
Digestive and Immune Health
Fonterra Research Centre
Palmerston North, New Zealand

Sherwood L. Gorbach, MD (Chapter 16)
Distinguished Professor, Departments of
Public Health & Medicine
Tufts University School of Medicine
Attending Physician
Division of Infectious Diseases
Tufts Medical Center
Boston, MA

Stefano Guandalini, MD (Chapter 13)
Professor and Chief
Section of Pediatric Gastroenterology
University of Chicago
Founder and Medical Director
Celiac Disease Center
Chicago, IL

Mario Guslandi, MD, FACG (Chapter 19)
Head, Clinical Hepato-Gastroenterology
Unit
Gastroenterology Division
S. Raffaele University Hospital
Milan, Italy

Ailsa Hart, PhD (Chapter 2)
Consultant Gastroenterologist
St. Mark's Hospital
Clinical Senior Lecturer
Imperial College London
London, UK

Laurel H. Hartwell, MD (Chapter 14)
Department of Medicine
Oregon Health and Science University
Portland, OR

Erika Isolauri, MD, PhD (Chapter 4)
Professor (Pediatrics)
University of Turku
Department of Pediatrics
Turku University Hospital
Turku, Finland

Karen Kroeker, MD, FRCP(C) (Chapters 17,
18)
University of Alberta
Edmonton, AB, Canada

Kirsi Laitinen, PhD (Chapter 4)
Senior Lecturer
Department of Biochemistry and
Food Chemistry
Functional Foods Forum
University of Turku
Turku, Finland

George T. Macfarlane, BSc, PhD (Chapter 7)
Professor of Bacteriology
University of Dundee
Centre for Oncology and Molecular
Medicine
Ninewells Hospital Medical School
Dundee, UK

Sandra Macfarlane, BSc, PhD (Chapter 7)
Senior Research Scientist
University of Dundee
Centre for Oncology and Molecular
Medicine
Ninewells Hospital Medical School
Dundee, UK

Karen L. Madsen, PhD (Chapter 3)
Professor, Department of Medicine
Division of Gastroenterology
University of Alberta
Edmonton, AB, Canada

Paola Mastromarino, PhD (Chapter 24)
Department of Public Health Sciences
Section of Microbiology
Sapienza University School of Medicine
Rome, Italy

Daniel Merenstein, MD (Chapter 8)
Assistant Professor
Director of Research Programs
Department of Family Medicine
Georgetown University Medical Center
Washington, DC

Giovanni Minisola, MD (Chapter 21)
Department of Internal Medicine,
Rheumatology Unit
San Camillo Hospital
Rome, Italy

Luciana Mosca, PhD (Chapters 21, 24)
Department of Biochemical Sciences
Sapienza University School of Medicine
Rome, Italy

Peter Neuhaus, PhD (Chapter 15)
Department of General, Visceral, and
Transplant Surgery
Charité Campus Virchow Clinic
Berlin, Germany

Siew C. Ng, PhD (Chapter 2)
Institute of Digestive Disease
Prince of Wales Hospital
Chinese University of Hong Kong
Shatin, Hong Kong

Eamonn M. M. Quigley, MD, FRCP, FACP,
FACG, FRCPI (Chapter 20)
Alimentary Pharmabiotic Centre
Department of Medicine
University College Cork
Cork, Ireland

Samuli Rautava, MD, PhD (Chapter 4)
Department of Pediatrics
Turku University Hospital
University of Turku
Turku, Finland

Nada Rayes, MD (Chapter 15)
Department of General, Visceral, and
Transplant Surgery
Charité Campus Virchow Clinic
Berlin, Germany

Yehuda Ringel, MD (Chapter 5)
Associate Professor of Medicine
Division of Gastroenterology
and Hepatology
University of North Carolina
Chapel Hill, NC

Tamar Ringel-Kulka, MD, MPH (Chapter 5)
Department of Maternal and Child Health
Gillings School of Global Public Health
University of North Carolina
Chapel Hill, NC

Jose M. Saavedra, MD, FAAP (Chapter 11)
Medical and Scientific Director
Nestlé Nutrition North America
Associate Professor of Pediatrics
Johns Hopkins University School of Medicine
Baltimore, MD

Seppo Salminen, PhD (Chapter 4)
Professor (Food Development)
Director, Functional Foods Forum
University of Turku
Turku, Finland

Mary Ellen Sanders, PhD (Chapter 8)
Consultant, Dairy & Food Culture
Technologies
Executive Director, International Scientific
Association for Probiotics and Prebiotics
Centennial, CO

Daniel Seehofer, MD (Chapter 15)
Department of General, Visceral, and
Transplant Surgery
Charité Campus Virchow Clinic
Berlin, Germany

Anish Sheth, MD (Chapter 23)
Assistant Professor
Director, Gastrointestinal
Motility Program
Yale University School of Medicine
Division of Digestive Diseases
New Haven, CT

Christina M. Surawicz, MD, MACG
(Chapter 14)
Professor of Medicine
Assistant Dean for Faculty Development
University of Washington School of Medicine
Section Chief of Gastroenterology
Harborview Medical Center
Seattle, WA

Gerald W. Tannock, PhD (Chapter 9)
Professor in Microbiology
Department of Microbiology & Immunology
University of Otago
Dunedin, New Zealand

Vito Trinchieri, MD (Chapter 21)
Infectious Diseases
University La Sapienza
Rome, Italy

Beatrice Vitali, PhD (Chapter 24)
Department of Pharmaceutical Sciences
University of Bologna
Bologna, Italy

W. Allan Walker, MD (Chapter 12)
Conrad Taff Professor of Nutrition
Harvard Medical School
Chief, Mucosal Immunology Laboratory
Pediatric Gastroenterology and Nutrition
Massachusetts General Hospital
for Children
Charlestown, MA

PREFACE

My experiences in the field of microbiology began while I was a graduate student at the University of New Hampshire, continued as a laboratory assistant at New York Medical College, and throughout my medical school training. With this gastroenterology training and U.S. Army Research Command active duty, I obtained an NIH grant in 1967 as a faculty member of Yale and began to study the importance of the anaerobic flora in the gastrointestinal tract. Stimulated by the works of Dubos and Shaedler, and Moore and Holdeman, we began to identify the human fecal anaerobic flora. The predominance of anaerobes was established in the tract. In those years, the anaerobic flora was identified by difficult growth and biochemical techniques. It was common for us to identify those organisms by their short-chain fatty acid production. At that point in time, we did not realize the importance of probiotics. However, those culture identification techniques have proven significant. Probiotics, as part of the anaerobic and gut flora, were clearly defined and their importance accepted by world authorities in 1990 to 2000.

This past year, SLACK asked me whether I thought it was time to bring out a book on "human" probiotic use. I could not resist the opportunity and, hence, this book was born.

The book is divided into two parts. Basic physiology is covered in the first half of the book. We attempt to explain the role of the microbiota and discuss the role of host physiology in intestinal microecology and the effects of the microbiota on the host. In the next chapters, Drs. Hart and Ng review intraluminal defenses, and Dr. Madsen the barrier function and the immune response. The allergic response is reviewed by Drs. Isolauri and Rautava, Laitinen and Salminen. Drs. Carroll, Ringel-Kulka, and Ringel describe the methods for identifying the microbiota and probiotic organisms. Drs. Flint and Duncan and Drs. George Macfarlane, Sandra Macfarlane and Blackett describe the importance of intestinal nutrients and fermentation in the gut. Since probiotics are widely administered in yogurts, Drs. Sanders and Merenstein explain yogurts as a vehicle, and Dr. Freitas reviews the methods employed by industry in the production of quality yogurts. Dr. Tannock, who edited the first important books on probiotics in this era, is joined by Dr. Gopal to elaborate on the problem of administration of single or multiple strains in probiotic supplements.

In the second part of the book, we have been fortunate to involve the experienced clinicians and prominent authors of probiotic therapy to review the literature on the clinical use of probiotics and make clinical recommendations where they are applicable. Dr. Saavedra, who is vastly experienced in this field, is joined by Dr. Dattilo to elaborate on the clinical application of probiotics in pediatrics. Drs. Walker and Claud review their exciting work in enterocolitis. Dr. Guandalini discusses and reviews the entire literature on probiotic use in diarrheal diseases, and Drs. Surawicz and Hartwell review the problems of antibiotic-associated diarrhea and *Clostridium difficile* infection. The use, treatment, and prevention of surgical infections, a clinical situation which is very important to practitioners, is reviewed by Dr. Rayes. Drs. Doran and Gorbach discuss the extensive opinions regarding the clinical use of probiotics in allergic disorders. Inflammatory bowel disease is a major treatment problem for patients and gastroenterologists, and Drs. Kroeker and Dieleman discuss the use of probiotics in ulcerative colitis, Drs. Kroeker and Fedorak in Crohn's disease, and Dr. Guslandi in pouchitis. Irritable bowel syndrome is becoming one of the most difficult problems to treat in primary care medicine and gastroenterology practice. Probiotic therapy for IBS is discussed and reviewed by Dr. Quigley. The use of radiation for pelvic or abdominal cancers is now a preferred therapy. Consequently, the evolving role of radiation enteritis is a problem. The use of probiotics in this situation may be helpful and is reviewed by Drs. Famularo, Trinchieri, Mosca, and Minisola. Helicobacter pylori is one of the most common infections in humans worldwide. Although it is treated with antibiotics, there are patients with resistant strains, and it appears that probiotics can assist in the effectiveness of antibiotics. This literature is reviewed by Dr. Kim. Drs. Kim and Sheth discuss the potential emerging role in chronic liver disease. The use in vaginal infections is extensively reviewed by Drs. Mastromarino, Vitali and Mosca.

I am grateful to all of these authors for their thorough and extensive contributions. We all hope this book helps clinicians in their understanding of probiotics and helps them make the best possible recommendations for their use.

We are grateful to the staff at SLACK, especially Carrie Kotlar, who brought this idea to us and helped design the book.

Martin H. Floch, MD, MACG, FACP, AGAF

INTRODUCTION

There are numerous topics covered in this book that are defined by many groups differently. In order to try to clarify some varying opinions, this Introduction attempts to define some terms used in accordance with standard references.

Probiotics

The Food and Agriculture Organization (FAO) of the United Nations defines probiotics as "Live microorganisms which, when administered in adequate amounts, confer a health benefit on the host."[1] Fuller's original definition was "live microbial food supplements which beneficially affect the host animal by improving its intestinal microbial balance."[2] Metchnikoff's original theories stated that probiotics were bacteria and came from the human large bowel. Other definitions included the terms "human" and "bacteria" in the definition; but at this time, with the inclusion of certain fungi and the fact that probiotics are used extensively in veterinary medicine, the definition of the FAO/WHO is the best definition to be used.

Strains

It is also important to emphasize the fact that strains of probiotic organisms have very specific proteins, enzymes, and biochemical reactions. Certainly, they may overlap—eg, they produce lactic acid but in varying amounts. However, their effect on specific functions of the intestinal mucosa, such as toll-like receptors and stimulation of dendritic cells, may well depend completely on a specific strain's chemical makeup. Therefore, we strongly recommend that only strains that have demonstrated effectiveness via clinical controlled studies should be used in an attempt to replicate a clinical response. This information is stressed in the chapters on basic physiology, and in the chapters recommending use of specific strains in a specific disorder or disease.

Prebiotics

The original definition of probiotics as presented by Gibson and Roberfroid in 1995 has persisted: "Non-digestible dietary ingredients that beneficially affect the host by selectively stimulating the growth and/or activity of one or a limited number of bacteria in the colon, thus improving host health."[3] This definition includes substances that are natural as well as those produced chemically. The concept is important, and the definition originally proposed by Gibson and Roberfroid is still accepted. Therefore, certain dietary fiber substances would be included under this definition.

Dietary Fiber

There are numerous definitions in the literature for dietary fiber. It is difficult to define because it depends on the chemical analysis employed and the substances that result from that analysis. However, certain generalities can be made.

The classic definition put forth by Trowell could be summarized as "plant non-starch polysaccharides that are not digested by human enzymes." This is a simple definition, but still a good one and it includes cell wall substances such as cellulose, semi-celluloses, pectin, and lignin, as well intracellular polysaccharides such as gums and mucilages.[4] More complex definitions are available, but they are detailed and described carefully by Spiller.[5] Regardless of the definition, the concept of dietary fiber is that they are plant polysaccharides that are poorly digested by human enzymes. The details of other definitions depend on the chemical analyses.

Resistant Starch

Resistant starch is a term that has gathered momentum and is used in experiments. Based on the chemical analysis of Englyst, it is defined as "starch that is not digested by human enzymes that reach the colon."[5]

Safety and Complications

Probiotics are sold without prescription and are also widely used in clinical practice. They are considered safe and complications are rare. However, there have been a few reports of associated sepsis. Boyle, Robins-Brown and Tang published a review article in 2006 in which they proposed risk factors for probiotic sepsis.[6] Major risk factors were the immune compromised and premature infants. Minor risk factors were central venous catheters, impaired intestinal epithelial barriers, administration of probiotic by jejunostomy, concomitant administration of broad spectrum antibiotics to which a probiotic may be resistant, probiotics with properties of high mucosal adherence of known pathogenicity, and cardiac valve disease (for *Lactobacillus* probiotics only). These risk factors have not been widely used but, nevertheless, when the authors reviewed the literature, they felt that these were important. They reviewed all of the cases available until 2005 and found 7 reports in which probiotic use may have been related to bacterial sepsis. The organisms identified were either *Lactobacillus rhamnosus* or *Bacillus subtilis.* They also reviewed the cases of fungal sepsis temporarily related to probiotic use in humans. There were 16 such reports containing 24 cases. In all of those, the organism identified was *Saccharomyces boulardii.* Many of these were controversial reports. That is the extent of the entire negative literature. Most clinicians, as well as the US Food and Drug Administration, feel that probiotics are extremely safe but that there must be caution whenever the subject is severely immunocompromised.[7] This occurs in cases with very low lymphocyte counts and in infants. The major concern is that probiotics adhere to the intestinal mucosa and can break through the barrier to be absorbed and create a sepsis situation. So this question should be addressed by clinicians when treating a patient at high risk. However, there should be emphasis on stressing that probiotics are safe in ordinary individuals who are not at high risk. The rare reports of sepsis or fungemia in high-risk patients have occurred with Lactobacilli or Saccharomyces. To the best of our knowledge, there have been no reports of sepsis or bacterium with Bifidobacteria or other commonly used probiotic organisms.

Most recently, a report was published in which patients with severe pancreatitis had developed sepsis and did much poorer on a probiotic than those not receiving probiotics in intensive care units. Therefore, there is now caution in treating severe pancreatitis with a probiotic. However, this was only one report in a limited number of patients and it is reviewed in Chapter 15.

REFERENCES

1. Report of Joint FAO/WHO Expert Consultation on Evaluation of Health and Nutritional Properties of Probiotics in Food Including Powder Milk with Live Lactic Acid Bacteria, October 2001.
2. Fuller R. Probiotics in man and animals. *J Appl Bacteriol.* 1989;66:365-378.
3. Gibson CR, Roberfroid MB. Dietary modulation of the human colonic microflora: introducing the concept of prebiotics. *J Nutr.* 1995;125:401.
4. Trowell H, Burkitt D, Heaton K. *Dietary Fibre, Fibre-Depleted Foods and Disease.* London:Academic Press; 1985.
5. Spiller GA. *CRC Handbook of Dietary Fiber in Human Nutrition.* 2nd ed. Boca Raton, FL: CRC Press; 1992:15-18.
6. Boyle RJ, Robins-Browne RM, Tang MLK. Probiotic use in clinical practice: what are the risks? *Am J Clin Nutr.* 2006;83:1256-1264.
7. Donohue D. Safety of probiotic organisms. In: Lee YK, Salminen S. *Handbook of Probiotics and Prebiotics.* 2nd ed. Hoboken, NJ: John Wiley & Sons, Inc; 2009:75-95.

SECTION I

BASIC PHYSIOLOGY

Intestinal Microecology

Martin H. Floch, MD, MACG, FACP, AGAF

DEFINITION AND HISTORY

Intestinal microecology is the relationship of organisms to their animate and inanimate environment within the intestine. The concept of intestinal microecology originates in modern times with the work of Metchnikoff. His classic thesis on aging and intestinal putrefaction won the Nobel Prize late in the 19th century.[1] In 1960, Haenel published a paper referring to the intestinal microflora and their effects on the host.[2] However, it was not until 1970 that Luckey began to emphasize the importance of the intestinal flora within the ecology that exists within the gastrointestinal lumen.[3,4] In 1970, 1972, and 1974, this author had the opportunity to be involved in three symposia that were held at the University of Missouri, the proceedings of which were published in the *American Journal of Clinical Nutrition*. Those symposia published almost 90 manuscripts on the subject. The data and concepts were enlightening and they furthered the theory and importance of intestinal microecology.[5-7]

These initial efforts to obtain information on the intestinal microflora and its relationships in the gastrointestinal tract were extensive. The depth of the field developed further with the burgeoning interest in and understanding of the role of dietary fiber and more recently prebiotic substances within the gastrointestinal tract. The evolution and our understanding of these factors were important in understanding the ecologic relationships between foods and the flora.[8-11]

ANIMATE PARTS OF INTESTINAL MICROECOLOGY

The host's intestinal wall and bacteria are the animate part of the ecology. In the proximal small bowel, the lumen contains numerous secretions entering it from the bile and pancreatic ducts and the cells lining the wall that mix with the food and flora. As

Floch MH, Kim AS, eds.
Probiotics: A Clinical Guide (pp 3-12)
© 2010 Taylor & Francis Group

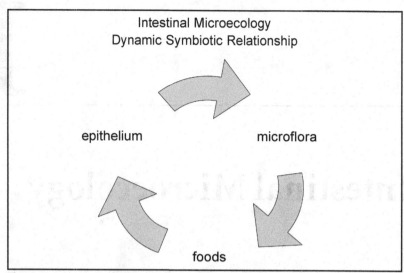

Intestinal Microecology
Dynamic Symbiotic Relationship

epithelium   microflora

foods

Figure 1-1. Intestinal microbiology: dynamic symbiotic relationship.

we proceed down the small intestine, the lumen contains secretions from the wall, as well as the modified food products and products of bacterial fermentation and metabolism.[10] The flora in the colon affects the contents of the lumen and the cells lining the lumen. It is a dynamic process (Figure 1-1). Our understanding has now grown to where scientists accept that microecology is responsible for major processes involved in both maintaining our health and causing disease.[10,11]

In this chapter, the action of the intestinal microflora and the major foods that are involved in this environment will be described. Examples of resultant products and functions of ecology as they affect the host will also be described. Figure 1-1 graphically depicts the reactions and the function of this ecology. The intestinal microflora is composed of more than 400 species and 10^{13} or 10^{14} organisms per gram of content. Depending on the amount of the content (eg, feces in the colon), the number of organisms will vary tremendously. Nevertheless, this huge number of bacterial cells is greater than the number of cells that make up the human body.[12,13] Bacteria in the oral cavity may have as many as 200 species. Cultures from the esophagus reveal total counts to be no more than 10^2. It is presumed that gastric acid keeps the flora counts low in the stomach. In the duodenum and proximal jejunum, the counts rise to 10^2 to 10^5, but the content of the ileum begins to harbor counts at 10^6 and 10^8. When we reach the colon, the counts range between 10^{10} and 10^{13}.

The species in the ileum are primarily a mix of aerobes and anaerobes, but when one reaches the colon, 99.99% of the content are anaerobes. The most common species are *Bacteroides*, clostridia, peptostreptococci, peptococci, bifidobacteria, lactobacilli, *Bacillus*, fusobacteria, *Enterococcus*, and *Enterobacter*.[12-17] Almost all of these values are based on the culture of the material. However, the most recent, sophisticated RNA and DNA polymerase analyses are research techniques that evaluate the genetic makeup of various species. They have not elaborated new data on the counts or contents but have been very useful in analysis in specific research studies.[13]

A review of the probiotic literature reveals that most organisms used as probiotics belong to the *Lactobacillus* and *Bifidobacterium* groups.[18] Other lactic acid-producing bacteria (LAB) are enterococci and streptococci, and non-LAB and yeasts belong to the *Bacillus*, *Escherichia coli*, *Propionibacterium*, and *Saccharomyces* groups. There are approximately 20 organisms that have been recovered from human feces and commonly used as probiotic organisms.[18]

TABLE 1-1

EFFECTS OF THE MICROFLORA (MICROBIOTA) ON THE HUMAN HOST*

SMALL BOWEL	LARGE BOWEL
Immunity	Production of energy via SCFA (acetic, propionic, butyric)
Stimulate cytokine production	
Stimulate immunoglobulin production	Breakdown of dietary oxalate
Stimulate Paneth cells	Metabolism of drugs
Cross talk to dendritic cells	Digestion of polysaccharides
Cross talk to epithelial cells	Alteration of lipids
Infections	Production of vitamins B, K and folate
Stimulate WBC production	Digestion of prebiotics
Stimulate defensin production via paneth cells	Production of gases—CO_2, H_2, CH_4, N_2 and O_2
	Helps regulate fat storage

*Modified from Omahoney S, Shanahan F. Enteric bacterial flora and bacterial overgrowth. In: Feldman M, Friedman LS, Brant LJ, eds. *Gastrointestinal and Liver Disease*. 8th ed. Philadelphia, PA: Saunders/Elsevier; 2006;2244-2256.

EFFECT OF THE MICROECOLOGY ON THE HUMAN HOST

The major effects of the microflora on the host vary in the small intestine and the large intestine. Table 1-1 lists the role of bacteria in these physiologic events.

Small Intestine

Immune Response

In the small bowel, the microflora has a great effect on host immune processes (see Chapters 2 and 3). It is now well accepted that the intestinal microflora stimulates the mucosa of the small bowel to produce immunoglobulin A (IgA), the chemicals and processes of the whole cytokine cascade, and interfaces with Paneth and dendritic cells (DC) to affect the host's response.[19,20] The bacteria and foods help regulate ß-cell and T-cell immune function in the gut.[21] We understand that a symbiotic ecosystem exists in which intestinal bacteria provide the stimuli to the gut to maintain a natural, healthy maturation of the intestinal immune system. There is a cross talk between the host's mucosa and its contents, which is dynamic and ongoing and permits the changing environment to affect the host's responsive immune processes.[21,22] This is the ultimate demonstration of how the intestinal microecology affects the function and health of the host.[23]

Infections

When a hostile or invading organism enters the internal environment and reaches the wall of the small intestine, it stimulates selective immune responses, and is attacked by our defense system, as described by Hart and Ng in Chapter 2. The hostile organisms stimulate the production of specific substances such as defensins and other host responses that either ward off an organism or help the host respond to the toxic substances produced by the invading organisms.[19-23]

Large Intestine

Fermentation and Metabolism

The major part of fermentation and metabolism of food substances takes place in the colon, although some of this metabolic activity occurs in the distal ileum. This truly demonstrates the commensal relationship between bacteria and the host. Scientists have suggested that the bacteria or microbiome be included as part of the host's genetic makeup. Using very sophisticated DNA sequence techniques, Hooper and Gordon[23] have stressed the importance of bacterial flora in affecting our genome and microbiome. This commensal relationship between the intestinal microflora and the host is a functional dynamic process. It constantly changes when food substances and different bacteria enter the gut. Although the flora tends to be stable, it can change, and recently the introduction of probiotic therapy has stressed the importance of this change for possible therapeutic effects.

EFFECT OF FOODS AND PREBIOTICS

Changes in the food that enters the microecology can have a great effect on both the organism's and host's reaction and may change the makeup of the flora.[17,24] Prebiotics, probiotic organisms, and synbiotics (combination of prebiotics and probiotics) will affect the host's metabolism and the microflora. The main fermentable substrates in the adult gut are carbohydrates. Fibers, resistant starch, and nonabsorbable sugars, including oligosaccharides, are fermented and are preferred fuels of the flora.[24] In the neonate, bifidobacteria are the most common organisms from mothers delivering vaginally and breastfeeding.[25] The flora of the infant changes rapidly once formula is added. Dietary fiber and prebiotics, both of which contain nonstarch polysaccharides that are not fermented by human enzymes but by the bacterial enzymes, have a marked effect on the microflora and intestinal microecology.

DIABETES

Our present understanding has grown such that it is now suggested that type I diabetes may be a result of the interplay between the intestinal flora, gut permeability, and mucosal immunity.[26] It is thought that the intestinal flora occurs in the setting of a "leaky" intestinal mucosal barrier so that altered mucosal immunity occurs, permitting the development of glucose intolerance and its consequences.[26] Vaarala et al reviewed the microflora and biochemical data available, which indicated that the setting of a leaky intestinal mucosa with a weakened mucosal barrier and loosening of the tight junctions permits a change in the immunologic response and makes a host susceptible to type I diabetes.[26] It is well known that high-carbohydrate, high-fiber diets can improve glucose tolerance in diabetic subjects, and that the addition to the diet of substances such as guar and pectin can further improve glucose tolerance.[27,28] There is evidence to indicate that the microflora, structural changes, and foods that make up the ecology can be related to the cause and course of diabetes.

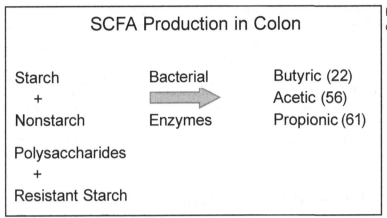

Figure 1-2. SCFA production in colon.

SHORT-CHAIN FATTY ACIDS

Short-chain fatty acids (SCFA) represent the best example of bacterial effect on the host's metabolism. Starch and nonstarch polysaccharides are fermented in the distal ileum and colon. Fiber, nonstarch polysaccharides (soluble fiber from fruits and vegetables), and prebiotics[29] are fermented primarily by bacterial enzymes (Figure 1-2). Humans have essentially no enzymes that permit their production, whereas bacteria extensively ferment and produce them in the molecular ratio of approximately 60:20:20 for acetic, butyric, and propionic. The amount produced varies with different organisms and the availability of different substrates.[17,30] Butyric acid is the main fuel for the colonocytes. The colon epithelial cells use butyric acid before they use glucose as a nutrient. Acetic acid is the building block for cholesterol. The functions of propionic acid are not well understood.[17,30] However, they seem to affect the rate of cholesterol metabolism. It is suggested that substrates that can decrease the acetic acid and propionic acid ratio may actually improve lipid risk factors.[31] Furthermore, as much as 5% to 10% of absorbed energy can come from SCFA metabolism.[17]

Butyrate has been studied as a possible therapeutic agent in the treatment of colitis. It is definitely helpful in the treatment of divergent colitis, where the colon has no nutrients; but if it is fed butyrate, it will heal colitis.[32] Furthermore, the energy derived from the SCFA can be beneficial to patients with a short bowel when carbohydrates are metabolized by the flora to produce SCFA and then absorbed.[33] The entire subject of organisms producing substances such as SCFA that are beneficial to the host requires further experimentation to see the therapeutic and beneficial effects.

Not only acetic and propionic acids have been demonstrated to effect lipid metabolism, but a newer avenue of experimentation that feeds probiotics has shown interesting results. Wall and associates fed a probiotic *Bifidobacterium* to mice and pigs and altered the lipid profile and the fatty acid composition in the liver tissue after administration of the bifidobacteria. This suggests that the microflora, and possibly the probiotic, has a marked effect on lipid production and deposition in the liver and in the host. Experiments in this area should be very fruitful in the future.[34]

ENTEROHEPATIC CIRCULATION

The microflora is essential in maintaining the enterohepatic circulation.[35] Bile salts are conjugated with either taurine or glycine in the liver and secreted in the bile into the upper small intestine where they are pivotal in assisting in fat absorption. Further down in the small bowel, bacterial enzymes degrade the conjugated bile acids, freeing up simple bile acids, which are then reabsorbed into the circulation and proceed to the liver where they are once again conjugated. This is an essential process in normal fat absorption. When it is impaired, disease and steatorrhea occur. It is also known that simple bile acids can have a negative effect on aerobic organisms, but do not appear to impair the growth of anaerobes or the probiotic organisms that belong to the anaerobic flora.[36] Therefore, the microflora is essential in maintaining a normal enterohepatic circulation and assisting in maintaining a homeostatic balance of the flora through bile acids.

FIBER AND PREBIOTICS

Dietary fiber as a part of the microecology is important in maintaining metabolism and health. It is now well accepted that deficiencies result in disease.[17] Theories and research brought forth by Cleave et al,[37] Burkitt and Trowell,[38] and Walker[39] have established that fiber deficiency can result in malfunction and degenerative disorders such as diverticular disease, constipation, diabetes mellitus, and disorders of the biliary tract. Dietary fiber is nonstarch polysaccharide of plant food, which is poorly digested by human enzymes.[17] Most clinicians and physicians working in this field classify dietary fiber as soluble and insoluble on the basis of a chemical reaction—not merely on the basis of its ability to dissolve in water. Insoluble fibers are mainly lignin and bran, or the wall of plant foods made up of cellulose and lignins and some hemicelluloses. Soluble fiber is primarily hemicelluloses, but also includes substances such as guar.[17] Of note is the fact that soluble fibers are digested by the bacterial flora enzymes producing volatile SCFA (as discussed above), whereas insoluble fibers are very poorly digested—if at all—and bind to water, leaving the gastrointestinal tract just as they enter it. In the chemical analysis of fiber, a nondigestible resistant starch is identified regularly, which is an important component of plant food.[40]

The fiber substances have physiologic effects in the gut; they slow motility, they transiently bind to minerals and transport them through the tract, and they tend to slow transit, hold on to water, and affect lipid metabolism.[17] Their action on lipid and glucose metabolism is accepted.[17] There is a large amount of literature on this, which is not reviewed here; but it is important to keep in mind that these changes in liver lipids occur as a manipulation of the intestinal microecology.[17,27-31]

When studying intestinal microecology, it is important to remember that nonstarch polysaccharides are a part of dietary fiber and are the main nutrient for the intestinal flora.[17,40,41] It is accepted that we have a healthier bowel if we eat enough fiber to nurture the normal microflora, whereas we have a less healthy bowel or host if there is a deficiency from eating inadequate amounts of fiber.[17,30,31,37-39]

PREBIOTICS

Prebiotics are nonstarch polysaccharides that are usually synthetic and not metabolized by human enzymes but by the bacterial flora.[9,17,29] Most of the prebiotics produced are oligosaccharides, and there is a whole host of modified oligosaccharides—such as fructooligosaccharides (FOS) and xylooligosaccharides—that have been created and used in experiments and as additions to food supplements. They are often combined with a probiotic and used as a synbiotic.[42]

Other prebiotic substances that are used extensively are inulin and lactulose. When these are administered, they can change the microflora; it has been shown that lactulose as a therapeutic agent in hepatic encephalopathy will alter the flora.[43,44] Inulin used as an agent in constipation in the elderly will also affect the flora and decrease constipation.[17,45] It also has been used successfully to increase calcium absorption for bone mineral density.[46]

These are clear examples of how dietary substances (here a prebiotic) affect microecology and, in turn, the bacterial content and the host's metabolism, hence improving the host's health.

Scientists or clinicians using prebiotics hope that probiotics will have a functional effect in the small or large bowel. It is assumed that the effect will alter the microflora and benefit the host.

PROBIOTICS

Probiotics are live organisms administered in capsules or foods in order to benefit the host. The logical interpretation is that the administered organisms will become part of the intestinal flora or in some way change it to benefit the host. The intestinal microflora is made up of commensal organisms that have a symbiotic relationship with the host.[17,22-24] The intent behind administering probiotics is that they will benefit the host by improving the contents and action of the intestinal microecology. The intake of dietary fiber is less in the Western, developed world; hence, intestinal growth of the anaerobic LAB is less. Therefore, the Western world has embraced the use of probiotics that have LAB in the hope of improving the microflora for maintaining health. A US study in 1983 revealed that *Lactobacillus plantarum* is found in only approximately 25% of Americans and about two-thirds of vegetarian Americans.[16] A Scandinavian study suggested the most common colonic lactic acid-producing organisms were present in only 50% of individuals. Since culture techniques are so difficult, only about one-third of the organisms can be cultured. Recent studies using RNA and DNA polymerase and genetic techniques should help evaluate the normal flora, but the results are yet to be published.

Administration of probiotics is gaining widespread appeal. In addition, prebiotics are being used more frequently, and it is suggested that combining them with a probiotic would give a so-called synbiotic that would be even more helpful than either alone. Public health efforts have gone as far as to link the gut microbiota to the clinical problems of stress[47] and obesity.[48,49]

Yogurts and drinks containing probiotics and synbiotics have also gained popularity with the hope that they are effective in altering the flora and improving health. The clinical use of probiotics are reviewed in detail in the second half of this book.

CONCLUSION

Intestinal microecology is the relationship of organisms to their animate and inanimate environment within the intestine. Intestinal microflora consists of bacteria, yeasts, and parasites that live in the small and large bowel and are nurtured by the host and the foods it eats. The microflora lives within the lumen of the small and large bowel. In the small bowel, the foods and host secretions nurture the flora, and the flora interacts with the epithelium and the subepithelial structures of the ileum. Immune processes are stimulated, and host defenses are continually developed depending on the changes in the flora and the foods. The flora is also responsible for key physiologic processes such as maintaining the enterohepatic circulation. In the colon, the flora metabolizes the foods, primarily soluble fiber and prebiotics if they are administered. They produce SCFA in varying amounts depending on what food is fed and what organisms are present. They affect the stability of the lipid process by producing the building blocks for cholesterol and probably for its control. It is a dynamic process in which any change in the ecology, either by changing the food or by changing the organisms, will change the host's response. Invasion by organisms or failure to maintain homeostasis results in disease.

During the last few decades we have learned a great deal, but more is to be discovered on how the intestinal ecology and its function is important with respect to basic physiology and disease processes. New techniques of identifying the microbiota and the genome should help in understanding and gaining more information.

REFERENCES

1. Metchnikoff E. *The Prolongation of Life: Optimistic Studies*. London: Butterworth-Heinemann; 1907.
2. Haenel H, Gruetzner L, Henneberg G. On the microecology of the intestinal canal of rhesus monkeys (*Simia rhesus*). *Zentralb Bakteriol*. 1960;178:42-50.
3. Luckey TD. Introduction to the ecology of the intestinal flora. *Am J Clin Nutr*. 1970;23:1430-1432.
4. Luckey TD. Introduction to intestinal microecology. *Am J Clin Nutr*. 1972;25:1292-1294.
5. Floch MH, Gorbach SL, Luckey TD. Intestinal microflora. *Am J Clin Nutr*. 1970;23:1425-1426.
6. Luckey TD, Floch MH. Intestinal microecology. *Am J Clin Nutr*. 1972;25:1291-1494.
7. Floch MH, Hentges DJ. Intestinal microecology. *Am J Clin Nutr*. 1974;27:1265-1485.
8. Floch MH, Wolfman M. Doyle R. Fiber and gastrointestinal microecology. *J Clin Gastroenterol*. 1980;2:175-184.
9. Collins MD, Gibson GR. Probiotics, prebiotics, and synbiotics: approaches for modulating the microbial ecology of the gut. *Am J Clin Nutr*. 1999;69:1052S-1057S.
10. Park J, Floch MH. Prebiotics, probiotics, and dietary fiber in gastrointestinal disease. *Gastroenterol Clin North Am*. 2007;36:47-63.
11. Neish AS. Microbes in gastrointestinal health and disease. *Gastroenterology*. 2009;136:65-80.
12. Hart AI, Stagg AJ, Groffner H, et al. *Gut Ecology*. London: Martin Duntiz Ltd.; 2002.
13. Omahoney S, Shanahan F. Enteric bacterial flora and bacterial overgrowth. In: Feldman M, Friedman LS, Brant LJ, eds. *Gastrointestinal and Liver Disease*. 8th ed. Philadelphia, PA: Saunders/Elsevier; 2006;2244-2256.
14. Moore WEC, Holdeman LV. Human fecal flora: the normal flora of 20 Japanese-Hawaiians. *Appl Microbiol*. 1974;27:961-979.
15. Finegold SM, Sutter VL, Sugihara PT, Elder HA, Lehmann SM, Phillips RL. Fecal microbial flora in Seventh Day Adventists population and control subjects. *Am J Clin Nutr*. 1977;30:1781-1792.
16. Guerrant RL, Steiner TS. Principles and syndromes of enteric infection. In: Mandell FL, Bennett JE, Dolin R, eds. *Principles and Practices of Infectious Disease*. 6th ed. Philadelphia, PA: Elsevier/Churchill Liustine; 2005:1217-1231.
17. Floch MH. Prebiotics, probiotics and dietary fiber. In: Buchman AL, ed. *Clinical Nutrition in Gastrointestinal Disease*. Thorofare, NJ: SLACK Incorporated; 2006:123-139.
18. Montrose D, Floch MH. Probiotics used in human studies. *J Clin Gastroenterol*. 2005;39:469-484.
19. Madsen K. Probiotics and the immune response. *J Clin Gastroenterol*. 2006;40:232-234.
20. Isolauri E, Salminen S. Probiotics, gut inflammation and barrier function. *Gastroenterol Clin North Am*. 2005;34:437-450.
21. MacDonald TT, Monteleone G. Bacteria and the regulation of T-cell immune function in the gut. In: Hart AI, Stagg AJ, Groffner H, et al. *Gut Ecology*. London: Martin Dunitz Ltd.; 2002;57-65.
22. Rautava S, Walker, WA. Commensal bacteria and epithelial cross talk in the developing intestine. *Curr Gastroenterol Rep*. 2007;9:385-392.
23. Hooper LV, Gordon JI. Commensal host-bacterial relationships in the gut. *Science*. 2001;292:1115-1118.
24. Collins MD, Gibson GR. Probiotics, prebiotics, and synbiotics: approaches for modulating the microbial ecology of the gut. *Am J Clin Nutr*. 1999;69:1052S-1057S.

25. Benno Y, Sawada K, Mitsuoka T. The intestinal microflora of infants: composition of fecal flora in breast-fed and bottle-fed infants. *Microbiol Immunol.* 1984;28:975-986.
26. Vaarala O, Atkinson MA, Neu J. The "perfect storm" for type 1 diabetes. *Diabetes.* 2008;57:2555-2562.
27. Kiehm TG, Anderson JW, Ward K. Beneficial effects of a high carbohydrate, high fiber diet on hyperglycemic diabetic men. *Am J Clin Nutr.* 1976;29:895-899.
28. Jenkins DJA, Leeds AR, Gassull MA, et al. Decrease in postprandial insulin and glucose concentration by guar and pectin. *Ann Intern Med.* 1977;86:20-23.
29. Gibson GR. Prebiotics as gut microflora management tools. *J Clin Gastroenterol.* 2008;42:S75-S79.
30. Wong JMW, de Souza R, Kendall CWC, et al. Colonic health: fermentation and short chain fatty acids. *J Clin Gastroenterol.* 2006;40:235-243.
31. Jenkins DJA, Wolever TMS, Jenkins A, et al. Specific types of colonic fermentation may raise low-density-lipoprotein-cholesterol concentrations. *Am J Clin Nutr.* 1991;54:141-147.
32. Harig JM, Soergel KH, Komorowski RA, et al. Treatment of diversion colitis with short-chain fatty acid irrigation. *New Eng J Med.* 1989;320:23-28.
33. Nordgaard I, Hansen BS, Mortensen PB. Colon as a digestive organ in patients with short bowel. *Lancet.* 1994;343:373-376.
34. Wall RA, Ross RP, Shanahan F, et al. The metabolic activity of the enteric microbiota influences the fatty acid composition of murine and porcine liver and adipose tissues. *Am J Clin Nutr.* 2009;89(5):1393-1401.
35. Dawson PA. Bile secretion and the enterohepatic circulation. In: Feldman M, Friedman LS, Brandt LJ, eds. *Gastroenterology and Liver Disease.* 8th ed. Philadelphia, PA: Saunders/Elsevier; 2006; 1369-1385.
36. Floch MH, Gershengoren W, Elliot, Spiro HM. Bile acid inhibition of intestinal microflora—a function for simple bile acids? *Gastroenterology.* 1971;61:228-233.
37. Cleave TL, Campbell GD, Painter NS. *Diabetes, Coronary Thrombosis and the Saccharine Disease.* 2nd ed. Bristol: John Wright; 1969.
38. Burkitt DP, Trowell HC. *Refined Carbohydrate Foods and Disease.* New York: Academic Press; 1975.
39. Walker ARP. Colon cancer and diet, with special reference to intakes of fat and fiber. *Am J Clin Nutr.* 1976;29:1417-1426.
40. Murphy MM, Douglass JS, Birkett A. Resistant starch intakes in the United States. *J Am Diet Assoc.* 2008;108:67-78.
41. Englyst KN, Liu S, Englyst HN. Nutritional characterization and measurement of dietary carbohydrates. *Eur J Clin Nutr.* 2007;61:S19-S39.
42. Spinkler-Vesel A, Bengmark S, Vovk I, et al. Synbiotics, prebiotics, glutamine, or peptide in early enteral nutrition: a randomized study in trauma patients. *J Parenter Enteral Nutr.* 2007;31:119-126.
43. Elkington SC, Floch MH, Conn HO. Lactulose in the treatment of chronic portal-systemic encephalopathy. A double-blind clinical trial. *New Eng J Med.* 1969;281:408-412.
44. Conn HO, Floch MH. Effects of lactulose and *Lactobacillus acidophilus* on the fecal flora. *Am J Clin Nutr.* 1970;23:1588-1594.
45. Klessen B, Sykura B, Zunfit HJ. Effects of inulin and lactose on fecal microflora, microbial activity, and bowel habit in elderly constipated persons. *Am J Clin Nutr.* 1997;65:1397-1402.
46. Abrams SA, Griffin IJ, Hawthorne KM, et al. A combination of prebiotic short- and long-chain inulin-type fructans enhances calcium absorption and bone mineralization in young adolescents. *Am J Clin Nutr.* 2005;82:471-476.
47. Eutamene H, Bueno L. Role of probiotics in correcting abnormalities of colonic flora induced by stress. *Gut.* 2007;56:1495-1497.
48. Turnbaugh PJ, Ley RE, Mahowald MA, et al. An obesity-associated gut microbiome with increased capacity for energy harvest. *Nature.* 2006;444:1027-1031.
49. DiBaise JK, Zhang H, Crowell MD, et al. Gut microbiota and its possible relationship with obesity. *Mayo Clin Proc.* 2008;83:460-469.

2

Intraluminal Defenses

Ailsa Hart, PhD and Siew C. Ng, PhD

The human gastrointestinal (GI) tract represents the largest surface area of the body that is colonized by a diverse and dynamic microbial community. It is constantly exposed to large numbers of bacteria, including the resident microbiota as well as foreign bacteria. The mucosal immune system is poised to sense the local environment and needs to avoid potentially harmful responses to dietary antigens and the resident microbiota while responding rapidly to challenges from pathogens. There is a constant level of highly regulated physiological inflammation in operation involving a network of connectivity between intraluminal defenses, the epithelial barrier, and the cells of the innate and adaptive immune systems in addition to neurons, muscles, fibroblasts, and endothelial cells. This chapter will focus on intraluminal defenses.

LUMINAL ENVIRONMENT

Intestinal secretions, peristalsis, and secretory IgA have long been shown to provide protection against pathogenic bacteria in the GI tract. Another mechanism by which the normal gut flora resists colonization by pathogenic bacteria is by the production of a physiologically restrictive environment, with respect to luminal pH (many LAB produce organic acids), redox potential, and hydrogen sulfide production.

ANTIMICROBIAL PEPTIDES

Antimicrobial peptides and proteins have emerged as key components of innate immunity that provide host defense against pathogen invasion at mucosal surfaces. Antimicrobial peptides are part of an ancient immunological system. Hundreds have been found in plants and animals, from mollusks to humans. As a class, the peptides are diverse and range from linear α-helical molecules to disulfide-bonded

Floch MH, Kim AS, eds.
Probiotics: A Clinical Guide (pp 13-20)
© 2010 Taylor & Francis Group

β-sheet-containing peptides. The peptides are usually cationic with spatially separated hydrophobic and charged regions. This arrangement allows them to insert into phospholipid membranes and form pores. They have an affinity for disrupting microbial membranes rich in anionic phospholipids, and in this way the host cells may be protected from concomitant damage. Other mechanisms of microbicidal activity include disruption of bacterial energy metabolism and interference with biosynthetic pathways.

IMMUNE CELLS AND ANTIMICROBIAL PEPTIDES

Antimicrobial peptides are expressed by phagocytic cells and epithelial cells. They provide early broad-spectrum antimicrobial protection against invading microorganisms at epithelial cell surfaces. The best characterized of all antimicrobial peptides in mammals and humans are the defensins and cathelicidins.[1] Other antimicrobial protein families include the peptidoglycan recognition proteins, S-100 family proteins, calcium-dependent lectins (c-type lectins), magainins, and cecropins. In the human small intestine, specialized secretory epithelial cells or Paneth cells express the antimicrobials α-defensin-5 (HD5), HD6, lysozyme, and secretory phospholipase A(2) (sPLA2),[2] all of which are part of the host defense against microorganisms.

DEFENSINS

In mammals, defensins are one of the major families of antimicrobial peptides. They fall into different structural classes, in particular α and β. Their 3-dimensional structure is similar, but their disulfide linkages differ, and their genes reside in the same gene cluster on the short arm of chromosome 8 (8p23). The α-defensins are a major constituent of neutrophils. In humans, the α-defensins (human neutrophil peptides 1 to 4) account for 5% of the total cellular protein of neutrophils. Other α-defensins are expressed in Paneth cells in the small intestine. β-Defensins are present in the epithelial cells of human skin, kidneys, and GI tract. Intestinal epithelial cells constitutively produce human β-defensin (hBD)-1, whereas other β-defensins are inducibly upregulated in response to "danger" signals such as infections or cytokines.

DISTRIBUTION, LOCALIZATION, AND REGIONAL VARIATION OF ANTIMICROBIAL PEPTIDES

Within the small intestine of the mouse, antimicrobial peptides are found in the intestinal crypts, the luminal content, and the surface mucus. Most of these proteins are retained by the surface mucus with only small amounts detected in the luminal content; this provides a physical and antibacterial barrier to prevent pathogen attachment and invasion.[3] In conventionally reared mice, the repertoire of antimicrobial peptides changes along the small intestine. Expression of Paneth cell antimicrobials, cryptdin 4 and cryptdin-related sequences (CRS)-4C peptides, is higher in the ileum compared with that in the duodenum, but expression is not altered in response to the challenge that enteric bacterial pathogens present, supporting the constitutive nature of the innate defensive system.[4] Other host factors that may influence colonization include pH, peristalsis, and glycans.

REGULATION AND FUNCTIONS
OF ANTIMICROBIAL PEPTIDES

Several factors influence the expression of antimicrobial peptides in the GI tract, including the type and numbers of antimicrobial peptide-expressing epithelial cells, their state of differentiation, and the interaction of epithelial cells with pathogens and commensals. Expression of antimicrobial peptides during the steady state may also be different from that in the disease state, especially in chronic inflammatory conditions such as inflammatory bowel disease (IBD). In the inflamed tissue, there may be infiltration or recruitment of antimicrobial peptide expressing polymorphonuclear leukocytes from the circulation.

Apart from their direct antimicrobial function through bacterial membrane permeabilization, antimicrobial peptides can function as opsonins,[5] chemokines,[6] and modulators of cytokine production. Recent evidence suggested that antimicrobial peptides can be regulated by cytokines of the innate and adaptive immune systems, particularly those of the Th17-cell subset (particularly involved in Crohn's disease), IL-17, and IL-22.[7] Th17-derived cytokines have an essential role in upregulating humoral antimicrobial factors that act locally to limit infection or inflammation. For instance, in the mouse GI tract, IL-22 is required for the expression of other c-type lectins to generate protein 3B (REG3B) and REG3γ (a soluble c-type protein produced by Paneth cells) after challenge with *Citrobacter rodentium*.[8]

Cytokine products traditionally associated with T-cell immunity can also regulate antimicrobial protein expression at mucosal surfaces. One such example is demonstrated by the antimicrobial protein lactoferrin that induces natural killer cell activity via the increased production of IL-18 and type 1 interferons in the small intestine of mice.[9] Wilson et al[10] showed that metalloproteinase matrilysin-7, the enzyme responsible for processing of the precursor forms of cryptdins to the active mature peptide, regulates activation of α-defensins in murine Paneth cells. Gene transfer mice expressing the human cathelicidin antimicrobial peptide LL37 had increased resistance to experimental respiratory and systemic bacterial infections, whereas gene knockout mice lacking matrilysin and only synthesizing the inactive cryptdin precursors appeared more susceptible to infections with lower doses of *S. typhimurium,* compared to their wild-type littermates.[10] A recent study has shown that HD-5 is an effective luminal antimicrobial; transgenic mice expressing HD-5 and cryptdins in the Paneth cells were resistant to oral infections due to *S. typhimurium* compared with nontransgenic controls.[11]

Furthermore, antimicrobial proteins may become prototypes of innovative drugs that can potentially be used as antibiotics, antilipopolysaccharide drugs, or modifiers of inflammation.[12]

MICROBIOTA-PRODUCED ANTIMICROBIAL PEPTIDES

Antimicrobial peptides or bacteriocins can be produced by the intestinal microbiota. Several bacteriocins produced by different species from the genus *Lactobacillus* have been described.[13] The activity of these bacteriocins varies; some inhibit other lactobacilli or taxonomically related species and some are active against a wider range of Gram-positive and Gram-negative bacteria as well as yeasts and molds.[14] *Enterococcus faecium* produces an antimicrobial substance showing activity against *Enterococcus*, *Lactobacillus*, *Listeria*, *Corynebacterium*, and *Staphylococcus aureus*.[15] The human probiotic bacterium, *Lactobacillus salivarius* ssp. *salivarius*, produces a bacteriocin with activity against *Bacillus*, *Listeria*, *Enterococcus*, and *Staphylococcus* species, and this antimicrobial peptide has been characterized at the genetic level.[16] Lacticin 3147, a broad-spectrum bacteriocin produced by *Lactococcus lactis* ssp., inhibits a range of genetically distinct *Clostridium difficile* isolates from healthy subjects and patients with IBD.[17] A further example is the antimicrobial effect of *Lactobacillus* species on *Helicobacter pylori* infection of gastric mucosa, achieved by the release of bacteriocins and the ability of *Lactobacillus* to decrease adherence of this pathogen to epithelial cells.[18]

INFLAMMATORY BOWEL DISEASES AND INTRALUMINAL DEFENSES

In IBD, there is impaired antimicrobial peptide expression, resulting in the breakdown of antimicrobial defenses in maintaining intestinal homeostasis.[19] The nucleotide-binding oligomerization protein 2 (NOD2) is a sensor for bacterial muramyl dipeptide, which is linked with ileal expression of antimicrobial peptides (α-defensins) and promotes cytokine and chemokine production by immunocytes and enterocytes. Ileal CD has been linked with a mutation in NOD2,[20] and a reduction in Paneth cell α-defensins has been implicated as a key contributor to the innate immune dysfunction in patients with Crohn's ileitis.[21] Furthermore, ileal expression of HD-5 and HD-6, but not sPLA2 or lysozyme, was less in affected ileum of CD patients, and the decrease was significantly more pronounced in patients with NOD2 mutations.[22] Simms et al recently showed that a reduction in α-defensin expression is independent of NOD2 status and is due to loss of surface epithelium as a consequence of inflammatory changes rather than being the inciting event prior to inflammation in ileal Crohn's disease (CD).[23]

MODIFICATION OF THE INTESTINAL LUMINAL MICROBIOTA IN HOST DEFENSE

Experiments in murine models and clinical observations in man suggest that luminal contents provide the constant antigenic stimulus for intestinal inflammation.[24,25] Manipulating the microbiota with probiotics can therefore influence the host. In germ-free mice, *Bifidobacterium longum* (a commonly used probiotic) can repress *B. thetaiotaomicron* (a prominent component of the adult human gut microbiota) expression of antibacterial proteins that may promote its own survival in the gut, as well as influence the composition, structure, and function of its microbial community. A single microbial molecule from *Bacteroides fragilis* has also been shown to protect its host from inflammatory disease caused by *H. hepaticus* in an animal model of experimental colitis, suggesting that natural anti-inflammatory molecules from the bacteria microbiota can actively promote human health, and may potentially be therapies for human inflammatory disorders.[26]

Recent illuminating work from Gordon's laboratory has shown that the intestinal environment affects microbial genome evolution; bacteroides are able to adapt to the distal human intestine via lateral gene transfer, a process that allows rapid transfer of genes under strong selection.[27]

Probiotic bacteria can antagonize pathogenic bacteria by reducing luminal pH, inhibiting bacterial adherence and translocation, or producing antibacterial substances and defensins. Reduction in the luminal pH by probiotic bacteria has been demonstrated in patients with ulcerative colitis (UC) following ingestion of the probiotic preparation VSL#3, which includes 8 different strains of bacteria (4 strains of lactobacilli, 3 strains of bifidobacteria, and a *Streptococcus thermophilus*).[28] In a fatal mouse model for Shiga toxin-producing *Escherichia coli* O157:H7 infection, the probiotic *B. breve* produced a high concentration of acetic acid, consequently lowering the luminal pH. This pH reduction was associated with increased animal survival.[29]

Lactobacilli have been shown to induce antimicrobial peptides such as defensins to stabilize gut barrier function.[30] Probiotics can also reduce the epithelial injury that follows due to exposure to *Escherichia coli* O157:H7 and *E. coli* O127:H6. The pretreatment of intestinal (T84) cells with LAB reduced the ability of pathogenic *E. coli* to inject virulence factors into the cells or to breach the intracellular tight junctions.[31] These findings demonstrate that probiotics prevent epithelial injury induced by attaching-effacing bacteria.[32,33]

The probiotic *E. coli* strain Nissle 1917 induced expression of hBD-2 in Caco-2 intestinal epithelial cells.[34] This type of effect may contribute to an improved mucosal barrier and provide a means of limiting access of enteric pathogens. Induction of hBD-2 by *E. coli* Nissle 1917 is dependent on the NF-κB and AP-1-pathways, mediated through bacterial flagellin.[35]

DENDRITIC CELLS AND INTRALUMINAL DEFENSES

Dendritic cells are professional antigen-presenting cells important in bacterial recognition and in shaping subsequent T-cell responses. In the intestine, DC have specialized functions. They contribute to oral tolerance induction by generating regulatory T cells and IgA-producing B cells through the production of cytokines such as IL-10 and TGF-β.[36,37] Intestinal DC sample luminal bacteria by passing their dendrites between epithelial tight junctions into the gut lumen[38] and indirectly with bacteria via M cells.[39] These findings suggest that DC may have a role in luminal gut defenses possibly via interaction with antimicrobial peptides. In a previous study,[40] it has been shown that intestinal DC are altered and more activated in IBD.

DC can influence the balance between a variety of effector and regulatory lymphocyte responses with different outcomes produced due to exposure of DC to different microbial products.[41,42] The regulatory functions of DC are particularly important at mucosal surfaces where the immune system interfaces with the external antigenic environment. The ability of intestinal DC to sample and respond to gut bacteria suggests that they may be targets for probiotic bacteria. In vitro, VSL#3 generates DC that produce the cytokine IL-10 and have regulatory or anti-inflammatory properties. Individual strains within VSL#3 displayed distinct immunomodulatory effects on DC; the most marked anti-inflammatory effects were produced by bifidobacteria strains (*B. longum*, *B. infantis*, and *B. breve*).[41] In UC patients treated with VSL#3, colonic DC produce more IL-10 and less IL-12p40, suggesting that the in vitro findings can be extrapolated into the in vivo settings.[43] Anti-inflammatory effects of bifidobacteria strains have been described in other studies. Rigby et al[44] showed that murine, freshly isolated lamina propria DC incubated with *B. longum* secreted IL-10 and IL-12, but a greater proportion of DC secreted IL-10 than IL-12.

Human β-defensins have been shown to be chemotactic for immature DC and memory T cells. Thus, they may not only mediate innate immunity but also regulate adaptive immune responses in IBD.[45] The endogenous antimicrobial peptide LL-37/hCAP-18 inhibits the activation of monocyte-derived DC by Toll-like receptor ligands. Exposure of DC to LL-37 during LPS exposure resulted in reduced production of proinflammatory cytokines, IL-6, IL-12p70, and TNF-α, decreased expression of DC activation markers, and reduced naive T-cell proliferation.[46]

CONCLUSION

There is a network of systems in operation within the intestinal lumen to defend the host. Antimicrobial peptides are produced by the resident microbiota itself in addition to immune cells. Disruption of such intraluminal defense mechanisms can contribute to disease states such as intestinal inflammation. The use of probiotics as therapeutic strategies in such conditions may be beneficial, and one of the mechanisms of action of probiotics may relate to their ability to fortify the intraluminal defense system, for example, through defensins production.

REFERENCES

1. Cunliffe RN, Mahida YR. Expression and regulation of antimicrobial peptides in the gastrointestinal tract. *J Leukoc Biol.* 2004;75(1):49-58.
2. Salzman NH, Underwood MA, Bevins CL. Paneth cells, defensins, and the commensal microbiota: a hypothesis on intimate interplay at the intestinal mucosa. *Semin Immunol.* 2007;19(2):70-83.
3. Meyer-Hoffert U, Hornef MW, Henriques-Normark B, et al. Secreted enteric antimicrobial activity localises to the mucus surface layer. *Gut.* 2008;57(6):764-771.
4. Karlsson J, Pütsep K, Chu H, Kays RJ, Bevins CL, Andersson M. Regional variations in Paneth cell antimicrobial peptide expression along the mouse intestinal tract. *BMC Immunol.* 2008;9:37.
5. Zelensky AN, Gready JE. The C-type lectin-like domain superfamily. *FEBS J.* 2005;272(24):6179-6217.
6. Soruri A, Grigat J, Forssmann U, Riggert J, Zwirner J. beta-Defensins chemoattract macrophages and mast cells but not lymphocytes and dendritic cells: CCR6 is not involved. *Eur J Immunol.* 2007;37(9):2474-2486.
7. Kolls JK, McCray PB Jr, Chan YR. Cytokine-mediated regulation of antimicrobial proteins. *Nat Rev Immunol.* 2008;8(11):829-835.
8. Zheng Y, Valdez PA, Danilenko DM, et al. Interleukin-22 mediates early host defense against attaching and effacing bacterial pathogens. *Nat Med.* 2008;14(3):282-289.
9. Kuhara T, Yamauchi K, Tamura Y, Okamura H. Oral administration of lactoferrin increases NK cell activity in mice via increased production of IL-18 and type I IFN in the small intestine. *J Interferon Cytokine Res.* 2006;26(7):489-499.
10. Wilson CL, Ouellette AJ, Satchell DP, et al. Regulation of intestinal alpha-defensin activation by the metalloproteinase matrilysin in innate host defense. *Science.* 1999;286(5437):113-117.
11. Salzman NH, Chou MM, de Jong H, Liu L, Porter EM, Paterson Y. Enteric salmonella infection inhibits Paneth cell antimicrobial peptide expression. *Infect Immun.* 2003;71(3):1109-1115.
12. Beisswenger C, Bals R. Functions of antimicrobial peptides in host defense and immunity. *Curr Protein Pept Sci.* 2005;6(3):255-264.
13. Klaenhammer TR. Bacteriocins of lactic acid bacteria. *Biochimie.* 1988;70(3):337-349.
14. Nemcova R. Criteria for selection of lactobacilli for probiotic use. *Vet Med (Praha).* 1997;42(1):19-27.
15. Lemos Miguel MA, Dias de Castro AC, Ferreira Gomes LS. Inhibition of vancomycin and high-level aminoglycoside-resistant enterococci strains and *Listeria* monocytogenes by bacteriocin-like substance produced by *Enterococcus faecium* E86. *Curr Microbiol.* 2008;57(5):429-436.
16. Flynn S, van Sinderen D, Thornton GM, Holo H, Nes IF, Collins JK. Characterization of the genetic locus responsible for the production of ABP-118, a novel bacteriocin produced by the probiotic bacterium *Lactobacillus salivarius* subsp. *salivarius* UCC118. *Microbiology.* 2002;148(pt 4):973-984.
17. Rea MC, Clayton E, O'Connor PM, et al. Antimicrobial activity of lacticin 3,147 against clinical *Clostridium difficile* strains. *J Med Microbiol.* 2007;56(Pt 7):940-946.
18. Gotteland M, Brunser O, Cruchet S. Systematic review: are probiotics useful in controlling gastric colonization by *Helicobacter pylori*? *Aliment Pharmacol Ther.* 2006;23(8):1077-1086.
19. Mukherjee S, Vaishnava S, Hooper LV. Multi-layered regulation of intestinal antimicrobial defense. *Cell Mol Life Sci.* 2008;65(19):3019-3027.

20. Wehkamp J, Chu H, Shen B, et al. Paneth cell antimicrobial peptides: topographical distribution and quantification in human gastrointestinal tissues. *FEBS Lett.* 2006;580(22):5344-5350.

21. Wehkamp J, Salzman NH, Porter E, et al. Reduced Paneth cell alpha-defensins in ileal Crohn's disease. *Proc Natl Acad Sci U S A.* 2005;102(50):18129-18134.

22. Wehkamp J, Harder J, Weichenthal M, et al. NOD2 (CARD15) mutations in Crohn's disease are associated with diminished mucosal alpha-defensin expression. *Gut.* 2004;53(11):1658-1664.

23. Simms LA, Doecke JD, Walsh MD, Huang N, Fowler EV, Radford-Smith GL. Reduced alpha-defensin expression is associated with inflammation and not NOD2 mutation status in ileal Crohn's disease. *Gut.* 2008;57(7):903-910.

24. Sartor RB. The influence of normal microbial flora on the development of chronic mucosal inflammation. *Res Immunol.* 1997;148(8-9):567-576.

25. Sellon RK, Tonkonogy S, Schultz M, et al. Resident enteric bacteria are necessary for development of spontaneous colitis and immune system activation in interleukin-10-deficient mice. *Infect Immun.* 1998;66(11):5224-5231.

26. Mazmanian SK, Round JL, Kasper DL. A microbial symbiosis factor prevents intestinal inflammatory disease. *Nature.* 2008;453(7195):620-625.

27. Xu J, Mahowald MA, Ley RE, et al. Evolution of symbiotic bacteria in the distal human intestine. *PLoS Biol.* 2007;5(7):e156.

28. Venturi A, Gionchetti P, Rizzello F, et al. Impact on the composition of the faecal flora by a new probiotic preparation: preliminary data on maintenance treatment of patients with ulcerative colitis. *Aliment Pharmacol Ther.* 1999;13(8):1103-1108.

29. Asahara T, Shimizu K, Nomoto K, Hamabata T, Ozawa A, Takeda Y. Probiotic bifidobacteria protect mice from lethal infection with Shiga toxin-producing *Escherichia coli* O157:H7. *Infect Immun.* 2004;72(4):2240-2247.

30. Schlee M, Harder J, Köten B, Stange EF, Wehkamp J, Fellermann K. Probiotic lactobacilli and VSL#3 induce enterocyte beta-defensin 2. *Clin Exp Immunol.* 2008;151(3):528-535.

31. Sherman PM, Johnson-Henry KC, Yeung HP, Ngo PS, Goulet J, Tompkins TA. Probiotics reduce enterohemorrhagic *Escherichia coli* O157:H7- and enteropathogenic *E. coli* O127:H6-induced changes in polarized T84 epithelial cell monolayers by reducing bacterial adhesion and cytoskeletal rearrangements. *Infect Immun.* 2005;73(8):5183-5188.

32. Malchow HA. Crohn's disease and *Escherichia coli*. A new approach in therapy to maintain remission of colonic Crohn's disease? *J Clin Gastroenterol.* 1997;25(4):653-658.

33. Rembacken BJ, Snelling AM, Hawkey PM, Chalmers DM, Axon AT. Non-pathogenic *Escherichia coli* versus mesalazine for the treatment of ulcerative colitis: a randomised trial. *Lancet.* 1999;354(9179):635-639.

34. Wehkamp J, Harder J, Wehkamp K, et al. NF-kappaB- and AP-1-mediated induction of human beta defensin-2 in intestinal epithelial cells by *Escherichia coli* Nissle 1917: a novel effect of a probiotic bacterium. *Infect Immun.* 2004;72(10):5750-5758.

35. Schlee M, Wehkamp J, Altenhoefer A, Oelschlaeger TA, Stange EF, Fellermann K. Induction of human beta-defensin 2 by the probiotic *Escherichia coli* Nissle 1917 is mediated through flagellin. *Infect Immun.* 2007;75(5):2399-2407.

36. Akbari O, DeKruyff RH, Umetsu DT. Pulmonary dendritic cells producing IL-10 mediate tolerance induced by respiratory exposure to antigen. *Nat Immunol.* 2001;2(8):725-731.

37. Iwasaki A, Kelsall BL. Freshly isolated Peyer's patch, but not spleen, dendritic cells produce interleukin 10 and induce the differentiation of T helper type 2 cells. *J Exp Med.* 1999;190(2):229-239.

38. Rescigno M, Urbano M, Valzasina B, et al. Dendritic cells express tight junction proteins and penetrate gut epithelial monolayers to sample bacteria. *Nat Immunol.* 2001;2(4):361-367.

39. Stagg AJ, Hart AL, Knight SC, Kamm MA. The dendritic cell: its role in intestinal inflammation and relationship with gut bacteria. *Gut.* 2003;52(10):1522-1529.

40. Hart AL, Al Hassi HO, Rigby RJ, et al. Characteristics of intestinal dendritic cells in inflammatory bowel diseases. *Gastroenterology.* 2005;129(1):50-65.

41. Hart AL, Lammers K, Brigidi P, et al. Modulation of human dendritic cell phenotype and function by probiotic bacteria. *Gut.* 2004;53(11):1602-1609.

42. Stagg AJ, Hart AL, Knight SC, Kamm MA. Microbial-gut interactions in health and disease. Interactions between dendritic cells and bacteria in the regulation of intestinal immunity. *Best Pract Res Clin Gastroenterol.* 2004;18(2):255-270.

43. Ng SC, Plamondon S, Hart AL, et al. Effective probiotic treatment (VSL#3), but not placebo, in acute ulcerative colitis is associated with downregulation of inflammatory intestinal dendritic cells. *Gut.* 2008;57(suppl 1):96.

44. Rigby R, Kamm MA, Knight SC, et al. Pathogenic bacteria stimulate colonic dendritic cells to produce pro-inflammatory IL-12 while the response to probiotic bacteria is to produce anti-inflammatory IL-10. *Gut.* 2002;50:A70.
45. Mahida YR, Cunliffe RN. Defensins and mucosal protection. *Novartis Found Symp.* 2004;263:71-77.
46. Kandler K, Shaykhiev R, Kleemann P, et al. The anti-microbial peptide LL-37 inhibits the activation of dendritic cells by TLR ligands. *Int Immunol.* 2006;18(12):1729-1736.

3

Barrier Function and the Immune Response

Karen L. Madsen, PhD

The ability of the intestinal tract to act as a barrier between the external environment and the closely regulated internal milieu is absolutely essential for human health. In our evolution as vertebrates, we have developed elegant mechanisms to coexist with bacteria. Colonization of the intestine with bacteria begins during the birth process, and within several months a relatively stable bacterial population resides in our intestines. Although humans are highly adapted to coexisting with bacteria, confining their existence to the lumen of the GI tract and restricting immune responses to the immense bacterial antigenic load in the gut is critical to the well-being of the host. Mucosal surfaces are continuously exposed to both pathogens and beneficial commensal microbes, which represents a challenge to the mucosal immune system to maintain homeostatic balance between tolerance and immunity. The intestinal epithelium serves as a protective barrier separating luminal contents from the underlying tissue. However, in addition to acting as a barrier, the epithelium, which consists of enterocytes, intraepithelial lymphocytes, goblet cells, microfold cells, and DCs, also has a critical role in linking innate and adaptive immune response and maintaining homeostasis within the intestinal tract. This chapter reviews the components of intestinal barrier function and discusses the impacts of probiotics on barrier and immune function.

BARRIER FUNCTION OF THE GUT

Epithelial Cells and Tight Junctions

Epithelial cells are polarized cells specialized for the vectorial transport of nutrients and are the predominant cell type lining the intestine. In terms of surface area, the apical brush border membrane of epithelial cells comprises the largest portion of the epithelial barrier. The membrane is covered by a 400- to 500-nm thick glycocalyx composed of filamentous transmembrane glycoproteins.[1-3] While the plasma membrane of intestinal epithelial cells is an effective barrier to hydrophilic substances,

Floch MH, Kim AS, eds.
Probiotics: A Clinical Guide (pp 21-40)
© 2010 Taylor & Francis Group

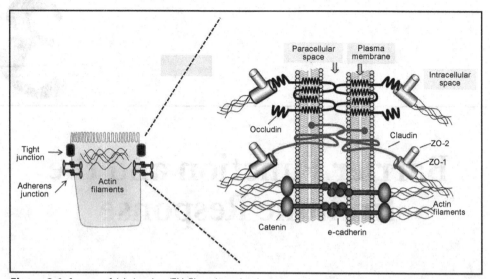

Figure 3-1. Structure of tight junctions (TJs). TJs are located at the most apical part of lateral membranes. TJ proteins interact with the actomyosin ring that surrounds the enterocyte at the level of the TJ via zonula occludens proteins (ZO-1, ZO-2, and ZO-3.) Claudins are a multigene family consisting of more than 20 different members shown to impart resistance and ion selectivity to epithelial paracellular pathways. Other proteins associated with the TJ and adherens junction (AJ) include cingulin, junctional adhesion molecules (JAMs), the Coxsackie adenovirus receptor, catenin, and E-cadherin.

the paracellular spaces are also joined together by a series of intercellular junctions along their lateral membranes.[4] At the uppermost apical surface, the junctional complex is composed of a tight junction (TJ) and an adherens junction (AJ). Both junctions are made up of complex lipoprotein structures that form fibrils that traverse the lateral plasma membrane to interact with proteins from the adjacent cell. TJ proteins also interact intracellularly with the actomyosin ring that surrounds the enterocyte at the level of the TJ via zonula occludens proteins ZO-1, ZO-2, and ZO-3 (Figure 3-1).[5,6] To date, the primary proteins identified as TJ-specific integral transmembrane proteins are the claudins and occludin. Claudins are a multigene family consisting of more than 20 different members shown to impart resistance and ion selectivity to epithelial paracellular pathways.[7] Other proteins associated with the TJ and AJ include cingulin,[8] junctional adhesion molecules (JAMs),[9] the Coxsackie adenovirus receptor,[10] catenin,[11] and E-cadherin.[12] TJ protein interactions establish a charge and size selectivity to the junctions.[13] In addition to their role in maintaining a barrier, TJs also play a key role in the control of cell polarity, differentiation, and maturation.[7]

Regulation of Tight Junctions

TJs are not static, impermeable structures, but demonstrate fluidity and enough permeability to allow leukocytes to pass through.[14,15] DCs also send dendrites through TJ to sample bacteria in the lumen and maintain the barrier by expressing TJ proteins to establish TJ-like structures with adjacent epithelial cells.[16] The Rho family of small guanosine triphosphate (GTP)-binding proteins (Rho, Rac, Cdc42) has been shown to be involved in the regulation of epithelial TJ organization and function.[17-19] F-actin organization is regulated by Rho GTPases, and the apical actin cytoskeleton is fundamental to the regulation of TJ function. Rho kinase has also been shown to regulate TJ structure and is essential for assembly of the apical junctional proteins and the F-actin cytoskeleton organization during junctional formation.[20] GTPase regulators, including GEF-H1 and Smurf1, modify epithelial barrier function.[21,22]

Opening of the TJ is driven, in part, by myosin light chain (MLC) phosphorylation, an event dependent on the activation of MLC kinase (MLCK)[23,24] through a NF-κB-dependent mechanism.[25] MLC phosphorylation occurs within the perijunctional actomyosin ring and colocalizes with the TJ.[24] MLCK-mediated regulation of TJ opening also seems to be a common intermediate in a variety of pathways related to altered paracellular permeability both in vitro and in vivo.[26-28]

Disruption of the epithelial barrier by the proinflammatory cytokines tumor necrosis factor (TNF)-α and interferon (IFN)-γ likely plays an important role in the pathogenesis of IBD and other GI diseases. IFN-γ and TNF-α have been shown to alter barrier function in an apoptosis-independent manner by inducing an internalization of TJ transmembrane proteins, rearranging the internal actin cytoskeleton, causing a redistribution of JAM-1 from membrane raft-containing fractions, and inducing a redistribution of the AJ protein E-cadherin.[29] IFN-γ and TNF-α have also been shown to induce a reduction in occludin and ZO-1 gene expression in HT-29/B6 cells, suggesting that cytokines can also modulate barrier function at gene level.[30] In addition to their effects on TJs, IFN-γ and TNF-α induce apoptosis by increasing Fas ligand sensitivity of colonic epithelial cells.[31] IFN-γ causes an increase in bacterial translocation in Caco-2 and T84 epithelial monolayers by the exploitation of lipid raft-mediated transcytotic pathways, which may precede cytokine-induced disruption of TJs.[32]

MLCK has also been shown to play a role in the breakdown of intestinal permeability. MLCK expression and MLC phosphorylation are increased in IBD and may contribute to barrier dysfunction and pathogenesis of the disease.[33] TNFα-induced increases in intestinal epithelial permeability are mediated by NF-κ-B binding and activation of the MLCK promoter and thereby an increase in TJ permeability.[25] T-cell-derived LIGHT (lymphotoxin-like inducible protein that competes with glycoprotein D for herpes virus entry on T-cells) also disrupts barrier function via MLCK.[34] TJ disassembly in response to IFN-γ occurs through macropinocytosis of TJ proteins, not through clathrin- or caveolar-mediated endocytosis.[35] IFN-γ-induced TJ uptake has also been shown to result from activation of Rho GTPase by Rho-associated kinase, and not from MLCK activation.[36]

Barrier Restitution

The repair and rapid resealing of the epithelial barrier after injury is a highly regulated process involving epithelial restitution, cell proliferation and maturation, and migration of cells.[37] Once intestinal epithelial injury occurs, numerous growth factors and cytokines, including epidermal growth factor, hepatocyte growth factor, trefoil peptides, keratinocyte growth factor, endothelial growth factor, transforming growth factor (TGF)-β, interleukin-1 (IL-1), IL-2, glucagon-like peptide-2, and bombesin,[38,39] are induced in both the intestinal lumen and submucosa, and these factors cooperatively stimulate epithelial mucosal repair. Lipidic structures such as lysophosphatidic acid[40] and prostaglandins[41] also contribute to epithelial restitution.

Mucus and Goblet Cells

Goblet cells are polarized, mucus-secreting cells present throughout the intestinal epithelium. Mucus is released constitutively and also in response to various stimuli, including bacterial enterotoxins and probiotics.[42] Mucin monomers are synthesized as apomucin cores that are posttranslationally modified by glycosylation.[43] The glycosylation of mucins increases their water-holding characteristics and also renders them resilient to proteolysis. At least 9 human mucin (MUC) genes have been identified, and MUC1, MUC2, MUC3, MUC4, and MUC5AC are expressed in the human colon.[44] MUC2 is the major gel-forming mucin of the small and large intestines and is the main structural component of the mucus gel.[45] The protective layer of mucus acts as both a lubricant for intestinal contents and as a barrier between the body and the external environment.[46] Mucins, along with secretory IgA and lysozyme, interact with microbes and microbial toxins and prevent them from reaching epithelial surfaces. The mucus layer is in a constant state of flux, whereby production of mucins by goblet cells is balanced by continual degradation by luminal microbes. Trefoil peptides are small peptides that are packaged with mucins and secreted along the entire intestinal tract.[47] Three types of trefoil peptides have been described: TFF1 in the proximal stomach; TFF2 expressed in the distal stomach, biliary tract, and pancreas; and TFF3 in the intestine and colon.[47] Trefoil peptides appear to have 2 primary functions: mucosal protection and mucosal repair.[48-50] Trefoil peptides act in synergy with mucin glycoproteins to enhance mucosal barrier function.[51] There is some evidence that trefoil factors alter the biophysical barrier properties of mucus by increasing mucus viscosity.[52] The effects of trefoil factors on epithelial restitution may be mediated through basolateral receptors and modulation of intracellular signaling pathways.[47]

Paneth Cells

Paneth cells are formed in the base of the crypts and can extend as high as halfway up the lateral walls of the crypts.[53] The innate immune defense function of Paneth cells is mediated in part by secretion of products including lysozyme,[54] angiogenin-4,[55] defensins,[56] and immunoglobulin.[57] Defensins have been shown to be not only antimicrobial, but also chemotactic and corticostatic.[58] α-Defensins, but not β-defensins, also regulate intestinal homeostasis by controlling IL-1β production.[59]

Probiotic Enhancement of Barrier Function

Probiotic bacteria have demonstrated numerous beneficial effects, including enhancing epithelial barrier function through effects on TJ proteins,[60] increasing mucus and defensin production,[61,62] and preventing pathogenic bacterial adhesion. Several strains of *Lactobacillus* and *Bifidobacterium* are able to compete with pathogens (*Bacteroides vulgatus*, *Clostridium histolyticum*, *C. difficile*, *Listeria monocytogenes*, *Staphylococcus aureus*, *Salmonella enterica*, *Yersinia enterocolitica*, enterotoxigenic *Escherichia coli*, enteropathogenic *E. coli*) for binding to intestinal epithelial cells and are able to displace pathogens even if the pathogens have already attached.[63-66] Probiotics also induce mucus secretion, which would aid in preventing pathogenic bacterial adhesion. Several strains of lactobacilli upregulate MUC2 and MUC3 mRNA expression,[61,67] while VSL#3 and *E. coli* Nissle both increase MUC2, MUC3, and MUC5AC gene and protein expression.[68,69] Probiotic inhibition of pathogen adherence to epithelial cells is mediated partially by competition for lectin-binding sites on glycoconjugate receptors on the brush border surface.[70,71]

In addition to their effects on preventing pathogen adherence, probiotics also modulate epithelial cell TJs, enhance restitution of damaged epithelium, increase production of antimicrobial molecules and cell protective proteins, and prevent cytokine-induced epithelial cell apoptosis. Oral administration of numerous probiotic strains (VSL#3; *Lactobacillus acidophilus*, *L. plantarum*, *Lactobacillus casei*, *Lactobacillus bulgaricus*, *B. infantis*, *B. breve*, *B. longum*, *Streptococcus thermophilus*; *E. coli* Nissle) has been shown to normalize barrier function in various rodent models of disease, involving a breakdown in gut permeability, and to protect against the onset of inflammation.[47,72-74] In one study, the ability to enhance barrier function was found to be associated with the secretion of a bioactive peptide from *B. infantis* that acted on epithelial cells to alter TJ protein expression.[75] Other probiotic strains, such as *Streptococcus thermophilus* and *L. acidophilus*, have been shown to enhance phosphorylation of actinin and occludin in the TJ, thereby inhibiting the invasion of strains of *E. coli* into human intestinal epithelial cell lines.[76] Probiotics are also able to protect TJs from disruptions induced by proinflammatory cytokines. Several studies have demonstrated that strains such as *B. thetaiotaomicron*, *Streptococcus thermophilus*, and *L. acidophilus* are able to prevent oxidant or cytokine-induced reductions in transepithelial resistance and increase in permeability.[68,77] *E. coli* Nissle 1917 promotes TJ barrier function following enteropathogenic *E. coli*-induced disruption in T84 cells by overexpression and redistribution of the TJ proteins ZO-2 and protein kinase C to the cell surface.[74] *Lactobacillus* GG (LGG) and LGG-derived soluble proteins (p40 and p75) can maintain epithelial barrier function from hydrogen peroxide-induced disruption by increasing membrane translocation of ZO-1, occludin, PKCβ1, and PKCE in an extracellular signal-related kinase (ERK1/2) and mitogen-activated protein kinase (MAPK)-dependent manner.[78]

Another mechanism by which probiotics can enhance gut barrier function is via enhanced production of cytoprotective molecules. Heat shock proteins are constitutively expressed in epithelial cells and are induced in cells by stress in order to help maintain homeostasis.[79] Soluble factors released from LGG induce cytoprotective heat shock protein synthesis in intestinal epithelial cells in a p38- and c-Jun *N*-terminal kinase (JNK)/MAPK-dependent manner.[80] Quorum-sensing molecules secreted by *Bacillus subtilis* also induce epithelial expression of cytoprotective heat shock proteins.[81] Probiotics also prevent cytokine- and oxidant-induced epithelial damage by promoting cell survival. LGG and soluble factors (p75 and p40) released from LGG prevent epithelial cell apoptosis through activating antiapoptotic Akt in a phosphatidylinositol-3'-kinase (PI3K)-dependent manner and inhibiting proapoptotic p38/MAPK activation.[82,83] This reduction in apoptosis may help in maintaining epithelial barrier integrity and increasing resistance to toxic agents and pathogens by reducing breaks in the mucosal barrier. Finally, some probiotics stimulate release of defensins from epithelial and Paneth cells. *L. fermentum* and *E. coli* Nissle 1917 both stimulate β-defensin mRNA and protein secretion in a time- and dose-dependent manner through regulation of NF-κB- and AP-1-dependent pathways.[84,85]

IMMUNE FUNCTION OF THE GUT

Dysregulated innate and adaptive immune responses in the gut play key roles in the pathogenesis of several diseases. Gut-associated lymphoid tissue (GALT) is the largest lymphoid tissue of the body and is extremely immunologically active. GALT consists of organized lymphoid tissues, including Peyer's patches and mesenteric lymph nodes, along with areas where lymphocytes are scattered throughout the epithelium and lamina propria. Peyer's patches have the highest density in the ileum and comprise 10 to 1000 individual follicles arranged into distinct lymphoid structures covered with follicle-associated epithelium.[86] Peyer's patches differ from the epithelium covering the villi in a paucity of goblet cells and abundance of lymphoepithelial microfold- or membranous-cells (M-cells). M-cells function to sample proteins and other antigens from the lumen of the GI tract and present them to underlying B- and T-lymphocytes, macrophages, and DCs.[87,88] Probiotic bacteria are internalized by M-cells to interact with DCs and epithelial cells, resulting in the initiation of responses mediated by macrophages and T- and B-lymphocytes.

Peyer's patches are also an important source of secretory IgA (sIgA) induction. Secretory IgA functions to neutralize toxins and pathogenic microbes, as well as

Figure 3-2. Toll-like receptor structure. The mammalian TLRs are type I transmembrane proteins with multiple leucine-rich repeats and 1-2 cysteine-rich regions in the ligand-binding ecto-main, a short transmembrane region, and a conserved cytoplasmic domain that is highly homologous among the individual TLRs and contains a TIR domain similar to the cytoplasmic domain of the interleukin-1 receptor.

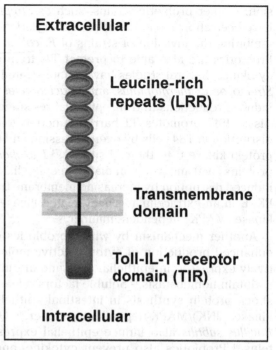

Extracellular

Leucine-rich repeats (LRR)

Transmembrane domain

Toll-IL-1 receptor domain (TIR)

Intracellular

acting to contain the commensal microbes within the intestinal lumen.[89] Peyer's patch germinal centers contain mostly B cells that are actively dividing, of which 70% are secreting IgA—a much higher frequency than peripheral lymphoid tissues, where most B cells switch to IgG subclasses.[89] In order to produce sIgA, B cells in Peyer's patches undergo a class switch recombination in response to antigen stimulation and TGF-β.[90] After IgA isotype switching, IgA-committed B cells migrate from the Peyer's patches to the intestinal lamina and become IgA plasma cells in the presence of cytokines such as IL-5 and IL-6.[91,92] IgA produced by these plasma cells then interacts with the poly-Ig receptor expressed on the basolateral membrane of intestinal epithelial cells and is transported to the apical membrane and secreted.[89] Some probiotic strains (VSL#3; *Bifidobacterium animalis*) promote the differentiation of B cells into plasma cells and increase the production of sIgA.[93,94] This probiotic-induced stimulation of sIgA would help reduce mucosal penetration by bacteria.

Toll-Like Receptors

The innate immune response is a rapid first line of defense against pathogens and is mediated primarily by macrophages, DCs, and epithelial cells. The innate immune response is not completely nonspecific, but rather discriminates between self and a variety of different pathogens. The innate immune system recognizes microbes via a limited number of germline-encoded pattern-recognition receptors that recognize conserved motifs referred to as microbe-associated molecular patterns (MAMPs).[95] These receptors recognize specific molecular patterns unique to bacteria, fungi, and viruses and include the Toll-like receptors (TLRs) and nucleotide-binding oligomerization domains (NODs). To date, 12 members of the of the TLR family have been identified in mammals (Table 3-1). TLRs are type 1 integral membrane glycoproteins that are characterized by extracellular domains containing varying numbers of leucine-rich repeat (LRR) motifs and a cytoplasmic signaling domain homologous to that of the IL-1 receptor, known as the Toll/IL-1R (TIR) domain (Figure 3-2).[96] TLRs can be divided into several subfamilies,

TABLE 3-1

TOLL-LIKE RECEPTORS AND THEIR LIGANDS

TLR	LIGAND(S)	REFERENCE
1	Triacyl lipoproteins	97
2	Lipoproteins	98-104
	Peptidoglycan	
	Lipoteichoic acid	
	Zymosan	
	Heat shock proteins	
	Lipoarabinomannan	
3	Double-stranded RNA	105
4	Lipopolysaccharide	106-115
	Taxol	
	Heat shock proteins	
	Fibronectin	
	Hyaluronic acid	
	Heparin sulfate	
	Fibrinogen	
	Respiratory syncytial virus fusion protein	
	Murine retroviral envelope protein	
5	Flagellin	116
6	Diacyl lipopeptides	117, 118
	Lipoteichoic acid	
	Zymosan	
7	Single-stranded RNA	119-121
	Imidazoquinoline	
8	Single-stranded RNA	120
	Imidazoquinoline	
9	Bacterial DNA	122
	Hemozoin	123
10	Unknown	
11	Profilin	124, 125
	Uropathogenic bacteria	

each of which recognizes related MAMPs. TLR1, TLR2, and TLR6 recognize lipids; TLR5 recognizes flagellen; and TLR7, TLR8, and TLR9 recognize nucleic acids (Table 3-1). TLR4 recognizes an extremely divergent collection of ligands, including lipopolysaccharide, the plant diterpene paclitaxel, the fusion protein of respiratory syncytial virus, fibronectin, and heat shock proteins, all of which have very different structures.

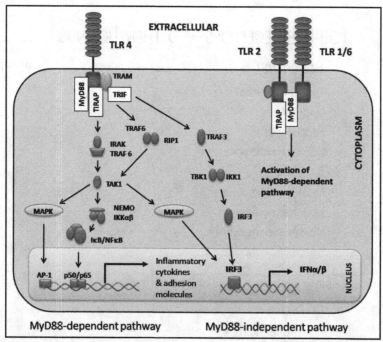

Figure 3-3. Toll-like receptor signaling. TLR1, 2, and 6 cooperate to recognize lipopeptides and lipoteichoic acid, found mainly in Gram-positive bacteria. TLR4 is the major receptor for LPS. Each TLR recruits a distinct set of TIR domain-containing adaptor molecules such as MyD88, TIRAP, TRIF, and TRAM. MyD88 binds to IRAK-4 and TRAF-6. TRIF binds receptor-interacting protein 1 and TRAF-6. TRAF-6 activates a complex containing TAK1, TAK1-binding protein 1 (TAB1), TAB2, and TAB3. TAK1 activates IKK complex consisting of IKKα, IKKβ, and Nemo, which results in the phosphorylation and proteasomal degradation of IκB proteins; p50/p65 transcription factors are released, which enter the nucleus to regulate expression of inflammatory cytokines and adhesion molecules. TAK1 simultaneously activates the MAPK (JNK, p38, and ERK) pathway, leading to activation of activator protein (AP-1). TRIF recruits TRAF3, which interacts with TANK-binding kinase 1 and IKK1. These kinases catalyze the phosphorylation of IRF3. Phosphorylated IRF3 forms a dimer, translocates into the nuclei, binds to DNA, and regulates the expression of IFN-β in collaboration with AP-1 and NF-κB.[124]

TLRs are expressed on a variety of myeloid (macrophages, DCs, neutrophils, B and T cells) and nonmyeloid (fibroblasts and epithelial) cells.[95] Expression and localization of TLRs is modulated rapidly in response to microbes, cytokines, and various environmental signals. A model showing TLR4 signaling is shown in Figure 3-3. All TLRs, with the exception of TLR3, signal through myeloid differentiation primary response protein 88 (MyD88).[126] Following ligand recognition, TIR domain-containing adapter protein (TIRAP)[127] and MyD88 interact with the cytoplasmic domain of the TLR and recruit IL-1R-associated kinase 4 (IRAK-4) and IRAK-1. IRAK-1 is phosphorylated by IRAK-4, which results in its activation and subsequent association with TNF receptor-associated factor 6 (TRAF-6).[128] TRAF-6 activates TGF-β-activating kinase 1 (TAK1) and TAK1 phosphorylates IκB kinase (IKK)-β, leading to the degradation of IκB and the nuclear translocation of NF-κB. This subsequently results in the induction of proinflammatory genes such as TNF-α, IL-1β, IL-6, and IL-10.[115,129] Activation of the MyD88 pathway also results in the activation of MAPKs, including JNK, p38 MAPK, and ERK, which leads to the activation of AP-1.[130] In addition, the MyD88 pathway can also activate a third transcription factor, IFN regulatory factor (IRF)-3, which can translocate into the nucleus and bind to IFN-stimulated response element motifs in the promoter region of various cytokine genes. TLR4 can also signal via an MyD88-independent pathway.[131] This pathway involves the activation of TRIF-related adaptor molecule (TRAM), a TIR domain-containing adapter molecule, which associates with and activates TIR-containing adaptor-inducing IFN-β (TRIF), another TIR domain-containing adapter protein.[132,133] TRIF then interacts with and activates TANK-binding kinase 1 and IKKζ,[134] which results in the phosphorylation of IRF-3 and subsequent translocation of IRF-3 into the nucleus, where it regulates the expression of the type 1 IFN family.[135] TRIF also interacts with TRAF-6 and receptor interacting protein 1, leading to the activation of NF-κB.[136]

The intracellular TLRs, including TLR3, TLR7, TLR8, and TLR9, are expressed on the endoplasmic reticulum (ER) in resting myeloid cells and trafficked to the endosomal compartment in response to MAMP-mediated stimulation.[137-139] The intracellular localization of these TLRs is primarily controlled by UNC93B, a membrane-spanning ER protein.[140] UNC93B interacts with the transmembrane regions of TLR3, TLR7, and TLR9 in the ER, and controls the trafficking of TLR7 and TLR9 from the ER to the endosome.[140] There is some evidence that proteolysis of TLR9 within the endosome is required for innate immune responses, as the ectodomain of TLR9 is cleaved by cathepsins, and the cleaved product can activate downstream signaling.[141] Binding of ligand by TLR7 and TLR9 can also result in the induction of IFN-α in an MyD88-dependent manner.[142] Upon activation, a complex consisting of MyD88, IRAK-4, IRAK-1, and TRAF-6 is formed at the TIR domain of TLR7 and TLR9, followed by the recruitment of IRF-7. The activation of IRF-7 by phosphorylation results in the translocation of IRF-7 into the nucleus and induction of the IFN response.

TLR Signaling in Epithelial Cells

In contrast to immune cells, intestinal epithelial cells express TLRs on their cell surfaces in a polarized fashion. While TLR2 and TLR4 are expressed on the apical surface,[68,143-145] TLR5 is primarily expressed on the basolateral surface,[146] and TLR 3, 7, and 8 are expressed intracellularly.[68] TLR9 is expressed on both the apical and basolateral surface, as well as intracellularly.[143,144] Depending on the stimulus, activation of TLRs in epithelial cells can result in changes in apoptosis and cellular proliferation,[147] paracellular permeability,[148,149] cytokine secretion,[68,144,150] and bacterial internalization and translocation,[151] suggesting that TLRs have extremely complex and critical roles in maintaining gut homeostasis while simultaneously protecting the host from pathogens. Regulation of TLR activation is critical in the gut, as mucosal surfaces are constantly bathed in bacteria, and inflammatory responses to these normal commensal bacteria must be prevented. The regulation of TLR activity in the gut involves altering TLR and adapter protein expression, localization, and levels of signaling intermediates, and negative regulatory proteins.[152] Probiotics can modulate gut permeability and inflammation through interactions with TLR2[148,149,153] through activation of protein kinase C and a tightening and sealing of TJ-associated ZO-1.[148]

NOD-Like Receptor Family

NOD-like receptor (NLR) family proteins consist of more than 20 identified members that appear to localize in the cytosol.[95] NLR proteins share a C-terminal LRR domain that recognizes conserved microbial patterns; a centrally located NACHT domain that mediates self-oligomerization; and an *N*-terminal effector domain responsible for protein-protein interactions with adapter molecules and signal transduction (Figure 3-4).[154,155] The NLRs can be divided into subfamilies on the basis of their *N*-terminal domains: the

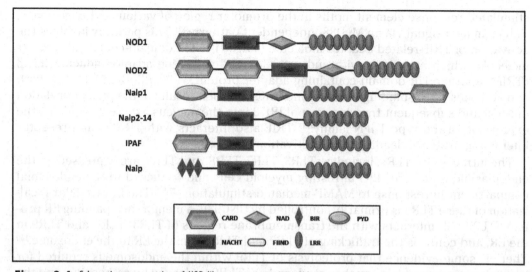

Figure 3-4. Schematic representation of NOD-like receptor proteins. *Abbreviations*: LRR = C-terminal leucine-rich repeat domain that is involved in recognition of conserved microbial patterns or other ligands; CARD = caspase activation and recruitment domain; NACHT = a central domain present in NAIP (neuronal apoptosis inhibitory protein); CIITA = Class II transactivator; HET-E = plant het product; and TP-1 = telomerase-associated protein that mediates self-oligomerization and is essential for activation; NAD = N-terminal effector domain responsible for protein-protein interaction with adapter molecules that results in signal transduction; PYD = pyrin domain; BIR = baculovirus inhibitor of apoptosis protein repeat domain.

NODs (NOD1 and NOD2) and IPAF contain a caspase activation and recruitment domain (CARD); the Nalps display a pyrin domain; and Naip presents a baculovirus inhibitor of apoptosis protein repeat domain (BIR).[154,155]

NOD1 and NOD2 recognize distinct structural motifs derived from peptidoglycan.[156-159] NOD1 recognizes the disaccharide of N-acetyl glucosamine-N-acetyl muramic acid linked to a tripeptide group, of which the terminal amino acid is *meso*-diaminopimelate (mDAP).[156] mDAP is a component of the bacterial cell wall of most Gram-negative species, with the exception of *mycoplasma* and a few other species.[160] NOD2 recognizes muramyl dipeptide, the largest component of peptidoglycan.[157] The presence of these microbial ligands within the cell stimulates NOD1 and NOD2 signaling and the induction of inflammatory cytokines and other antimicrobial genes via the NF-κB and MAPK pathways.[95] In DCs and macrophages, activation of NOD1 and NOD2 results primarily in secretion of proinflammatory cytokines (IL-1β, IL-6, TNF-α, CXCL8/IL-8, IL-18, IL-12p40, IL-12p70), nitric oxide, and the expression of costimulatory molecules and adhesion molecules.[161] In epithelial cells, stimulation of NOD pathways induces the secretion of proinflammatory mediators (TNF-α, IL-6, CXCL8/IL-8, MIP2, CCL2/MCP1, CXCL5/ENA78) and antimicrobial peptides (β-defensins),[161] resulting in the recruitment and activation of immune effector cells. Some studies have shown that NOD1 and NOD2 agonists can synergize with TLR agonists to induce proinflammatory responses and immune cell maturation and activation, while others have demonstrated that in certain cell types NODs and TLRs can antagonize each other.[161] Along with TLRs, NLRs not only have a role in initiating the innate immune response, but are also involved in driving adaptive immunity.[162]

Nalp-3 responds to agonists of both microbial and host origin, including bacterial RNA and imidazoquinolone compounds, dsRNA from viruses,[163] uric acid,[164] and K+ cellular efflux,[165] which can arise from the insertion of a bacterial toxin through the plasma membrane. Because Nalp-3 can be activated in response to host molecules that are released by necrotic cells, this would suggest that this NLR may act to detect host danger signals as well as microbial stimuli.[162] IPAF is another member of the NLR family that activates caspase-1 in response to intracellular infection with pathogens such as *Salmonella typhimurium* and *Legionella pneumophila*, and that appears to be critical for controlling the intracellular replication of bacteria.[166,167] Both IPAF and Naip5 are able to sense the presence of bacterial flagellin in a TLR5-independent manner, suggesting that the primary role of these proteins may be to act as sensors for surveillance of cytosolic flagellin.[166,167]

Probiotic Effects on Epithelial Cell Immune Function

Intestinal epithelial cells have an important immunomodulatory role in the gut through their interactions with and influence over underlying immune cells. Epithelial cells are able to modulate and induce appropriate innate and adaptive immune responses by releasing chemokines/cytokines to influence DC and macrophage functions.[152] Probiotic bacteria can interact with epithelial cells and alter cytokine/chemokine production through modulation of cellular signal transduction pathways.[68,168,169] Epithelial cells recognize and respond to whole bacteria and bacterial components from commensal and pathogenic microbes in a differential manner, releasing proinflammatory cytokines such as IL-8 in response to pathogenic bacteria, while showing no response to probiotic strains.[123,170] Certain probiotic strains can also elicit anti-inflammatory responses and/or inhibit the NF-κB pathway in epithelial cells through various mechanisms, including blocking IκB degradation by inhibiting ubiquination,[168] by inhibiting proteasome function,[123,171] and by regulating nuclear-cytoplasmic movement of RelA through a PPAR-γ-dependent pathway.[172] In addition, *Enterococcus faecalis* regulates the phosphorylation, expression, and transcription activity of PPAR-γ and increases expression of IL-10 by colonic epithelial cells.[173] However, anti-inflammatory effects of probiotics are not limited to live bacteria.[75,145] Bacterial DNA is also recognized in a differential manner by epithelial cells—with pathogenic strains evoking a phosphorylation of the ERK pathway and activation of AP-1.[174] DNA derived from the probiotic compound, VSL#3 delayed NF-κB activation, stabilized levels of IκB, and inhibited proteasome function.[150] Probiotic bacterial DNA can also suppress systemic inflammatory responses to pathogenic bacterial DNA.[118,150] Overall, these findings suggest that IKK/NFκB signaling in intestinal epithelial cells is an important factor for the maintenance of epithelial integrity and immune homeostasis in the gut, and that probiotics may be harnessed to modulate barrier and immune function through this signaling pathway.

Intestinal epithelial cells express several antigen-presenting molecules and costimulatory molecules and play a role in the activation and expansion of both CD4[+] and CD8[+] regulatory T-cell subsets.[175] Proteasomes have a key role in the degradation of endogenous and exogenous proteins for antigen presentation by both MHC class I and II molecules.[176] Probiotic bacteria modulate epithelial cell proteasomal activity,[123,171] thus providing a potential mechanism for probiotic-induced alterations in epithelial-driven T-cell activation in the gut.

Dendritic Cells and Microbes

DCs directly sample commensal and pathogenic bacteria in the intestinal lumen via transepithelial dendrites that pass through paracellular spaces between epithelial cells.[16] They have a key role in linking innate immune responses with adaptive responses in the intestine and are modulated by microbes and epithelial cells.[177] DCs are able to activate naïve T-cells and also direct helper T-cell responses toward Th1, Th2, Th17, or regulatory T-cells along with inducing IgA-producing B cells. Intestinal DCs differ phenotypically and functionally from peripheral DCs in that they preferentially prime antigen-specific CD4[+] T cells to produce Th2 cytokines or to differentiate into regulatory T cells and induce tolerance.[178,179] Probiotics induce distinct and strain-specific maturation and cytokine patterns in isolated DCs.[180,181] For instance, *Lactobacillus* strains can induce either a strong or a weak release of IL-12 and TNF-α, along with high levels of IL-10, while most *Bifidobacterium* strains stimulate the production of high levels of IL-10 and low levels of IL-12 and TNF-α.[182] However, the presence or absence of other strains can significantly alter the response of DCs to specific probiotic strains, suggesting that the particular microflora of the host may have a strong influence on the response to treatment with a specific probiotic strain.

Interactions Between Bacteria, Epithelial Cells, and Immune Cells

The presence of epithelial cells significantly modulates immune cell responses to microbes.[183] In the presence of epithelial cells, DCs and macrophages are profoundly noninflammatory.[184,185] In particular, the presence of intestinal epithelial cells alters the ability of bacteria to induce DC maturation and also modulates the ratio of IL-10 to IL-12 production. In addition, DCs that sample bacteria through paracellular spaces are activated to a much less degree than those that come into contact directly with microbes.[183,186] The release of retinoic acid, TGF-β, and thymic stromal lymphopoietin by intestinal epithelial cells has been implicated in the modulation of DC maturation and activation.[183] The type of T-cell response to microbial stimulation is controlled by interactions between epithelial cells, DC, and T-cells in the lamina propria and in Peyer's patches. It has been shown that probiotics induce T regulatory cells, decrease T-cell proliferation, and decrease T-cell cytokine production.[182] In addition, oral probiotics can also affect immune cell distribution by enhancing the ability of lymphatic endothelial cells to trap T lymphocytes; this is evidenced in studies showing that in *S. boulardii*-fed mice, IFN-γ production by CD4+ T-cells was reduced in the colon but increased in the mesenteric lymph nodes.[187]

CONCLUSION

The intestinal epithelium regulates interactions between commensal bacteria and the immune system through the provision of a physical barrier and by the expression and secretion of numerous immunomodulatory compounds and antimicrobial peptides. It is clear that because of their ability to discriminate pathogenic and commensal microbes, and influence the function of antigen-presenting cells and lymphocytes, intestinal epithelial cells are a critical component for maintaining intestinal immune homeostasis. Further, probiotics have the capacity to enhance gut barrier function and enhance local and systemic immunity through effects on the epithelium.

REFERENCES

1. Ito S. Form and function of the glycocalyx on free cell surfaces. *Philos Trans R Soc Lond B Biol Sci.* 1974;268(891):55-66.
2. Maury J, Nicoletti C, Guzzo-Chambraud L, Maroux S. The filamentous brush border glycocalyx, a mucin-like marker of enterocyte hyper-polarization. *Eur J Biochem.* 1995;228(2):323-331.
3. Maury J, Bernadac A, Rigal A, Maroux S. Expression and glycosylation of the filamentous brush border glycocalyx (FBBG) during rabbit enterocyte differentiation along the crypt-villus axis. *J Cell Sci.* 1995;108(Pt 7):2705-2713.

4. Van Itallie CM, Anderson JM. The molecular physiology of tight junction pores. *Physiology (Bethesda)*. 2004;19:331-338.
5. Jesaitis LA, Goodenough DA. Molecular characterization and tissue distribution of ZO-2, a tight junction protein homologous to ZO-1 and the *Drosophila* discs-large tumor suppressor protein. *J Cell Biol*. 1994;124(6):949-961.
6. Siliciano JD, Goodenough DA. Localization of the tight junction protein, ZO-1, is modulated by extracellular calcium and cell-cell contact in Madin-Darby canine kidney epithelial cells. *J Cell Biol*. 1988;107(6 Pt 1):2389-2399.
7. Anderson JM, Van Itallie CM. Tight junctions. *Curr Biol*. 2008;18(20):R941-R943.
8. Cordenonsi M, D'Atri F, Hammar E, et al. Cingulin contains globular and coiled-coil domains and interacts with ZO-1, ZO-2, ZO-3, and myosin. *J Cell Biol*. 1999;147(7):1569-1582.
9. Martìn-Padura I, Lostaglio S, Schneemann M, et al. Junctional adhesion molecule, a novel member of the immunoglobulin superfamily that distributes at intercellular junctions and modulates monocyte transmigration. *J Cell Biol*. 1998;142(1):117-127.
10. Philipson L, Pettersson RF. The Coxsackie-adenovirus receptor—a new receptor in the immunoglobulin family involved in cell adhesion. *Curr Top Microbiol Immunol*. 2004;273:87-111.
11. Rajasekaran AK, Hojo M, Huima T, Rodriguez-Boulan E. Catenins and zonula occludens-1 form a complex during early stages in the assembly of tight junctions. *J Cell Biol*. 1996;132(3):451-463.
12. Nagafuchi A, Shirayoshi Y, Okazaki K, et al. Transformation of cell adhesion properties by exogenously introduced E-cadherin cDNA. *Nature*. 1987;329(6137):341-343.
13. Van Itallie CM, Holmes J, Bridges A, et al. The density of small tight junction pores varies among cell types and is increased by expression of claudin-2. *J Cell Sci*. 2008;121:298-305.
14. Burns AR, Bowden RA, MacDonell SD, et al. Analysis of tight junctions during neutrophil transendothelial migration. *J Cell Sci*. 2000;113(Pt 1):45-57.
15. Sasaki H, Matsui C, Furuse K, Mimori-Kiyosue Y, Furuse M, Tsukita S. Dynamic behavior of paired claudin strands within apposing plasma membranes. *Proc Natl Acad Sci U S A*. 2003;100(7):3971-3976.
16. Rescigno M, Urbano M, Valzasina B, et al. Dendritic cells express tight junction proteins and penetrate gut epithelial monolayers to sample bacteria. *Nature Immunol*. 2001;2(4):361-367.
17. Weber E, Berta G, Tousson A, et al. Expression and polarized targeting of a rab3 isoform in epithelial cells. *J Cell Biol*. 1994;125(3):583-594.
18. Braga VMM, Machesky LM, Hall A, Hotchin NA. The small GTPases Rho and Rac are required for the establishment of cadherin-dependent cell-cell contacts. *J Cell Biol*. 1997;137(6):1421-1431.
19. Nusrat A, Giry M, Turner JR, et al. Rho protein regulates tight junctions and perijunctional actin organization in polarized epithelia. *Proc Natl Acad Sci USA*. 1995;92(23):10629-10633.
20. Walsh SV, Hopkins AM, Chen J, Narumiya S, Parkos CA, Nusrat A. Rho kinase regulates tight junction function and is necessary for tight junction assembly in polarized intestinal epithelia. *Gastroenterology*. 2001;21(3):566-579.
21. Wang HR, Ogunjimi AA, Zhang Y, Ozdamar B, Bose R, Wrana JL. Degradation of RhoA by Smurf1 ubiquitin ligase. *Methods Enzymol*. 2006;406:437-447.
22. Aijaz S, D'Atri F, Citi S, Balda M, Matter K. Binding of GEF-H1 to the tight junction-associated adaptor cingulin results in inhibition of Rho signaling and G1/S phase transition. *Dev Cell*. 2005;8(5):777-786.
23. Turner JR, Rill BK, Carlson SL, et al. Physiological regulation of epithelial tight junctions is associated with myosin light-chain phosphorylation. *Am J Physiol*. 1997;273(4 Pt 1):C1378-C1385.
24. Berglund JJ, Riegler M, Zolotarevsky Y, Wenz E, Turner JR. Regulation of human jejunal transmucosal resistance and MLC phosphorylation by Na(+)-glucose cotransport. *Am J Physiol Gastrointest Liver Physiol*. 2001;281(6):G1487-G1493.
25. Ye D, Ma I, Ma TY. Molecular mechanism of tumor necrosis factor-alpha modulation of intestinal epithelial tight junction barrier. *Am J Physiol Gastrointest Liver Physiol*. 2006;290(3):G496-G504.
26. Turner JR. 'Putting the squeeze' on the tight junction: understanding cytoskeletal regulation. *Semin Cell Dev Biol*. 2000;11(4):301-308.
27. Nusrat A, Turner JR, Madara JL. Molecular physiology and pathophysiology of tight junctions. IV. Regulation of tight junctions by extracellular stimuli: nutrients, cytokines, and immune cells. *Am J Physiol Gastrointest Liver Physiol*. 2000;279(5):G851-G857.
28. Wainwright MS, Rossi J, Schavocky J, et al. Protein kinase involved in lung injury susceptibility: evidence from enzyme isoform genetic knockout and in vivo inhibitor treatment. *Proc Natl Acad Sci U S A*. 2003;100(10):6233-6238.
29. Bruewer M, Luegering A, Kucharzik T, et al. Proinflammatory cytokines disrupt epithelial barrier function by apoptosis-independent mechanisms. *J Immunol*. 2003;171(11):6164-6172.
30. Mankertz J, Tavalali S, Schmitz H, et al. Expression from the human occludin promoter is affected by tumor necrosis factor alpha and interferon gamma. *J Cell Sci*. 2000;113(Pt 11):2085-2090.

31. Strater J, Wellisch I, Riedl S, et al. CD95 (APO-1/Fas)-mediated apoptosis in colon epithelial cells: a possible role in ulcerative colitis. *Gastroenterology.* 1997;113(1):160-167.

32. Clark E, Hoare C, Tanianis-Hughes J, Carlson GL, Warhurst G. Interferon gamma induces translocation of commensal *Escherichia coli* across gut epithelial cells via a lipid raft-mediated process. *Gastroenterology.* 2005;128(5):1258-1267.

33. Blair SA, Kane SV, Clayburgh DR, Turner JR. Epithelial myosin light chain kinase expression and activity are upregulated in inflammatory bowel disease. *Lab Invest.* 2006;86(2):191-201.

34. Schwarz BT, Wang F, Shen L, et al. LIGHT signals directly to intestinal epithelia to cause barrier dysfunction via cytoskeletal and endocytic mechanisms. *Gastroenterology.* 2007;132(7):2383-2394.

35. Bruewer M, Utech M, Ivanov AI, Hopkins AM, Parkos CA, Nusrat A. Interferon-gamma induces internalization of epithelial tight junction proteins via a macropinocytosis-like process. *FASEB J.* 2005;19(8):923-933.

36. Utech M, Ivanov AI, Samarin SN, et al. Mechanism of IFN-gamma-induced endocytosis of tight junction proteins: myosin II-dependent vacuolarization of the apical plasma membrane. *Mol Biol Cell.* 2005;16(10):5040-5052.

37. Sturm A, Dignass AU. Epithelial restitution and wound healing in inflammatory bowel disease. *World J Gastroenterol.* 2008;14(3):348-353.

38. Kinoshita K, Taupin DR, Itoh H, Podolsky DK. Distinct pathways of cell migration and antiapoptotic response to epithelial injury: structure-function analysis of human intestinal trefoil factor. *Mol Cell Biol.* 2000;20(13):4680-4690.

39. Chen LW, Hsu CM, Huang JK, Chen JS, Chen SC. Effects of bombesin on gut mucosal immunity in rats after thermal injury. *J Formos Med Assoc.* 2000;99(6):491-498.

40. Hines OJ, Ryder N, Chu J, McFadden D. Lysophosphatidic acid stimulates intestinal restitution via cytoskeletal activation and remodeling. *J Surg Res.* 2000;92(1):23-28.

41. Zushi S, Shinomura Y, Kiyohara T, et al. Role of prostaglandins in intestinal epithelial restitution stimulated by growth factors. *Am J Physiol.* 1996;270(5 Pt 1):G757-G762.

42. Moon HW, Whipp SC, Baetz AL. Comparative effects of enterotoxins from *Escherichia coli* and *Vibrio cholerae* on rabbit and swine small intestine. *Lab Invest.* 1971;25:133-140.

43. McCool DJ, Forstner JF, Forstner GG. Synthesis and secretion of mucin by the human colonic tumour cell line LS180. *Biochem J.* 1994;302(Pt 1):111-118.

44. Aksoy N, Akinci OF. Mucin macromolecules in normal, adenomatous, and carcinomatous colon: evidence for the neotransformation. *Macromol Biosci.* 2004;4(5):483-496.

45. Deplancke B, Gaskins HR. Microbial modulation of innate defense: goblet cells and the intestinal mucus layer. *Am J Clin Nutr.* 2001;73(6):1131S-1141S.

46. Bansil R, Stanley E, LaMont JT. Mucin biophysics. *Annu Rev Physiol.* 1995;57:635-657.

47. Hoffmann W. Trefoil factors TFF (trefoil factor family) peptide-triggered signals promoting mucosal restitution. *Cell Mol Life Sci.* 2005;62(24):2932-2938.

48. Soriano-Izquierdo A, Gironella M, Massaguer A, et al. Trefoil peptide TFF2 treatment reduces VCAM-1 expression and leukocyte recruitment in experimental intestinal inflammation. *J Leukocyte Biol.* 2004;75(2):214-223.

49. FitzGerald AJ, Pu M, Marchbank T, et al. Synergistic effects of systemic trefoil factor family 1 (TFF1) peptide and epidermal growth factor in a rat model of colitis. *Peptides.* 2004;25(5):793-801.

50. Zhang BH, Yu HG, Sheng ZX, et al. The therapeutic effect of recombinant human trefoil factor 3 on hypoxia-induced necrotizing enterocolitis in immature rat. *Regul Pept.* 2003;116(1-3):53-60.

51. McKenzie C, Thim L, Parsons ME. Topical and intravenous administration of trefoil factors protect the gastric mucosa from ethanol-induced injury in the rat. *Aliment Pharmacol Ther.* 2000;14(8):1033-1040.

52. Babyatsky MW, deBeaumont M, Thim L, Podolsky DK. Oral trefoil peptides protect against ethanol- and indomethacin-induced gastric injury in rats. *Gastroenterology.* 1996;110(2):489-497.

53. Cheng H, Merzel J, Leblond CP. Renewal of Paneth cells in the small intestine of the mouse. *Am J Anat.* 1969;126(4):507-525.

54. Peeters T, Vantrappen G. The Paneth cell: a source of intestinal lysozyme. *Gut.* 1975;16(7):553-558.

55. Hooper LV, Stappenbeck TS, Hong CV, Gordon JI. Angiogenins: a new class of microbicidal proteins involved in innate immunity. *Nat Immunol.* 2003;4(3):269-273.

56. Bevins CL. Paneth cell defensins: key effector molecules of innate immunity. *Biochem Soc Trans.* 2006;34(Pt 2):263-266.

57. Erlandsen SL, Chase DG. Paneth cell function: phagocytosis and intracellular digestion of intestinal microorganisms. I. Hexamita muris. *J Ultrastruct Res.* 1972;41(3):296-318.

58. Taylor K, Clarke DJ, McCullough B, et al. Analysis and separation of residues important for the chemoattractant and antimicrobial activities of beta-defensin 3. *J Biol Chem.* 2008;283(11):6631-6639.

59. Shi J, Aono S, Lu W, et al. A novel role for defensins in intestinal homeostasis: regulation of IL-1beta secretion. *J Immunol.* 2007;179(2):1245-1253.

60. Montalto M, Maggiano N, Ricci R, et al. *Lactobacillus acidophilus* protects tight junctions from aspirin damage in HT-29 cells. *Digestion.* 2004;69(4):225-228.

61. Mack DR, Ahrne S, Hyde L, Wei S, Hollingsworth MA. Extracellular MUC3 mucin secretion follows adherence of *Lactobacillus* strains to intestinal epithelial cells in vitro. *Gut.* 2003;52(6):827-833.

62. Mondel M, Schroeder BO, Zimmermann K, et al. Probiotic *E. coli* treatment mediates antimicrobial human beta-defensin synthesis and fecal excretion in humans. *Mucosal Immunol.* 2009;2(2):166-172.

63. Collado MC, Meriluoto J, Salminen S. Role of commercial probiotic strains against human pathogen adhesion to intestinal mucus. *Lett Appl Microbiol.* 2007;45(4):454-460.

64. Candela M, Seibold G, Vitali B, Lachenmaier S, Eikmanns BJ, Brigidi P. Real-time PCR quantification of bacterial adhesion to Caco-2 cells: competition between bifidobacteria and enteropathogens. *Res Microbiol.* 2005;156(8):887-895.

65. Roselli M, Finamore A, Britti MS, Mengheri E. Probiotic bacteria *Bifidobacterium animalis* MB5 and *Lactobacillus rhamnosus* GG protect intestinal Caco-2 cells from the inflammation-associated response induced by enterotoxigenic *Escherichia coli* K88. *Brit J Nutr.* 2006;95(6):1177-1184.

66. Sherman PM, Johnson-Henry KC, Yeung HP, Ngo PSC, Goulet J, Tompkins TA. Probiotics reduce enterohemorrhagic *Escherichia coli* O157:H7- and enteropathogenic *E. coli* O127:H6-induced changes in polarized T84 epithelial cell monolayers by reducing bacterial adhesion and cytoskeletal rearrangements. *Infect Immun.* 2005;73(8):5183-5188.

67. Mack DR, Michail S, Wei S, McDougall L, Hollingsworth MA. Probiotics inhibit enteropathogenic *E. coli* adherence in vitro by inducing intestinal mucin gene expression. *Am J Physiol.* 1999;276(4 Pt 1):G941-G950.

68. Otte JM, Podolsky DK. Functional modulation of enterocytes by gram-positive and gram-negative microorganisms. *Am J Physiol Gastrointest Liver Physiol.* 2004;286(4):G613-G626.

69. Caballero-Franco C, Keller K, De Simone C, Chadee K. The VSL#3 probiotic formula induces mucin gene expression and secretion in colonic epithelial cells. *Am J Physiol Gastrointest Liver Physiol.* 2007;292(1): G315-G322.

70. Mukai T, Kaneko S, Matsumoto M, Ohori H. Binding of *Bifidobacterium bifidum* and *Lactobacillus reuteri* to the carbohydrate moieties of intestinal glycolipids recognized by peanut agglutinin. *Int J Food Microbiol.* 2004;90(3):357-362.

71. Tallon R, Arias S, Bressolier P, Urdaci MC. Strain- and matrix-dependent adhesion of *Lactobacillus plantarum* is mediated by proteinaceous bacterial compounds. *J Appl Microbiol.* 2007;102(2):442-451.

72. Madsen K, Cornish A, Soper P, et al. Probiotic bacteria enhance murine and human intestinal epithelial barrier function. *Gastroenterology.* 2001;121(3):580-591.

73. Mao Y, Nobaek S, Kasravi B, et al. The effects of *Lactobacillus* strains and oat fiber on methotrexate-induced enterocolitis in rats. *Gastroenterology.* 1996;111(2):334-344.

74. Zyrek AA, Cichon C, Helms S, Enders C, Sonnenborn U, Schmidt MA. Molecular mechanisms underlying the probiotic effects of *Escherichia coli* Nissle 1917 involve ZO-2 and PKCzeta redistribution resulting in tight junction and epithelial barrier repair. *Cell Microbiol.* 2007;9(3):804-816.

75. Ewaschuk JB, Diaz H, Meddings L, et al. Secreted bioactive factors from *Bifidobacterium infantis* enhance epithelial cell barrier function. *Am J Physiol Gastrointest Liver Physiol.* 2008;295(5):G1025-G1034.

76. Resta-Lenert S, Barrett KE. Live probiotics protect intestinal epithelial cells from the effects of infection with enteroinvasive *Escherichia coli* (EIEC). *Gut.* 2003;52(7):988-997.

77. Resta-Lenert S, Barrett KE. Probiotics and commensals reverse TNF-alpha- and IFN-gamma-induced dysfunction in human intestinal epithelial cells. *Gastroenterology.* 2006;130(3):731-746.

78. Seth A, Yan F, Polk DB, Rao RK. Probiotics ameliorate the hydrogen peroxide-induced epithelial barrier disruption by a PKC- and MAP kinase-dependent mechanism. *Am J Physiol Gastrointest Liver Physiol.* 2008;294(4):G1060-G1069.

79. Petrof EO, Ciancio MJ, Chang EB. Role and regulation of intestinal epithelial heat shock proteins in health and disease. *Chin J Dig Dis.* 2004;5(2):45-50.

80. Tao Y, Drabik KA, Waypa TS, et al. Soluble factors from *Lactobacillus* GG activate MAPKs and induce cytoprotective heat shock proteins in intestinal epithelial cells [erratum appears in *Am J Physiol Cell Physiol.* 2006;291(1):C194]. *Am J Physiol Cell Physiol.* 2006;290(4):C1018-C1030.

81. Fujiya M, Musch MW, Nakagawa Y, et al. The Bacillus subtilis quorum-sensing molecule CSF contributes to intestinal homeostasis via OCTN2, a host cell membrane transporter. *Cell Host Microbe.* 2007;1(4):299-308.

82. Yan F, Polk DB. Probiotic bacterium prevents cytokine-induced apoptosis in intestinal epithelial cells. *J Biol Chem.* 2002;277(52):50959-50965.

83. Yan F, Cao H, Cover TL, Whitehead R, Washington MK, Polk DB. Soluble proteins produced by probiotic bacteria regulate intestinal epithelial cell survival and growth. *Gastroenterology.* 2007;132(2):562-575.

84. Schlee M, Harder J, Köten B, Stange EF, Wehkamp J, Fellermann K. Probiotic lactobacilli and VSL#3 induce enterocyte beta-defensin 2. *Clin Exp Immunol.* 2008;151(3):528-535.

85. Wehkamp J, Harder J, Wehkamp K, et al. NF-kappaB- and AP-1-mediated induction of human beta defensin-2 in intestinal epithelial cells by *Escherichia coli* Nissle 1917: a novel effect of a probiotic bacterium. *Infect Immun.* 2004;72(10):5750-5758.
86. Cornes JS. Peyer's patches in the human gut. *Proc R Soc Med.* 1965;58(9):716.
87. Keljo DJ, Hamilton JR. Quantitative determination of macromolecular transport rate across intestinal Peyer's patches. *Am J Physiol.* 1983;244(6):G637-G644.
88. Kim B, Bowersock T, Griebel P, et al. Mucosal immune responses following oral immunization with rotavirus antigens encapsulated in alginate microspheres. *J Controlled Release.* 2002;85(1-3):191-202.
89. Macpherson A, McCoy KD, Johansen FE, Brandtzaeg P. The immune geography of IgA induction and function. *Mucosal Immunol.* 2008;1(1):11-22.
90. Cazac BB, Roes J. TGF-beta receptor controls B cell responsiveness and induction of IgA in vivo. *Immunity.* 2000;13(4):443-451.
91. Takatsu K, Tominaga A, Harada N, et al. T cell-replacing factor (TRF)/interleukin 5 (IL-5): molecular and functional properties. *Immunol Rev.* 1988;102:107-135.
92. McGhee JR, Fujihashi K, Beagley KW, Kiyono H. Role of interleukin-6 in human and mouse mucosal IgA plasma cell responses. *Immunol Res.* 1991;10(3-4):418-422.
93. Bakker-Zierikzee AM, Tol EA, Kroes H, Alles MS, Kok FJ, Bindels JG. Faecal SIgA secretion in infants fed on pre- or probiotic infant formula. *Pediatr Allergy Immunol.* 2006;17(2):134-140.
94. Alberda C, Gramlich L, Meddings J, et al. Effects of probiotic therapy in critically ill patients: a randomized, double-blind, placebo-controlled trial. *Am J Clin Nutr.* 2007;85(3):816-823.
95. Kawai T, Akira S. The roles of TLRs, RLRs, and NLRs in pathogen recognition. *Int Immunol.* 2009;21(4):317-337.
96. Medzhitov R, Preston-Hurlburt P, Janeway CA Jr. A human homologue of the *Drosophila* Toll protein signals activation of adaptive immunity. *Nature.* 1997;388(6640):394-397.
97. Takeuchi O, Sato S, Horiuchi T, et al. Cutting edge: role of Toll-like receptor 1 in mediating immune response to microbial lipoproteins. *J Immunol.* 2002;169(1):10-14.
98. Aliprantis AO, Yang RB, Mark MR, et al. Cell activation and apoptosis by bacterial lipoproteins through toll-like receptor-2. *Science.* 1999;285(5428):736-739.
99. Schwandner R, Dziarski R, Wesche H, Rothe M, Kirschning CJ. Peptidoglycan- and lipoteichoic acid-induced cell activation is mediated by toll-like receptor 2. *J Biol Chem.* 1999;274(25):17406-17409.
100. Takeuchi O, Hoshino K, Kawai T, et al. Differential roles of TLR2 and TLR4 in recognition of gram-negative and gram-positive bacterial cell wall components. *Immunity.* 1999;11(4):443-451.
101. Underhill DM, Ozinsky A, Smith KD, Aderem A. Toll-like receptor-2 mediates mycobacteria-induced proinflammatory signaling in macrophages. *Proc Natl Acad Sci U S A.* 1999;96(25):14459-14463.
102. Vabulas RM, Ahmad-Nejad P, Ghose S, Kirschning CJ, Issels RD, Wagner H. HSP70 as endogenous stimulus of the Toll/interleukin-1 receptor signal pathway. *J Biol Chem.* 2002;277(17):15107-15112.
103. Asea A, Rehli M, Kabingu E, et al. Novel signal transduction pathway utilized by extracellular HSP70: role of toll-like receptor (TLR) 2 and TLR4. *J Biol Chem.* 2002;277(17):15028-15034.
104. Tapping RI, Tobias PS. Mycobacterial lipoarabinomannan mediates physical interactions between TLR1 and TLR2 to induce signaling. *J Endotoxin Res.* 2003;9(4):264-268.
105. Alexopoulou L, Holt AC, Medzhitov R, Flavell RA. Recognition of double-stranded RNA and activation of NF-kappaB by Toll-like receptor 3. *Nature.* 2001;413(6857):732-738.
106. Kawasaki K, Akashi S, Shimazu R, Yoshida T, Miyake K, Nishijima M. Mouse toll-like receptor 4.MD-2 complex mediates lipopolysaccharide-mimetic signal transduction by Taxol. *J Biol Chem.* 2000;275(4):2251-2254.
107. Bulut Y, Faure E, Thomas L, et al. Chlamydial heat shock protein 60 activates macrophages and endothelial cells through Toll-like receptor 4 and MD2 in a MyD88-dependent pathway. *J Immunol.* 2002;168(3):1435-1440.
108. Ohashi K, Burkart V, Flohé S, Kolb H. Cutting edge: heat shock protein 60 is a putative endogenous ligand of the toll-like receptor-4 complex. *J Immunol.* 2000;164(2):558-561.
109. Okamura Y, Watari M, Jerud ES, et al. The extra domain A of fibronectin activates Toll-like receptor 4. *J Biol Chem.* 2001;276(13):10229-10233.
110. Termeer C, Benedix F, Sleeman J, et al. Oligosaccharides of Hyaluronan activate dendritic cells via toll-like receptor 4. *J Exp Med.* 2002;195(1):99-111.
111. Johnson GB, Brunn GJ, Kodaira Y, Platt JL. Receptor-mediated monitoring of tissue well-being via detection of soluble heparan sulfate by Toll-like receptor 4. *J Immunol.* 2002;168(10):5233-5239.
112. Smiley ST, King JA, Hancock WW. Fibrinogen stimulates macrophage chemokine secretion through toll-like receptor 4. *J Immunol.* 2001;167(5):2887-2894.
113. Kurt-Jones EA, Popova L, Kwinn L, et al. Pattern recognition receptors TLR4 and CD14 mediate response to respiratory syncytial virus. *Nature Immunol.* 2000;1(5):398-401.
114. Rassa JC, Meyers JL, Zhang Y, Kudaravalli R, Ross SR. Murine retroviruses activate B cells via interaction with toll-like receptor 4. *Proc Natl Acad Sci U S A.* 2002;99(4):2281-2286.

115. Kawai T, Adachi O, Ogawa T, Takeda K, Akira S. Unresponsiveness of MyD88-deficient mice to endotoxin. *Immunity.* 1999;11(1):115-122.
116. Hayashi F, Smith KD, Ozinsky A, et al. The innate immune response to bacterial flagellin is mediated by Toll-like receptor 5. *Nature.* 2001;410(6832):1099-1103.
117. Takeuchi O, Kawai T, Mühlradt PF, et al. Discrimination of bacterial lipoproteins by Toll-like receptor 6. *Int Immunol.* 2001;13(7):933-940.
118. Ozinsky A, Underhill DM, Fontenot JD, et al. The repertoire for pattern recognition of pathogens by the innate immune system is defined by cooperation between toll-like receptors. *Proc Natl Acad Sci U S A.* 2000;97(25):13766-13771.
119. Diebold SS, Kaisho T, Hemmi H, Akira S, Reis e Sousa C. Innate antiviral responses by means of TLR7-mediated recognition of single-stranded RNA. *Science.* 2004;303(5663):1529-1531.
120. Heil F, Hemmi H, Hochrein H, et al. Species-specific recognition of single-stranded RNA via toll-like receptor 7 and 8. *Science.* 2004;303(5663):1526-1529.
121. Hemmi H, Kaisho T, Takeuchi O, et al. Small anti-viral compounds activate immune cells via the TLR7 MyD88-dependent signaling pathway. *Nature Immunol.* 2002;3(2):196-200.
122. Hemmi H, Takeuchi O, Kawai T, et al. A Toll-like receptor recognizes bacterial DNA. *Nature.* 2000;408(6813):740-745.
123. Coban C, Ishii KJ, Kawai T, et al. Toll-like receptor 9 mediates innate immune activation by the malaria pigment hemozoin. *J Exp Med.* 2005;201(1):19-25.
124. Yarovinsky F, Zhang D, Andersen JF, et al. TLR11 activation of dendritic cells by a protozoan profilin-like protein. *Science.* 2005;308(5728):1626-1629.
125. Zhang D, Zhang G, Hayden MS, et al. A toll-like receptor that prevents infection by uropathogenic bacteria. *Science.* 2004;303(5663):1522-1526.
126. Adachi O, Kawai T, Takeda K, et al. Targeted disruption of the MyD88 gene results in loss of IL-1- and IL-18-mediated function. *Immunity.* 1998;9(1):143-150.
127. Kagan JC, Medzhitov R. Phosphoinositide-mediated adaptor recruitment controls Toll-like receptor signaling. *Cell.* 2006;125(5):943-955.
128. Gohda J, Matsumura T, Inoue J. Cutting edge: TNFR-associated factor (TRAF) 6 is essential for MyD88-dependent pathway but not toll/IL-1 receptor domain-containing adaptor-inducing IFN-beta (TRIF)-dependent pathway in TLR signaling. *J Immunol.* 2004;173(5):2913-2917.
129. Hoshino K, Takeuchi O, Kawai T, et al. Cutting edge: Toll-like receptor 4 (TLR4)-deficient mice are hyporesponsive to lipopolysaccharide: evidence for TLR4 as the Lps gene product. *J Immunol.* 1999;162(7):3749-3752.
130. An H, Yu Y, Zhang M, et al. Involvement of ERK, p38 and NF-kappaB signal transduction in regulation of TLR2, TLR4 and TLR9 gene expression induced by lipopolysaccharide in mouse dendritic cells. *Immunology.* 2002;106(1):38-45.
131. Kawai T, Takeuchi O, Fujita T, et al. Lipopolysaccharide stimulates the MyD88-independent pathway and results in activation of IFN-regulatory factor 3 and the expression of a subset of lipopolysaccharide-inducible genes. *J Immunol.* 2001;167(10):5887-5894.
132. Yamamoto M, Sato S, Hemmi H, et al. Role of adaptor TRIF in the MyD88-independent toll-like receptor signaling pathway. *Science.* 2003;301(5633):640-643.
133. Yamamoto M, Sato S, Hemmi H, et al. TRAM is specifically involved in the Toll-like receptor 4-mediated MyD88-independent signaling pathway. *Nature Immunol.* 2003;4(11):1144-1150.
134. Fitzgerald KA, McWhirter SM, Faia KL, et al. IKKepsilon and TBK1 are essential components of the IRF3 signaling pathway. *Nature Immunol.* 2003;4(5):491-496.
135. Nakaya T, Sato M, Hata N, et al. Gene induction pathways mediated by distinct IRFs during viral infection. *Biochem Biophys Res Commun.* 2001;283(5):1150-1156.
136. Sato S, Sugiyama M, Yamamoto M, et al. Toll/IL-1 receptor domain-containing adaptor inducing IFN-beta (TRIF) associates with TNF receptor-associated factor 6 and TANK-binding kinase 1, and activates two distinct transcription factors, NF-kappa B and IFN-regulatory factor-3, in the Toll-like receptor signaling. *J Immunol.* 2003;171(8):4304-4310.
137. Latz E, Schoenemeyer A, Visintin A, et al. TLR9 signals after translocating from the ER to CpG DNA in the lysosome. *Nature Immunol.* 2004;5(2):190-198.
138. Latz E, Latz E, Visintin A, Espevik T, Golenbock DT. Mechanisms of TLR9 activation. *J Endotoxin Res.* 2004;10(6):406-412.
139. Nishiya T, Nishiya T, Kajita E, Miwa S, Defranco AL. TLR3 and TLR7 are targeted to the same intracellular compartments by distinct regulatory elements. *J Biol Chem.* 2005;280(44):37107-37117.
140. Kim YM, Brinkmann MM, Paquet ME, Ploegh HL. UNC93B1 delivers nucleotide-sensing toll-like receptors to endolysosomes. *Nature.* 2008;452(7184):234-238.
141. Ewald SE, Lee BL, Lau L, et al. The ectodomain of Toll-like receptor 9 is cleaved to generate a functional receptor. *Nature.* 2008;456(7222):658-662.

142. Schulz O, Diebold SS, Chen M, et al. Toll-like receptor 3 promotes cross-priming to virus-infected cells. *Nature.* 2005;433(7028):887-892.

143. Ewaschuk JB, Backer JL, Churchill TA, Obermeier F, Krause DO, Madsen KL. Surface expression of Toll-like receptor 9 is upregulated on intestinal epithelial cells in response to pathogenic bacterial DNA. *Infect Immun.* 2007;75(5):2572-2579.

144. Lee J, Mo JH, Katakura K, et al. Maintenance of colonic homeostasis by distinctive apical TLR9 signalling in intestinal epithelial cells. *Nature Cell Biol.* 2006;8(12):1327-1336.

145. Lee J, Rachmilewitz D, Raz E. Homeostatic effects of TLR9 signaling in experimental colitis. *Ann N Y Acad Sci.* 2006;1072:351-355.

146. Gewirtz AT, Navas TA, Lyons S, Godowski PJ, Madara JL. Cutting edge: bacterial flagellin activates basolaterally expressed TLR5 to induce epithelial proinflammatory gene expression. *J Immunol.* 2001;167(4):1882-1885.

147. Ruemmele FM, Beaulieu JF, Dionne S, et al. Lipopolysaccharide modulation of normal enterocyte turnover by toll-like receptors is mediated by endogenously produced tumour necrosis factor alpha [erratum appears in *Gut.* 2003;52(1):157]. *Gut.* 2002;51(6):842-848.

148. Cario E, Gerken G, Podolsky DK. Toll-like receptor 2 enhances ZO-1-associated intestinal epithelial barrier integrity via protein kinase C. *Gastroenterology.* 2004;127(1):224-238.

149. Cario E, Gerken G, Podolsky DK. Toll-like receptor 2 controls mucosal inflammation by regulating epithelial barrier function. *Gastroenterology.* 2007;132(4):1359-1374.

150. Jijon H, Backer J, Diaz H, et al. DNA from probiotic bacteria modulates murine and human epithelial and immune function. *Gastroenterology.* 2004;126(5):1358-1373.

151. Neal MD, Leaphart C, Levy R, et al. Enterocyte TLR4 mediates phagocytosis and translocation of bacteria across the intestinal barrier. *J Immunol.* 2006;176(5):3070-3079.

152. Gribar SC, Richardson WM, Sodhi CP, Hackam DJ. No longer an innocent bystander: epithelial toll-like receptor signaling in the development of mucosal inflammation. *Mol Med.* 2008;14(9-10):645-659.

153. Grabig A, Paclik D, Guzy C, et al. *Escherichia coli* strain Nissle 1917 ameliorates experimental colitis via toll-like receptor 2- and toll-like receptor 4-dependent pathways. *Infect Immun.* 2006;74(7):4075-4082.

154. Ting JP, Lovering RC, Alnemri ES, et al. The NLR gene family: a standard nomenclature. *Immunity.* 2008;28(3):285-287.

155. Ye Z, Ting JP. NLR, the nucleotide-binding domain leucine-rich repeat containing gene family. *Curr Opin Immunol.* 2008;20(1):3-9.

156. Girardin SE, Boneca IG, Carneiro LA, et al. Nod1 detects a unique muropeptide from gram-negative bacterial peptidoglycan. *Science.* 2003;300(5625):1584-1587.

157. Girardin SE, Boneca IG, Viala J, et al. Nod2 is a general sensor of peptidoglycan through muramyl dipeptide (MDP) detection. *J Biol Chem.* 2003;278(11):8869-8872.

158. Girardin SE, Travassos LH, Hervé M, et al. Peptidoglycan molecular requirements allowing detection by Nod1 and Nod2. *J Biol Chem.* 2003;278(43):41702-41708.

159. Inohara N, Koseki T, del Peso L, et al. Nod1, an Apaf-1-like activator of caspase-9 and nuclear factor-kappaB. *J Biol Chem.* 1999;274(21):14560-14567.

160. Chamaillard M, Girardin SE, Viala J, Philpott DJ. Nods, Nalps and Naip: intracellular regulators of bacterial-induced inflammation. *Cell Microbiol.* 2003;5(9):581-592.

161. Carneiro LA, Magalhaes JG, Tattoli I, Philpott DJ, Travassos LH. Nod-like proteins in inflammation and disease. *J Pathol.* 2008;214(2):136-148.

162. Martinon F, Tschopp J. NLRs join TLRs as innate sensors of pathogens. *Trends Immunol.* 2005;26(8):447-454.

163. Kanneganti TD, Ozören N, Body-Malapel M, et al. Bacterial RNA and small antiviral compounds activate caspase-1 through cryopyrin/Nalp3. *Nature.* 2006;440(7081):233-236.

164. Martinon F, Pétrilli V, Mayor A, Tardivel A, Tschopp J. Gout-associated uric acid crystals activate the NALP3 inflammasome. *Nature.* 2006;440(7081):237-241.

165. Mariathasan S, Weiss DS, Newton K, et al. Cryopyrin activates the inflammasome in response to toxins and ATP. *Nature.* 2006;440(7081):228-232.

166. Amer A, Franchi L, Kanneganti TD, et al. Regulation of *Legionella* phagosome maturation and infection through flagellin and host Ipaf. *J Biol Chem.* 2006;281(46):35217-35223.

167. Franchi L, Amer A, Body-Malapel M, et al. Cytosolic flagellin requires Ipaf for activation of caspase-1 and interleukin 1beta in *Salmonella*-infected macrophages. *Nature Immunol.* 2006;7(6):576-582.

168. Neish AS. Bacterial inhibition of eukaryotic pro-inflammatory pathways. *Immunol Res.* 2004;29(1-3):175-186.

169. Ruiz PA, Hoffmann M, Szcesny S, Blaut M, Haller D. Innate mechanisms for *Bifidobacterium lactis* to activate transient pro-inflammatory host responses in intestinal epithelial cells after the colonization of germ-free rats. *Immunology*. 2005;115(4):441-450.

170. Lammers KM, Helwig U, Swennen E, et al. Effect of probiotic strains on interleukin 8 production by HT29/19A cells. *Am J Gastroenterol*. 2002;97(5):1182-1186.

171. Petrof EO, Kojima K, Ropeleski MJ, et al. Probiotics inhibit nuclear factor-kappaB and induce heat shock proteins in colonic epithelial cells through proteasome inhibition. *Gastroenterology*. 2004;127(5):1474-1487.

172. Kelly D, Campbell JI, King TP, et al. Commensal anaerobic gut bacteria attenuate inflammation by regulating nuclear-cytoplasmic shuttling of PPAR-gamma and RelA. *Nature Immunol*. 2004;5(1):104-112.

173. Are A, Aronsson L, Wang S, et al. *Enterococcus faecalis* from newborn babies regulate endogenous PPARgamma activity and IL-10 levels in colonic epithelial cells. *Proc Natl Acad Sci U S A*. 2008;105(6):1943-1948.

174. Akhtar M, Watson JL, Nazli A, McKay DM. Bacterial DNA evokes epithelial IL-8 production by a MAPK-dependent, NF-kappaB-independent pathway. *FASEB J*. 2003;17(10):1319-1321.

175. Dahan S, Roth-Walter F, Arnaboldi P, Agarwal S, Mayer L. Epithelia: lymphocyte interactions in the gut. *Immunol Rev*. 2007;215:243-253.

176. Mukherjee P, Dani A, Bhatia S, et al. Efficient presentation of both cytosolic and endogenous transmembrane protein antigens on MHC class II is dependent on cytoplasmic proteolysis. *J Immunol*. 2001;167(5):2632-2641.

177. Rescigno M, Borrow P. The host-pathogen interaction: new themes from dendritic cell biology. *Cell*. 2001;106(3):267-270.

178. Iwasaki A, Kelsall BL. Freshly isolated Peyer's patch, but not spleen, dendritic cells produce interleukin 10 and induce the differentiation of T helper type 2 cells. *J Exp Med*. 1999;190(2):229-239.

179. Iwasaki A, Kelsall BL. Mucosal immunity and inflammation. I. Mucosal dendritic cells: their specialized role in initiating T cell responses. *Am J Physiol*. 1999;276(5 Pt 1):G1074-G1078.

180. Hart AL, Lammers K, Brigidi P, et al. Modulation of human dendritic cell phenotype and function by probiotic bacteria. *Gut*. 2004;53(11):1602-1609.

181. Stagg AJ, Hart AL, Knight SC, Kamm MA. Microbial-gut interactions in health and disease. Interactions between dendritic cells and bacteria in the regulation of intestinal immunity. *Best Prac Res Clin Gastroenterol*. 2004;18(2):255-270.

182. Ng S, Hart AL, Kamm MA, et al. Mechanisms of action of probiotics: recent advances. *Inflamm Bowel Dis*. 2009;15(2):300-310.

183. Rimoldi M, Chieppa M, Salucci V, et al. Intestinal immune homeostasis is regulated by the crosstalk between epithelial cells and dendritic cells. *Nature Immunol*. 2005;6(5):507-514.

184. Smythies LE, Sellers M, Clements RH, et al. Human intestinal macrophages display profound inflammatory anergy despite avid phagocytic and bacteriocidal activity. *J Clin Invest*. 2005;115(1):66-75.

185. Monteleone I, Platt AM, Jaensson E, Agace WW, Mowat AM. IL-10-dependent partial refractoriness to Toll-like receptor stimulation modulates gut mucosal dendritic cell function. *Eur J Immunol*. 2008;38(6):1533-1547.

186. Rimoldi M, Chieppa M, Larghi P, Vulcano M, Allavena P, Rescigno M. Monocyte-derived dendritic cells activated by bacteria or by bacteria-stimulated epithelial cells are functionally different. *Blood*. 2005;106(8):2818-2826.

187. Dalmasso G, Cottrez F, Imbert V, et al. *Saccharomyces boulardii* inhibits inflammatory bowel disease by trapping T cells in mesenteric lymph nodes. *Gastroenterology*. 2006;131(6):1812-1825.

4

Probiotics and the Allergic Response

Erika Isolauri, MD, PhD; Samuli Rautava, MD, PhD;
Kirsi Laitinen, PhD; and Seppo Salminen, PhD

Allergic responses are characterized by the generation of T helper (Th) cell 2-type cytokines, including interleukin (IL)-4, IL-5, and IL-13, which promote IgE production and eosinophilia recruitment. Early events in the immunologic activation promote the generation of these cytokines. The Th2-skewed immune type may be balanced by cytokines secreted by Th1, Th3, and Tr1 cells, partially as a result of stimulation by the gut microbiota.[1] Allergic response, however, is not limited to IgE-associated immunologic processes,[2] which, again, are not directly causally linked to a clinical allergic condition.

Traditional thinking has focused on the antigens; consequently, antigen elimination has been the strategy to address the allergic response. Epidemiologic data, however, imply that eradication of allergens from the early environment may not neutralize the allergic response. Hence, the increased prevalence of allergic disease in industrialized countries cannot be explained by an increased number of dietary allergens or aeroallergens sensitizing the host. Rather, it would appear that the altered environment, devoid of the necessary balancing stimulation needed to hinder the consolidation of the atopic Th2-skewed immunity, more directly shapes the immune responder type of the host during a critical period of life (Figure 4-1). The environment can be taken to represent both the internal and external environments of the host, including the nutritional environment. The ubiquitous allergens, thus, may act as recipients of the altered immunologic responses and not as their causes.

EXPOSURE–SENSITIZATION–HYPERSENSITIVITY: WHAT IS THE SEQUENCE OF EVENTS?

Notwithstanding extensive scientific efforts, fundamental issues in allergic response remain unresolved. Specifically, the exact chain of pathologic events—ie, the cascade consisting of exposure, sensitization, and hypersensitivity—remains elusive. First,

Floch MH, Kim AS, eds.
Probiotics: A Clinical Guide (pp 41-54)
© 2010 Taylor & Francis Group

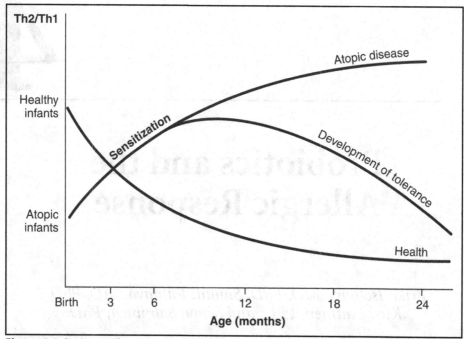

Figure 4-1. Development of immune responses in healthy and atopic infants. The T-helper cell 2 (Th2)-skewed immune type is prevalent in early life.

remarkable overlap in the concentrations of IgE antibodies between atopics and non-atopics occurs.[3] In healthy children, transient, asymptomatic increases in antigen-specific IgE antibodies prevail in up to 80% of cases during the first 5 years of life.[4] Second, exposure to allergens sensitizing the host immune system may not necessarily induce allergic disease,[2] but act as an essential initial step in tolerance induction. Third, reducing the risk of allergic disease does not necessitate reduction in sensitization.[5-7] In like manner, resolution or aggravation of clinical symptoms is not invariably associated with alteration in the allergic response.

Recent data of cohort studies evaluating the development of immune responses early in life have opened up new angles to aberrant immunologic maturation resulting in allergic responses. The immune responder type is physiologically Th2-dominated due to the immunologic balance prevailing in utero.[8] Furthermore, neonatal Th2 responses, including the production of IL-13[9] and IL-4,[10] are actually lower in infants who develop atopic disease as compared to those who remain healthy (Figure 4-1). It has been suggested that healthy infants exhibit an age-dependent decline in Th2 responses during the early postnatal period, whereas infants who develop atopic disease with initially lower Th2 responsiveness are characterized by a converse pattern.[10] It would thus appear that increased production of Th2 cytokines is the result of defective immune regulation associated with the development of atopic disease rather than a direct cause of such development.

According to the current perception, the dilemma of the host immune defense is to generate an effective response to pathogens while concomitantly maintaining unresponsiveness to antigens in food and environment. Indeed, the phenomenon of tolerance is crucial in avoiding local and peripheral inflammatory responses upon exposure to ubiquitous antigens.[2] Sustained inflammatory responses, again, may perturb mucosal integrity and thereby interfere with homeostatic mechanisms preserving normal immune regulation. As depicted in Figure 4-1, the question of current research interest is, could allergies be ascribed to a lack of physiologic anti-inflammatory processes?

EXTENDING THE HYGIENE HYPOTHESIS

The hygiene hypothesis contends that the allergic response is related to reduced exposure to microbes at an early age as a result of environmental changes in the industrialized world.[11] An important prerequisite is that the exposure occurs very early, as the first expression of the allergic responder type frequently occurs within the first months of life. Indeed, the collective composition and the compositional development of the gut microbiota provide the first massive source of microbial exposure. On the basis of this evidence, we currently consider that the gut microbiota may represent the most important foundation of maturational signals to the developing immune system, and propose an "extended hygiene hypothesis": Lifestyle-related changes in hygienic, dietary, and medical practices have altered the pattern of microbial exposure and particularly the compositional development of the gut microbiota. Thus, the modern infant is devoid of sufficient stimulation to generate a tolerogenic immune milieu and is prone to develop chronic inflammatory conditions, which may take the form of any Western lifestyle-related disease, including allergic or autoimmune disease, or a low-grade inflammatory state affecting energy metabolism that predisposes the child to obesity.

Traditionally, the intestinal tract colonization of the infant was considered to start at birth,[12] thus providing timely counter-regulatory signals against sustained Th2-skewed immunity. However, there is recent evidence of exposure to bacterial DNA and even bacteria prior to birth.[13] This inoculum is then expanded during delivery and breastfeeding with an uninterrupted exchange of microbes between the mother and infant. Introduction of new microbial species throughout breastfeeding and weaning proceeds in a stepwise manner with increasing diversity and metabolic activity.[14] Such tonic stimulation of the developing gut-associated lymphoid tissue may allow control over the metabolic activity and the immunologic balance within the intestinal tract.

ABERRANT COMPOSITIONAL DEVELOPMENT OF THE GUT MICROBIOTA AND THE ALLERGIC RESPONSE

The predominant intestinal organisms during the first weeks of life comprise enterobacteria, clostridia, bacteroides, and streptococci, followed by bifidobacteria and LAB, or mainly *Firmicutes*, *Bacteroidetes*, and *Actinobacteria*. Breastfed infants harbor a natural predominance of bifidobacteria with specific strains present, while the formula-fed infants have a more complex microbiota profile, with less bifidobacteria and greater proportion of enterobacteria, lactobacilli, bacteroides, clostridia, and streptococci. New methodology has revealed higher numbers of unculturable microbial phylotypes.[15] One intriguing new finding is the abundance of *Akkermansia muciniphila*, a microbe that utilizes intestinal mucus glycoproteins as a source of nutrition.[16,17]

The original inoculum and environmental factors direct the composition and activity of newborn microbiota. Indeed, early microbiota deviations appear to predispose infants to allergic responses,[18] and this tendency can be reversed by microbiota modulation.[5,19-21] The allergic response is reflected in altered *Bifidobacterium/Clostridium* ratios, which may further activate the gut barrier dysfunction. Hence, microbes directly disturbing the intestinal integrity or debilitating the healthy colonization can be identified; thus far, *Akkermansia* and altered *Bifidobacterium/Clostridium* ratios may exemplify new specific targets when addressing the allergic response.

In the context of inflammation, the altered rate, route, and mode of antigen presentation may lead to abrogation of tolerance. Intestinal permeability can be secondarily increased as a result of inflammation in the intestinal mucosa.[22] A greater amount of antigens may thus traverse the mucosal barrier, and the routes of transport may be altered. During the ensuing mucosal dysfunction caused by immaturity or hypersensitivity reaction, the normal pattern of antigen handling is impaired, which may evoke aberrant immune responses and lead to sensitization.[1] Therapeutically exploiting the intestine's endogenous defense mechanisms may provide a new direction in treating gastrointestinal disorders associated with intestinal inflammation. Thus far, specific probiotics have been shown to reinforce the different lines of gut defense: immune exclusion, immune elimination, and immune regulation.[23]

VALIDATION OF PROBIOTICS IN ALLERGIC RESPONSE: HITTING THE TARGETS?

Allergic response appears to result from an interplay between susceptibility genes, impaired barrier functions (including the skin, respiratory tract, and gut), aberrant gut microbiota, and immunological dysregulation. In addition, bacterial and viral infections, as well as other environmental factors, can play a role in the allergic response. On this basis, a working hypothesis for reducing the risk of sustained allergic inflammation could propose novel targets for intervention (Figure 4-2), including the barrier functions of the skin, respiratory tract, and gut epithelium (including the barrier effect of local microbiota), and the sustained inflammatory response.

The rationale of probiotic therapy in allergic response is, in the simplest terms, to provide an anti-inflammatory microbial stimulus for the host immune system by means of cultures of beneficial live microorganisms characteristic of the healthy breastfed infant gut microbiota. Timing is important, and microbiota modulation needs to be addressed already in mothers during pregnancy to influence the microbial inoculum. Modulation is continued in infants during breastfeeding and weaning to establish and maintain healthy development.

Specific Requirements for the Strains

The main selection criteria for bifidobacteria and LAB first focus on species and strains in the intestine of healthy breastfed infants, including *B. longum* and *B. infantis*. Second, lactobacilli favoring the development of *Bifidobacterium* microbiota should be considered.

Traditionally, adherence and colonization have been considered crucial for probiotic action. However, long-term intestinal colonization has not been demonstrated even after perinatal administration.[24] Nonetheless, transient colonization, together with antagonisms, competitive exclusion, or displacement of common proinflammatory strains within the gut, is an important criterion. On this basis, specific strains, or strain combinations, should have the ability to influence microbiota composition. For example, it has been demonstrated that LGG impacts the bifidobacterial microbiota composition and activity in infants,[25-27] and *B. lactis* affects the total clusters of both *Bifidobacterium* and *Clostridium*, in parallel with the stimulating effect on intestinal butyrate production.[28] The best-characterized probiotic effect on the intestinal micro-

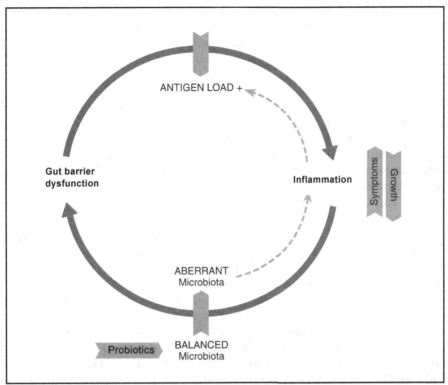

Figure 4-2. The targets of probiotic therapy in the prevention or treatment of allergic disease. Intraluminal antigens induce an immunoinflammatory response that impairs the intestine's barrier function. Mucosal dysfunction may lead to aberrant antigen absorption. Probiotics (1) degrade antigens, (2) terminate inflammatory response, (3) avert deviant microbiota development, and (4) normalize the barrier functions. The probiotics target allergic responses with intestinal involvement. (Modified from Isolauri E, Salminen S. Probiotics. In: Kleinman RE, Sanderson IR, Goulet O, Sherman PM, Mieli-Vergani G, Shneider BL, eds. *Walker's Pediatric Gastrointestinal Disease: Physiology, Diagnosis, Management.* Hamilton, Ontario: BC Decker Inc; 2008:391-398.)

ecology and mucus is competitive exclusion of pathogens.[29] Many probiotic effects, however, cannot be directly related to the intestinal microbiota changes, as measured by fecal cultures. Fecal recovery of ingested probiotics indicates that the strain is able to survive the passage through the intestinal tract, but there is no indication of adherence or transient colonization. For immune regulation, local epithelial or mucus adherence properties may be required.[30] In fact, colonization and the immunomodulatory effects of probiotics may be mutually exclusive. Sporadically intruding microorganisms may elicit specific responses in the gut-associated lymphoid tissue, whereas the potential to stimulate an immune response may be abolished at the time the strain is adopted by the normal microbiota.[31]

The probiotic performance has been shown to manifest itself in normalization of increased intestinal permeability,[22] also contributing to the capacity of specific strains to dampen inflammatory responses in the gut. LGG, *B. lactis*, and *B. infantis* have strengthening effects on the gut barrier,[22,32] potentially associated with the surface structure of the probiotic strain and the production of metabolites interacting with the detrimental or proinflammatory bacteria, modifying the gut immunologic milieu, as indicated further in the text. In the future, probiotic efficacy may also arise from the use of specifically selected natural bacteria or genetically modified bacteria evincing improved or added functional properties. These include probiotics engineered to produce anti-inflammatory cytokines.[33] While no such new probiotics or starters are yet available in food, basic research is active in the field.

Antigen Processing and Gut Barrier Functions

Degradation of antigens is a necessary initial step in controlling inflammatory responsiveness to dietary antigens.[34] Most antigens encountered are already processed when they contact the mucosal surface. Proteases of specific strains of the intestinal microbiota contribute to the processing of food antigens in the gut and modify their immunogenicity in vitro and in vivo. For example, caseins degraded by probiotic bacteria-derived enzymes have further been shown to modulate cytokine production by anti-CD3 antibody-induced peripheral blood mononuclear cells in atopic infants with cow milk allergy.[35-37]

As a token of probiotic effects on gut humoral defenses, it has been shown that the capacity to generate IgA-producing cells increases progressively in response to intestinal antigenic stimulation, particularly the establishment of the gut microbiota.[38] Probiotic supplementation in infancy has been reported to be associated with increased total IgA concentrations in both serum[39] and feces,[40] reflecting systemic and mucosal IgA production, respectively. In a prospective study of 72 formula-fed infants, supplementation with the probiotics LGG and *B. lactis* Bb-12 resulted in a significant increase in cells secreting IgA antibodies specific to cow milk antigens while total quantities of IgA-secreting cells remained unaltered.[41] On the basis of these data, it may be argued that the observed increase in humoral immune responses is attributable to IgA antibodies specific to antigens encountered during supplementation. Generation of an antigen-specific IgA response reflects development of specific immune memory, whereas an increase in total IgA may result from increased exposure to antigens through a compromised mucosal barrier. In line with this notion, probiotic supplementation has been demonstrated to be associated with increased rotavirus-specific IgA after rotavirus infection,[42] and has been shown to enhance antigen-specific IgA and IgG responses to vaccines,[43] while stabilizing the gut barrier function during infection and inflammation.[22]

LGG has been suggested to strengthen the epithelial barrier by several mechanisms such as the induction of mucin secretion, enhancement of tight-junction functioning,[44,45] upregulation of cytoprotective heat shock proteins,[46] and prevention of apoptosis of epithelial cells.[47] LGG was also shown to reverse the increased intestinal permeability induced by cow milk in suckling rats[22]; the permeability was measured by absorption of horseradish peroxidase across jejunal segments containing Peyer's patches and across patch-free segments. Targeting antigen transport to Peyer's patches may provide one explanation for the concomitant stimulation of the humoral immunity. The same method was used to show that antigen transfer across the gut mucosal barrier is increased in children with atopic eczema.[48] In theory, by reducing antigen transfer to the lamina propria, probiotics might reduce the antigenic load to the gut-associated lymphatic tissue in affected children, thereby controlling the allergic responses.

Anti-Inflammatory Potential

Establishment of the gut microbiota is an essential component of postnatal intestinal development because interaction with indigenous intestinal microbes, that is, "host-microbe crosstalk," is necessary for normal morphologic and functional maturation of the intestinal immune system.[49] The importance of specific intestinal microbes for development of oral tolerance in early infancy is demonstrated in a series of experiments conducted by Sudo and colleagues.[50] Mice reared in germ-free conditions and, thus, devoid of intestinal microbes displayed defective establishment of oral tolerance toward ovalbumin characterized by excessive IL-4 responsiveness and IgE production. Monocolonization of these mice with the commensal B. infantis restored normal oral tolerance formation. However, if B. infantis was introduced after the neonatal period, the mice remained intolerant. On the basis of these data, it may be suggested that initial signals to counter IL-4, and thereby IgE and atopy, and IL-5-generated eosinophilic inflammation may stem from components of the innate immunity triggered by microbe-associated molecular patterns.

Data from experimental animal models are consistent with the notion that specific probiotics are capable of inhibiting allergic-type immune responsiveness. In a murine model for allergic asthma, L. reuteri, acting via the innate immune receptor TLR9, attenuated Th2 cytokine production, the influx of eosinophils, and airway hyperresponsiveness.[51] In a similar fashion, supplementation with L. casei has been reported to inhibit IgE responses and systemic anaphylaxis in a murine food allergy model.[52] In a study conducted using peripheral blood mononuclear cells obtained from allergic individuals, lactobacilli reportedly inhibited allergen-specific secretion of the Th2 cytokines IL-4 and IL-5 in vitro.[53]

Recent advances in basic research suggest that the inhibition of allergic-type immune responsiveness may at least partially be mediated by induction of tolerogenic regulatory T cells. Regulatory T cells are central in the establishment and maintenance of immune tolerance toward both environmental and dietary allergens and indigenous microbes. The function of regulatory T cells is dependent on anti-inflammatory cytokines such as transforming growth factor-beta (TGF-β) and IL-10. In an in vitro study, the probiotic Lactobacillus paracasei has been reported to inhibit inflammatory responses of both Th1 and Th2 types by inducing a population of T cells that produce TGF-β and IL-10 and thus display some characteristics of regulatory T cells.[54] Using a murine model, Di Giacinto and coworkers have provided evidence to suggest that probiotic bacteria can induce regulatory T cells in vivo: A combination of the probiotic bacteria B. longum, B. breve, L. acidophilus, L. casei, Lactobacillus delbrueckii ssp. bulgaricus, L. plantarum, and S. salivarius ssp. thermophilus protected the animals from intestinal inflammation by inducing regulatory T cells with surface-bound TGF-β.[55] Oral administration of L. reuteri has recently been reported to attenuate airway inflammation and hyperresponsiveness in a murine asthma model by inducing non-antigen-specific regulatory T cells.[56] Importantly, according to a series of experiments conducted using a murine model, administration of the probiotic LGG during the neonatal period may enhance regulatory T-cell induction and inhibit subsequent sensitization and allergic airway response.[57] These data suggest that early probiotic supplementation has the potential to induce long-lasting immunomodulatory effects that may protect the infant from the development of an allergic immune responder phenotype.

As alluded to previously, TGF-β is a central cytokine in the establishment and maintenance of oral tolerance. According to a recent report by Verhasselt and colleagues, using a murine asthma model, maternal exposure to allergen during breastfeeding protects the offspring from allergic airway disease.[58] This induction of allergen-specific immune tolerance was dependent on TGF-β in breast milk together with small amounts of allergen transferred to breast milk. In a series of experiments conducted using a rat model, infant formula supplemented with TGF-β inhibited allergic immune responses such as production of IgE and cow milk-specific IgG1 antibodies.[59] Indeed, in human follow-up studies, TGF-β in breast milk has been associated with reduced risk of atopic eczema[60] and wheezing.[61] Maternal probiotic supplementation[62] has been reported to promote breast milk TGF-β1[63] and TGF-β2 concentrations,[64] and therefore consumption of probiotics by the breastfeeding mother may inhibit allergic responses in the infant by enhancing the tolerogenic properties inherent in breast milk. Perplexingly, however, Böttcher and coworkers recently reported that maternal supplementation with the probiotic *L. reuteri* resulted in a decrease in breast milk TGF-β2 that was associated with reduced risk of atopic sensitization in the infant.[65] These discrepant data may be explained not only by the strain-specific properties of probiotic microbes as well as differences in study populations and intervention protocols, but also by the fact that allergic responder type is not limited to sensitization, that is, generation of allergen-specific IgE antibodies.

Also, IL-10 is produced in response to microbial stimuli in experimental animals. Anti-inflammatory IL-10 responses are elicited in response to luminal microbiota in humans as well. In patients with pouchitis, a nonspecific inflammation of the ileal reservoir, reduced numbers of lactobacilli and bifidobacteria, and an increased number of *C. perfringens* in the reservoir microbiota have been observed.[66] The administration of a probiotic mixture resulted in a significant increase in IL-10 in biopsies.[67] In line with this observation, supplementation with the probiotic LGG has been reported to be associated with increased serum IL-10[68] in children, thus furnishing another mechanism for probiotics to counter the allergic response.

Indeed, a concise connection between the control of the inflammatory response and the antiallergic potential of specific probiotics is substantiated by studies in atopic infants. In these subjects, markers of systemic[69] and intestinal[70] allergic inflammation were significantly decreased, which parallels the clinical benefit. Therefore, a working target for reducing the risk of allergic response could be identified as impaired barrier functions of the skin epithelium and gut mucosa (see Figure 4-2), including the role of local microbiota in these functions. This hypothesis also offers one explanation for the variable clinical benefit; probiotics, with the main function within the gastrointestinal tract, indeed have appeared as potential therapeutic agents in the treatment of a variety of gastrointestinal disorders or allergic conditions due to intestinal involvement (Chapter 16).

PROBIOTICS INTERACT WITH OTHER DIETARY COMPONENTS

Studying the benefits of breastfeeding will help find the means of reducing the risk of allergic response. The protective effect of breastfeeding not only confers passive protection, but also actively stimulates the development of the infant's own immune system.

Enteral nutrition is vital for the maintenance of mucosal integrity; thus, assimilation of nutrients and endorsement of intestinal defenses against the constant presence of antigens from food and microorganisms in the gut lumen is important. Enteral nutrition is important, especially during the immediate postnatal period when an abrupt change in gut barrier function occurs as it is switched from processing amniotic fluid to digesting milk. Major changes also occur during the introduction of solid foods. The lack of nutrients or an imbalanced nutrition may result in both structural histologic defects and functional abnormalities, evinced as increased susceptibility to infection and inflammation. These may further deteriorate the gut barrier function due to increased cell turnover and, therefore, increased nutrient requirements.[71]

The key nutrients in gut function include glutamine, arginine, nucleotides, *n*-3 fatty acids, and vitamin A. Although these nutrients have immunomodulatory properties of their own, the interest here is in the potential interaction of these nutrients with probiotics. Undeniably, research focusing on single dietary compounds has resulted in major contributions to human health, including the identification of vitamins whose deficiency causes clinical symptoms and conditions. However, with the modern research, instead of a reductionistic approach, a holistic one is called for with the recognition that the whole may be more than the sum of its parts.[72] This strategy may reveal more about the relationship between the diet and health. We have raised this point by showing that the antiallergic mechanisms accredited to specific probiotics evolve in joint action with the dietary intake of particular nutrients;[73] increased intakes of vitamin A, calcium, and zinc, with perinatal administration of probiotics, reduced the infant's risk of atopic eczema.

Along with its impact on cell differentiation, vitamin A also affects the development of innate immunity, which is required for neutrophil, macrophage, and natural killer cell function, as well as antibody-mediated responses.[74] The cellular mechanisms relate to the regulation of function and gut-homing properties of T and B cells by retinoic acid, the oxidized form of vitamin A.[75] The formation of retinoic acid from retinaldehyde appears to be the limiting step. In addition to its formation in basophils, intestinal mucosa and Peyer's patch DC express the retinoic acid-synthesizing enzyme. By this route, dietary vitamin A concentration may control immune responses within the gut mucosa and provide the link for communication between basophils, mast cells, and T cells, as suggested by Bischoff.[75] Vitamin A is also important because of the antioxidant properties of its provitamins, carotenoids, which have the capacity to counteract oxidative stress and dampen the inflammatory response.[76] In murine models, inhibition of IgE production by vitamin A in peripheral blood mononuclear cells has been reported.[77] Additionally, vitamin A supplementation has resulted in a decrease in interferon-γ and IL-4 levels, the potential cytokines in allergic response, and an increase in mucosal IgA, with the capacity to protect mucosal surfaces.[78] β-Carotene and retinol may also alter the activation of the arachidonic acid cascade and, hence, suppress prostaglandin E2 production in vitro.[79]

Fatty acids are evidently important immune regulators because of their derivative eicosanoids, particularly prostaglandin E2, and consequent cytokine responses, as suggested by Black and Sharpe.[80] An increase in the consumption of polyunsaturated fat in the diet, particularly *n*-6 polyunsaturated fatty acids, results in conversion to prostaglandin E2, whereas *n*-3 series fatty acid-derived eicosapentaenoic acid inhibits the formation of prostaglandin E2. Prostaglandin E2 exerts its effect on the Th1/Th2 balance by decreasing the production of the Th1-type cytokines and enhances the production of Th2-type cytokines, thereby promoting IgE synthesis by B cells.[81] Recent studies propose that microbes and fatty acids engage the same signaling channels through Toll-like receptor 4[82] and soluble CD14[83] of innate immunity. The major function described for soluble CD14, a pattern recognition receptor, is binding of lipopolysaccharides, thus contributing to antimicrobial host defense.[84] However, the binding specificity is not restricted to bacteria. CD14 also binds phospholipids, thereby providing a lipid transfer system.[85] We showed that serum-soluble CD14 correlates with polyunsaturated fatty acids, the main correlations were with arachidonic acid (20:4*n*-6) and dihomo-γ-linolenic acid (20:3*n*-6). Prostaglandin E2, in turn, correlated positively with the ratio of *n*-6 to *n*-3 fatty acids and docosahexaenoic acid (22:6*n*-3) and negatively with the sum of *n*-3 fatty acid in serum.[83] It may thus be suggested that fatty acids contribute to the regulation of innate and adaptive immune responses and link the immune responses to intraluminal antigen exposures, both diet and microbes.

Nutrients and probiotics may exert immunoregulatory effects through several routes, including joint effects on the intestinal integrity and inflammation signaling routes and mediators. One such evidence is the effect of polyunsaturated fatty acids in growth medium on physicochemical surface properties of lactobacilli.[86] When culturing lactobacilli with various free polyunsaturated fatty acids, the incorporation of a given fatty acid into bacterial fatty acids was observed, and changes in the proportions of other fatty acids and interconversions of fatty acids were seen. Also, changes in the hydrophilic or hydrophobic characteristics of lactobacilli occurred, suggesting that the polyunsaturated fatty acids inhibit microbial adhesion to intestinal surfaces.[86]

SUMMARY

Our knowledge of the factors contributing to allergic response is by no means satisfactory. A more profound understanding is indeed needed, as it is likely that there are distinct etiologic factors and pathogenetic mechanisms underlying the heterogeneous manifestations of the disorder. In general, probiotic supplementation aims at providing safe yet sufficient bacterial exposure, with a subsequent immunologic stimulation, in order to avert aberrant compositional development of the gut microbiota and to control local and systemic inflammation when encountering new antigens. Hence, early modification of the diet toward a balanced intake of nutrients and taking account of interactions amongst nutrients and microbes may offer a tool for either prevention or management of allergic response.

Data from experimental models suggest that specific probiotics are capable of creating tolerogenic signals that inhibit allergic hypersensitivity reactions. In particular, accumulating evidence indicates that certain probiotic bacteria, possibly acting through innate pattern recognition receptors, may induce regulatory T cells that suppress both Th1- and Th2-type inflammatory responses and thus attenuate delayed-type hypersensitivity reactions as well as IgE production and eosinophilic inflammation, respectively. Intriguingly, novel data suggest that probiotic intervention in the neonatal period may have long-term programming effects on the immune responder type by, for example, inducing regulatory T cells capable of inhibiting inflammation, thereby reducing the risk of subsequent sensitization. This notion opens appealing avenues for the use of probiotics in not only treatment but also primary prevention of allergic response. Rigorous scientific effort is still required for the clinical validation and safety survey of specific strains of gut microbiota.

REFERENCES

1. Isolauri E, Sütas Y, Kankaanpää P, Arvilommi H, Salminen S. Probiotics: effects on immunity. *Am J Clin Nutr.* 2001;73(suppl 2):S444-S450.
2. Isolauri E, Rautava S, Kalliomäki M, Kirjavainen P, Salminen S. Role of probiotics in food hypersensitivity. *Curr Opin Allergy Clin Immunol.* 2002;2(3):263-271.
3. Nakagawa T, Nakagomi T, Hisamatsu S, Itaya H, Nakagomi O, Mizushima Y. Increased prevalence of elevated serum IgE and IgG4 antibodies in students over a decade. *J Allergy Clin Immunol.* 1996;97(5): 1165-1166.
4. Isolauri E, Huurre A, Salminen S, Impivaara O. The allergy epidemic extends beyond the past few decades. *Clin Exp Allergy.* 2004;34(7):1007-1010.
5. Kalliomäki M, Salminen S, Kero P, Arvilommi H, Koskinen P, Isolauri E. Probiotics in the primary prevention of atopic disease: a randomised, placebo-controlled trial. *Lancet.* 2001;357(9262):1076-1079.
6. Riedler J, Braun-Fahrländer C, Eder W, et al. Exposure to farming in early life and development of asthma and allergy: a cross-sectional survey. *Lancet.* 2001;358(9288):1129-1133.

7. Von Berg A, Koletzko S, Grübl A, et al. The effect of hydrolyzed cow's milk formula for allergy prevention in the first year of life: The German Infant Nutritional Intervention Study, a randomized double-blind trial. *J Allergy Clin Immunol.* 2003;111(3):533-540.

8. Piccinni MP, Beloni L, Livi C, Maggi E, Scarselli G, Romagnani S. Defective production of both leukemia inhibitory factor and type 2 T-helper cytokines by decidual T cells in unexplained recurrent abortions. *Nat Med.* 1998;4(9):1020-1024.

9. Williams TJ, Jones CA, Miles EA, Warner JO, Warner JA. Fetal and neonatal IL-13 production during pregnancy and at birth and subsequent development of atopic symptoms. *J Allergy Clin Immunol.* 2000;105(5):951-959.

10. Prescott SL, Macaubas C, Smallacombe T, Holt BJ, Sly PD, Holt PG. Development of allergen-specific T-cell memory in atopic and normal children. *Lancet.* 1999;353(9148):196-200.

11. Rautava S, Ruuskanen O, Ouwehand A, Salminen S, Isolauri E. The hygiene hypothesis of atopic disease—an extended version. *J Pediatr Gastroenterol Nutr.* 2004;38(4):378-388.

12. Penders J, Thijs C, Vink C, et al. Factors influencing the composition of the intestinal microbiota in early infancy. *Pediatrics.* 2006;118(2):511-521.

13. Satokari R, Grönroos T, Laitinen K, Salminen S, Isolauri E. *Bifidobacterium* and *Lactobacillus* DNA in the human placenta. *Lett Appl Microbiol.* 2009;48(1):8-12.

14. Amarri S, Benatti F, Callegari ML, et al. Changes of gut microbiota and immune markers during the complementary feeding period in healthy breast-fed infants. *J Pediatr Gastroenterol Nutr.* 2000;42(5): 488-495.

15. Eckburg PB, Bik EM, Bernstein CN, et al. Diversity of the human intestinal microbial flora. *Science.* 2005;308(5728):1635-1638.

16. Collado MC, Derrien M, Isolauri E, de Vos WM, Salminen S. Intestinal integrity and *Akkermansia muciniphila*, a mucin-degrading member of the intestinal microbiota present in infants, adults, and the elderly. *Appl Environ Microbiol.* 2007;73(23):7767-7770.

17. Derrien M, Collado MC, Ben-Amor K, Salminen S, de Vos WM. The mucin degrader *Akkermansia muciniphila* is an abundant resident of the human intestinal tract. *Appl Environ Microbiol.* 2008;74(5): 1646-1648.

18. Kalliomäki M, Kirjavainen P, Eerola E, Kero P, Salminen S, Isolauri E. Distinct patterns of neonatal gut microflora in infants in whom atopy was and was not developing. *J Allergy Clin Immunol.* 2001;107(1):129-134.

19. Kalliomäki M, Salminen S, Poussa T, Arvilommi H, Isolauri E. Probiotics and prevention of atopic disease: 4-year follow-up of a randomised placebo-controlled trial. *Lancet.* 2003;361(9372):1869-1871.

20. Kalliomäki M, Salminen S, Poussa T, Isolauri E. Probiotics during the first 7 years of life: a cumulative risk reduction of eczema in a randomized, placebo-controlled trial. *J Allergy Clin Immunol.* 2007;119(4):1019-1021.

21. Wickens K, Black PN, Stanley TV, et al. A differential effect of 2 probiotics in the prevention of eczema and atopy: a double-blind, randomized, placebo-controlled trial. *J Allergy Clin Immunol.* 2008;122(4):788-794.

22. Isolauri E, Majamaa H, Arvola T, Rantala I, Virtanen E, Arvilommi H. *Lactobacillus casei* strain GG reverses increased intestinal permeability induced by cow milk in suckling rats. *Gastroenterology.* 1993;105(6):1643-1650.

23. Isolauri E, Kalliomäki M, Laitinen K, Salminen S. Modulation of the maturing gut barrier and microbiota: a novel target in allergic disease. *Curr Pharm Des.* 2008;14(14):1368-1375.

24. Rinne M, Kalliomäki M, Salminen S, Isolauri E. Probiotic intervention in the first months of life: short-term effects on gastrointestinal symptoms and long-term effects on gut microbiota. *J Pediatr Gastroenterol Nutr.* 2006;43(2):200-205.

25. Benno Y, He F, Hosoda M, et al. Effects of *Lactobacillus* GG yogurt on human intestinal microecology in Japanese subjects. *Nutrition Today.* 1996;31:9-11.

26. Mah KW, Chin VI, Wong WS, et al. Effect of a milk formula containing probiotics on the fecal microbiota of Asian infants at risk of atopic diseases. *Pediatr Res.* 2007;62(6):674-679.

27. Grönlund MM, Gueimonde M, Laitinen K, et al. Maternal breast-milk and intestinal bifidobacteria guide the compositional development of the *Bifidobacterium* microbiota in infants at risk of allergic disease. *Clin Exp Allergy.* 2007;37(12):1764-1772.

28. Matsumoto M, Aranami A, Ishige A, Watanabe K, Benno Y. LKM512 yogurt consumption improves the intestinal environment and induces the T-helper type 1 cytokine in adult patients with intractable atopic dermatitis. *Clin Exp Allergy.* 2007;37(3):358-370.

29. Collado MC, Meriluoto J, Salminen S. Role of commercial probiotic strains against human pathogen adhesion to intestinal mucus. *Lett Appl Microbiol.* 2007;45(4):454-460.

30. Ibnou-Zekri N, Blum S, Schiffrin EJ, von der Weid T. Divergent patterns of colonization and immune response elicited from two intestinal *Lactobacillus* strains that display similar properties in vitro. *Infect Immun.* 2003;71(1):428-436.

31. Duchmann R, Kaiser I, Hermann E, Mayet W, Ewe K, Meyer zum Büschenfelde KH. Tolerance exists towards resident intestinal flora but is broken in active inflammatory bowel disease (IBD). *Clin Exp Immunol.* 1995;102(3):448-455.

32. Ewaschuk JB, Diaz H, Meddings L, et al. Secreted bioactive factors from *Bifidobacterium infantis* enhance epithelial cell barrier function. *Am J Physiol Gastrointest Liver Physiol.* 2008;295(5):G1025-G1034.

33. Steidler L, Hans W, Schotte L, et al. Treatment of murine colitis by *Lactococcus lactis* secreting interleukin-10. *Science.* 2000;289(5483):1352-1355.

34. Barone KS, Reilly MR, Flanagan MP, Michael JG. Abrogation of oral tolerance by feeding encapsulated antigen. *Cell Immunol.* 2000;199(2):65-72.

35. Sütas Y, Soppi E, Korhonen H, et al. Suppression of lymphocyte proliferation in vitro by bovine caseins hydrolysed with *Lactobacillus* GG-derived enzymes. *J Allergy Clin Immunol.* 1996;98(1):216-224.

36. Sütas Y, Hurme M, Isolauri E. Downregulation of antiCD3 antibody-induced IL-4 production by bovine caseins hydrolysed with *Lactobacillus* GG-derived enzymes. *Scand J Immunol.* 1996;43(6):687-689.

37. Pessi T, Sütas Y, Marttinen A, Isolauri E. Antiproliferative effects of homogenates derived from five strains of candidate probiotic bacteria. *Appl Environ Microbiol.* 1999;65(11):4725-4728.

38. Cebra JJ. Influences of microbiota on intestinal immune system development. *Am J Clin Nutr.* 1999;69(5): 1046-1051.

39. Marschan E, Kuitunen M, Kukkonen K, et al. Probiotics in infancy induce protective immune profiles that are characteristic for chronic low-grade inflammation. *Clin Exp Allergy.* 2008;38(4):611-618.

40. Viljanen M, Kuitunen M, Haahtela T, Juntunen-Backman K, Korpela R, Savilahti E. Probiotic effects on faecal inflammatory markers and on faecal IgA in food allergic atopic eczema/dermatitis syndrome infants. *Pediatr Allergy Immunol.* 2005;16(1):65-71.

41. Rautava S, Arvilommi H, Isolauri E. Specific probiotics in enhancing maturation of IgA responses in formula-fed infants. *Pediatr Res.* 2006;60(2):221-224.

42. Kaila M, Isolauri E, Soppi E, Virtanen E, Laine S, Arvilommi H. Enhancement of the circulating antibody secreting cell response in human diarrhea by a human *Lactobacillus* strain. *Pediatr Res.* 1992;32(2):141-144.

43. de Vrese M, Rautenberg P, Laue C, Koopmans M, Herremans T, Schrezenmeir J. Probiotic bacteria stimulate virus-specific neutralizing antibodies following a booster polio vaccination. *Eur J Nutr.* 2005;44(7):406-413.

44. Mack DR, Michail S, Wei S, McDougall L, Hollingsworth MA. Probiotics inhibit enteropathogenic E. coli adherence in vitro by inducing intestinal mucin gene expression. *Am J Physiol.* 1999;276(4 Pt 1):G941-G950.

45. Johnson-Henry KC, Donato KA, Shen-Tu G, Gordanpour M, Sherman PM. *Lactobacillus rhamnosus* strain GG prevents enterohemorrhagic *Escherichia coli* O157:H7-induced changes in epithelial barrier function. *Infect Immun.* 2008;76(4):1340-1348.

46. Tao Y, Drabik KA, Waypa TS, et al. Soluble factors from *Lactobacillus* GG activate MAPKs and induce cytoprotective heat shock proteins in intestinal epithelial cells. *Am J Physiol Cell Physiol.* 2006;290(4): C1018-C1030.

47. Yan F, Cao H, Cover TL, Whitehead R, Washington MK, Polk DB. Soluble proteins produced by probiotic bacteria regulate intestinal epithelial cell survival and growth. *Gastroenterology.* 2007;132(2): 562-575.

48. Majamaa H, Isolauri E. Evaluation of the gut mucosal barrier: evidence for increased antigen transfer in children with atopic eczema. *J Allergy Clin Immunol.* 1996;97(4):985-990.

49. Rautava S, Walker WA. Commensal bacteria and epithelial cross talk in the developing intestine. *Curr Gastroenterol Rep.* 2007;9(5):385-392.

50. Sudo N, Sawamura S, Tanaka K, Aiba Y, Kubo C, Koga Y. The requirement of intestinal bacterial flora for the development of an IgE production system fully susceptible to oral tolerance induction. *J Immunol.* 1997;159(4):1739-1745.

51. Forsythe P, Inman MD, Bienenstock J. Oral treatment with live *Lactobacillus reuteri* inhibits the allergic airway response in mice. *Am J Respir Crit Care Med.* 2007;175(6):561-569.

52. Shida K, Takahashi R, Iwadate E, et al. *Lactobacillus casei* strain Shirota suppresses serum immunoglobulin E and immunoglobulin G1 responses and systemic anaphylaxis in a food allergy model. *Clin Exp Allergy.* 2002;32(4):563-570.

53. Pochard P, Gosset P, Grangette C, et al. Lactic acid bacteria inhibit TH2 cytokine production by mononuclear cells from allergic patients. *J Allergy Clin Immunol.* 2002;110(4):617-623.

54. von der Weid T, Bulliard C, Schiffrin EJ. Induction by a lactic acid bacterium of a population of CD4(+) T cells with low proliferative capacity that produce transforming growth factor beta and interleukin-10. *Clin Diagn Lab Immunol.* 2001;8(4):695-701.

55. Di Giacinto C, Marinaro M, Sanchez M, Strober W, Boirivant M. Probiotics ameliorate recurrent Th1-mediated murine colitis by inducing IL-10 and IL-10-dependent TGF-beta-bearing regulatory cells. *J Immunol.* 2005;174(6):3237-3246.
56. Karimi K, Inman MD, Bienenstock J, Forsythe P. *Lactobacillus reuteri* induced regulatory T cells protect against an allergic airway response in mice. *Am J Respir Crit Care Med.* 2009;179(3):186-193.
57. Feleszko W, Jaworska J, Rha RD, et al. Probiotic-induced suppression of allergic sensitization and airway inflammation is associated with an increase of T regulatory-dependent mechanisms in a murine model of asthma. *Clin Exp Allergy.* 2007;37(4):498-505.
58. Verhasselt V, Milcent V, Cazareth J, et al. Breast milk-mediated transfer of an antigen induces tolerance and protection from allergic asthma. *Nat Med.* 2008;14(2):170-175.
59. Penttila I. Effects of transforming growth factor-beta and formula feeding on systemic immune responses to dietary beta-lactoglobulin in allergy-prone rats. *Pediatr Res.* 2006;59(5):650-655.
60. Kalliomäki M, Ouwehand A, Arvilommi H, Kero P, Isolauri E. Transforming growth factor beta in breast milk: a potential regulator of atopic disease at an early age. *J Allergy Clin Immunol.* 1999;104(6):1251-1257.
61. Oddy WH, Halonen M, Martinez FD, et al. TGF-beta in human milk is associated with wheeze in infancy. *J Allergy Clin Immunol.* 2003;112(4):723-728.
62. Gueimonde M, Sakata S, Kalliomäki M, Isolauri E, Benno Y, Salminen S. Effect of maternal consumption of *Lactobacillus* GG on transfer and establishment of fecal bifidobacterial microbiota in neonates. *J Pediatr Gastroenterol Nutr.* 2006;42(2):166-170.
63. Prescott SL, Wickens K, Westcott L, et al. Supplementation with *Lactobacillus rhamnosus* or *Bifidobacterium lactis* probiotics in pregnancy increases cord blood interferon-gamma and breast milk transforming growth factor-beta and immunoglobin A detection. *Clin Exp Allergy.* 2008;38(10):1606-1614.
64. Rautava S, Kalliomäki M, Isolauri E. Probiotics during pregnancy and breastfeeding may confer immunomodulatory protection against atopic disease in the infant. *J Allergy Clin Immunol.* 2002;109(1):119-121.
65. Böttcher MF, Abrahamsson TR, Fredriksson M, Jakobsson T, Björkstén B. Low breast milk TGF-beta2 is induced by *Lactobacillus reuteri* supplementation and associates with reduced risk of sensitization during infancy. *Pediatr Allergy Immunol.* 2008;19(6):497-504.
66. Ruseler-van-Embden JGH, Schouren WR, van Lieshout LMC. Pouchitis: result of microbial imbalance? *Gut.* 1994;35(5):658-664.
67. Ulisse S, Gionchetti P, D'Alò S, et al. Expression of cytokine, inducible nitric oxide synthase, and matrix metalloproteinases in pouchitis: effects of probiotic treatment. *Am J Gastroenterol.* 2001;96(9):2691-2699.
68. Pessi T, Sütas Y, Hurme M, Isolauri E. Interleukin-10 generation in atopic children following oral *Lactobacillus rhamnosus* GG. *Clin Exp Allergy.* 2000;30(12):1804-1808.
69. Majamaa H, Isolauri E. Probiotics: a novel approach in the management of food allergy. *J Allergy Clin Immunol.* 1997;99(2):179-186.
70. Isolauri E, Arvola T, Sütas Y, Moilanen E, Salminen S. Probiotics in the management of atopic eczema. *Clin Exp Allergy.* 2000;30(11):1605-1610.
71. Laiho K, Isolauri E. Biotherapeutic and nutraceutical agents. In: Guandalini S, ed. *Textbook of Pediatric Gastroenterology and Nutrition.* London, UK: Taylor & Francis; 2004:525-537.
72. Hoffmann I. Transcending reductionism in nutrition research. *Am J Clin Nutr.* 2003;78(suppl 3):514-516.
73. Laitinen K, Kalliomäki M, Poussa T, Lagström H, Isolauri E. Evaluation of diet and growth in children with and without atopic eczema: follow-up study from birth to four years. *Brit J Nutr.* 2005;94(4):565-574.
74. Stephensen CB. Vitamin A, infection, and immune function. *Annu Rev Nutr.* 2001;21:167-192.
75. Bischoff SC. 'Vitamin hypothesis' explanation for allergy increase. *Blood.* 2008;112(9):3535-3536.
76. Greene LS. Asthma, oxidant stress, and diet. *Nutrition.* 1999;15(11-12):899-907.
77. Worm M, Herz U, Krah JM, Renz H, Henz BM. Effects of retinoids on in vitro and in vivo IgE production. *Int Arch Allergy Immunol.* 2001;124(1-3):233-236.
78. Albers R, Bol M, Bleumink R, Willems AA, Pieters RH. Effects of supplementation with vitamins A, C, and E, selenium, and zinc on immune function in a murine sensitization model. *Nutrition.* 2003;19(1-2):940-946.
79. Halevy O, Sklan D. Inhibition of arachidonic acid oxidation by β-carotene, retinol, and alpha-tocopherol. *Biochim Biophys Acta.* 1987;918(3):304-307.
80. Black PN, Sharpe S. Dietary fat and asthma: is there a connection? *Eur Respir J.* 1997;10(1):6-12.
81. Gottrand F. Long-chain polyunsaturated fatty acids influence the immune system of infants. *J Nutr.* 2008;138(suppl 9);1807-1812.

82. Shi H, Kokoeva MV, Inouye K, Tzameli I, Yin H, Flier JS. TLR4 links innate immunity and fatty acid-induced insulin resistance. *J Clin Invest.* 2006;116(11):3015-3025.

83. Laitinen K, Hoppu U, Hämäläinen M, Linderborg K, Moilanen E, Isolauri E. Breast milk fatty acids may link innate and adaptive immune regulation: analysis of soluble CD14, prostaglandin E2 and fatty acids. *Pediatr Res.* 2006;59(5):723-727.

84. Goldblum SE, Grann TW, Ding X, Pugin J, Tobias PS. Lipopolysaccharide (LPS)-binding protein and soluble CD14 function as accessory molecules for LPS-induced changes in endothelial barrier function, in vitro. *J Clin Invest.* 1994;93(2):692-702.

85. Yu B, Hailman E, Wright SD. Lipopolysaccharides binding protein and soluble CD14 catalyze exchange of phospholipids. *J Clin Invest.* 1997;99(2):315-324.

86. Kankaanpää P, Yang B, Kallio H, Isolauri E, Salminen S. Effects of polyunsaturated fatty acids in growth medium on lipid composition and on physicochemical surface properties of lactobacilli. *Appl Environ Microbiol.* 2004;70(1):129-136.

5

Quantification and Identification of Probiotic Organisms in Humans

Ian M. Carroll, PhD; Tamar Ringel-Kulka, MD, MPH; and Yehuda Ringel, MD

The identification and quantification of microorganisms serve multiple purposes relating to the development, use, and evaluation of probiotics in clinical and commercial applications. Because probiotics can play an important role in maintaining health and in the prevention and treatment of disease,[1] it is imperative that researchers be able to track the presence, densities, and effects of these organisms in the complex host-microbial ecosystems of the human body. Most of the currently available applications of probiotics relate to oral administration of products with the belief that a probiotic can induce beneficial effects on the host when given in the right form and concentration. This chapter discusses the investigation of orally administered probiotics and their effect on the intestinal microbiota. The theories and methodologies described in this discussion can be extrapolated to research related to probiotics in other systems and organs.

With regard to probiotic research and the beneficial effects of probiotics, several points need to be emphasized. The full characterization of bacteria in the human body is yet to be completed.[2] Similarly, a complete understanding of changes in microbial ecosystems in relation to specific diseases is not yet known (eg, IBD vs healthy individuals). In addition, although significant advances in understanding the mechanisms by which probiotic bacteria exert their beneficial effects have been made,[3-5] more research is necessary to fully understand the molecular processes by which these microorganisms influence health. Furthermore, probiotics may have direct or indirect effects on host immune and metabolic systems, as well as the indigenous intestinal microbiota. Nevertheless, investigation of the identity, quantity, viability, survival, and colonization of probiotics is an important component of any clinical study examining the effect and benefits of probiotics. Additionally, it is important to identify the effect(s) of probiotics on other microbial communities in the relevant host-microbial ecosystem. These factors are important in order to ensure that the probiotic microorganisms under investigation are responsible for any observed effects on the host, as well as for evaluation of the safety and quality of probiotic end products.

Floch MH, Kim AS, eds.
Probiotics: A Clinical Guide (pp 55-70)
© 2010 Taylor & Francis Group

This chapter reviews both traditional bacteriology and culture techniques, as well as more recent molecular methodologies available to researchers for the quantification and identification of specific probiotics used in clinical settings. Additionally, methods for elucidating the effects of probiotics on the intestinal microbiota are discussed.

QUANTIFICATION AND IDENTIFICATION OF PROBIOTICS USING CULTURE TECHNIQUES

Culture Techniques

The most common probiotics used today are of bacterial (mainly *Lactobacillus* and *Bifidobacterium* species) or fungal (*Saccharomyces boulardii*) origin. Probiotics were initially characterized on the basis of their cell or colony morphology (eg, their appearance under a microscope—rod or coccoid shape), reaction to the Gram staining, fermentation profiles, and enzyme activity properties.[6] Early clinical studies utilized culture techniques to investigate the fate of probiotic bacteria consumed by subjects. This was achieved by the recovery of probiotic bacteria from different organs (eg, mouth[7] or vagina[8]), different parts of the GI tract (eg, fluid from the jejunum[9]), or in feces.[10] Classic nonselective culture techniques use defined media and conditions to cultivate all microorganisms within a sample. Conversely, selective culture techniques provide the medium and conditions that allow a specific probiotic of interest to flourish while inhibiting other organisms (Figure 5-1). For example, several selective media for enumerating *Lactobacillus* species have been developed (eg, Rogosa,[11] de-Man, Rogosa and Sharpe [MRS] agar[12]). Selective growth can also be achieved by adding sugars or an antibiotic to a defined medium.[13-15] For example, adding vancomycin to MRS agar will selectively enable the growth of *Lactobacillus* species that are resistant to this antibiotic, while inhibiting the growth of other bacteria that are sensitive to vancomycin.[15] Another example of selective culture conditions is the use of lactic acid and aerobic incubation to inhibit strict anaerobes (such as *Bifidobacterium* species) while enabling the growth of *Lactobacillus* species.[15] This technique was shown to be capable of differentiating and quantifying *Bifidobacterium* and *Lactobacillus* species within the microbiota of a developing infant.[15]

Selective culture techniques have several limitations. First, it is often difficult to culture all the microbes of interest from a sample containing complex bacterial communities. Second, other members within the genus of a probiotic of interest are difficult to inhibit as they may share characteristics (eg, fermentation profiles) similar to the organism to be investigated. Currently, there are several selective media that promote the growth of specific species of *Lactobacillus*.[16] However, there are no reliable media to selectively grow and differentiate *Bifidobacterium* species. Thus, in the case of *Bifidobacterium* species, it is not possible to detect and quantify all members of this genus using selective media. To overcome these limitations, selective differential media have been developed. Selective differential media can differentiate bacterial species of interest on the basis of unique characteristics that lead to a measurable biochemical reaction. For example, selective differential media have been used to select and differentiate *L. plantarum* from other LAB by using sorbitol as a carbon source and bromocresol purple as an indicator.[17] However, a significant pitfall of the selective media technique is that the interpretation of the bacterial growth on a selective/differential agar palate is somewhat subjective and needs skilled personnel in order to achieve reliable results. Moreover, selective culture techniques do not always provide an accurate

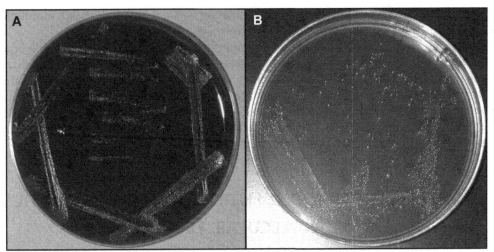

Figure 5-1. Different selective media used for the cultivation of intestinal bacteria. (A) *Bifidobacterium bifidum* grown on brain heart infusion (BHI) blood agar. (B) *Lactobacillus acidophilus* grown on MRS agar.

representation of all the bacterial species within a sample. This observation was highlighted in a study where culture techniques were compared to DNA techniques.[18]

Quantification of the concentrations of bacteria in a given sample is routinely achieved by counting the total number of colony-forming units (CFU) grown on an agar plate from a serially diluted sample. Culture values are expressed as CFU per gram of the original sample (eg, CFU/g of feces). The bacterial quality and quantity of a given sample can be assessed using multiple culture media that enable the calculation of the concentration of all bacteria, specific groups of bacteria (eg, aerobes or anaerobes), a particular genus (eg, *Lactobacillus* or *Bifidobacterium*), or a particular bacterial species (eg, *L. acidophilus* and *L. bulgaricus*).[9] The concentration of the bacteria of interest can then be expressed as the percentage of a particular organism relative to the total bacteria or total bacteria from a specific genus within a given sample.

The importance of the concentration of a probiotic bacterium within a sample can be demonstrated in a study in which patients with recurrent *Clostridium difficile* diarrhea (CDD) received a 10-day standard antibiotic regimen together with 28 days of *S. boulardii* or a placebo.[16] It was found that the mean concentration of *S. boulardii* in the stool from patients with recurrent CDD was significantly lower compared to samples from patients who did not have a recurrence (2.5×10^4 CFU/g of feces vs 1×10^6 CFU/g, respectively; $P = .02$). Similarly, the recurrence rate was significantly higher (93% vs 54%; $P = .007$) in patients with low stool concentrations of the probiotic *S. boulardii* ($<1 \times 10^4$/g of feces).[19]

Early studies used selective culture techniques to assess the survival of probiotics (eg, in the intestinal tract) by measuring their levels in relevant (eg, fecal) samples collected during a probiotic intervention.[10,19-23] Selective culture studies have also been used to investigate the postintervention persistence of probiotic bacteria/yeast over time. For example, one of the first human studies with *Lactobacillus rhamnosus* GG (LGG) used selective culture to demonstrate that the consumed LGG probiotic was recovered in all samples during the consumption period and persisted in fecal samples of 87% of subjects at 4 days and 33% of subjects at 7 days after the termination of probiotic feeding.[22] Additionally, culture techniques have been used to study the colonization and effect of probiotics on the intestinal microbiota. For example, a study in premature infants demonstrated that daily administration of LGG (1×10^8 CFUs) led to intestinal colonization of this probiotic bacterium. However, this colonization was not associated with a reduction in fecal pathogens, as was initially hypothesized.[23]

While a key advantage to cultivation techniques is the ability to identify viable organisms, these approaches have several limitations. Because these techniques are carried out manually, they are often time consuming, labor intensive, subject to contamination, and sensitive to the effects of environmental factors and therefore not always reproducible. In addition, due to the large diversity of bacterial strains and because most of the human-harbored bacteria are unculturable, these techniques can only identify a minor portion of organisms of the human microbiota.

QUANTIFICATION AND IDENTIFICATION OF PROBIOTICS USING MOLECULAR TECHNIQUES

The 16S rRNA Gene

Most molecular microbiology techniques are based on the bacterial small-subunit ribosomal rRNA gene, also known as the 16S rRNA gene. This gene codes for an rRNA that makes up part of the ribosome. The 16S rRNA gene is an ideal marker for molecular analysis of the intestinal microbiota, because it is contained within the genome of all bacteria and archaea and is distinct from eukaryotic organisms that harbor the 18S rRNA gene. As this gene is essential to a bacterium's survival, there are areas within the 16S rRNA gene that cannot be altered. Changes in the structure of these conserved regions would result in loss of the gene function, and the bacterium would not survive. However, there are areas within the gene that can be altered without the loss of function to the gene. These areas, known as variable regions, have been subject to evolutionary variation as different species of bacteria evolved from each other throughout time. The result is a prokaryotic 16S rRNA gene that contains 10 conserved regions and 9 variable regions. This phenomenon can be visualized when the 16S rRNA gene of different bacterial species are aligned (Figure 5-2).

While traditional culture techniques use phenotypic characteristics, such as morphologic, physiologic, and metabolic characteristics to classify bacteria, molecular techniques are built on the unique properties of the 16S rRNA to enable the classification of bacteria in a more reliable genetic-based method. Indeed, amplification of the 16S rRNA gene, using polymerase chain reaction (PCR) with "universal" primers, and subsequently sequencing the amplified gene allow for the identification/classification of an unknown bacterium detected within a sample. Additionally, specific nucleotide probes that can accurately identify the unique regional sequences of the 16S rRNA locus allow for identification and amplification of both total bacteria and specific bacteria of interest within a complex microbial community. Thus, the prokaryotic 16S rRNA gene has become an important molecule for current molecular microbiology techniques.

Quantitative Polymerase Chain Reaction

Real-time PCR, also referred to as quantitative PCR (qPCR), is a molecular technique that is used to quantitatively assess the levels of genes/gene transcripts in a given sample. qPCR in recent years has been employed to determine the concentrations of specific bacteria or bacterial groups in complex bacterial communities (eg, soil and marine environments). This technique is based on the phenomenon that all bacteria

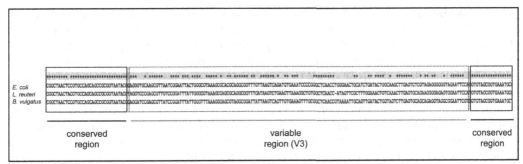

Figure 5-2. Aligned partial sequences of the 16S rRNA gene from *Escherichia coli*, *Lactobacillus reuteri*, and *Bacteroides vulgatus* using ClustalX. Conserved regions and the V3 variable region are shown. Sequences were retrieved at www.ncbi.nlm.nih.gov/.

have a 16S rRNA gene and that all bacteria can be differentiated and categorized on the basis of the sequence of their 16S rRNA gene regions. Indeed, a comprehensive list of 16S rRNA sequences from gut bacteria has been deposited and categorized in the Ribosomal Database Project II.[24] This database provides ribosome-related data and services to the scientific community. By determining the number of conserved 16S rRNA genes in a given sample, qPCR can indirectly indicate the number of bacteria present in that sample. Conversely, appropriate design of qPCR nucleotide primers allows for the detection and enumeration of a specific bacterium of interest, making qPCR a useful tool for quantifying specific bacteria in a complex microbial community. Indeed, there are several programs that facilitate the design of qPCR primers for this purpose. Examples of these programs are ARB,[25] primrose,[26] green genes,[27] and the RDP II.[24]

The sensitivity and accuracy of qPCR has revolutionized research relating to the gut microbiota, because it can detect and enumerate bacteria that are difficult to culture or are uncultivable. Nevertheless, although qPCR is a specific and sensitive molecular tool, it is not without limitations, and there are some caveats that need to be considered before using it to determine the concentrations of specific bacteria/bacterial groups within a sample. First, because the technique is based on measuring 16S rRNA genes, it cannot differentiate between live and dead bacteria. Second, it is important to recognize that the number of copies of the 16S rRNA gene varies between organisms. For example, *Escherichia coli* contains 7 copies of the 16S rRNA gene in its genome, whereas *Enterococcus faecalis* contains only 4 16S rRNA genes.[28] These numbers can differ between strains and fluctuate dramatically within a genus. Thus, if the number of copies of the 16S rRNA gene harbored within a specific bacterium's genome is known and one is assaying that specific organism, it is then possible to calculate the exact number of that organism within a sample. However, as the number of 16S rRNA gene varies between species within a genus, it is difficult to estimate the exact number of bacteria of a group/genus in a sample. Consequently, the quantities of groups of bacteria within a sample using qPCR will generally be expressed as the number of 16S genes per microgram of DNA/gram of feces. Third, the design of specific primers for qPCR assessment of gut microorganisms can sometimes be problematic despite various programs that are available to aid in the design of qPCR primers. The difficulty in achieving selective amplification of a specific bacterial group relates to the diversity of the human gut microbiota[29] and the fact that this technique is based around one genetic locus. As the design of qPCR primers broadens to encompass more bacteria within a family/genus, a minority of species from another genus are invariably amplified as well. Additionally, the attempt to make qPCR primers more specific for a particular genus reduces the number of species in the genus that can be detected. Indeed, many of the genus-specific qPCR primers that are reported in the literature do not encompass all the species from the listed genus.[30,31]

qPCR has been used for quantification of bacteria and determining alterations of specific bacteria and bacterial groups in relation to different GI illnesses.[32-34] In addition, qPCR has been useful in clinical trials using probiotics to monitor the persistence of a particular probiotic and compare the levels of different probiotics in the gut over time. For example, Bartosch et al[35] used qPCR to determine the levels of *Bifidobacterium bifidum*, *Bifidobacterium lactis*, and the *Bifidobacterium* genus in fecal DNA from a probiotic trial in which elderly subjects consumed *B. bifidum* BB-02, *B. lactis* BL-01, and an inulin-based prebiotic.[35] It was demonstrated that both administered probiotics and the whole *Bifidobacterium* genus increased in concentration during the feeding period in subjects receiving the probiotic mix, but not in the control group. Additionally, it was determined that at least one of the probiotic species (either *B. bifidum* BB-02 or *B. lactis* BL-01) was detectable in fecal samples from subjects in the probiotic group up to 3 weeks after cessation of the probiotic consumption.

qPCR can also be used to investigate the effect(s) of probiotics on other members of the GI microbiota by determining the levels of specific bacteria/bacterial groups pre- and postprobiotic intervention. For example, a recent study of VSL#3 to treat IBD patients with pouchitis used qPCR to demonstrate that daily consumption of this mix of probiotic bacteria increased the total number of bacteria and shifted the spectrum of the gut microbiota toward anaerobic species in these patients.[36] Additionally, qPCR has also been used to track the levels of *Lactobacillus* species in the gut during probiotic and prebiotic trials.[37,38] Haarman and Knol[38] demonstrated that the concentrations of members of the *Lactobacillus* genus were comparable between infants receiving a probiotic-supplemented formula- and breastfed infants; however, the levels of *L. delbrueckii* and *L. paracasei* differed between breastfed and standard formula-fed infants. These studies illustrate the usefulness of qPCR for tracking probiotics and their effects on the complex ecosystem of the gut microbiota.

Fluorescent In Situ Hybridization

Although enumeration of indigenous or supplemented bacteria within the gut microbiota is important, the localization of bacterial organisms is also important. The GI microbiota forms a biofilm that lines the GI tract, and careful processing of biopsy samples can preserve this biofilm. Fluorescent in situ hybridization (FISH) is a molecular technique that uses a single fluorescently labeled DNA probe (usually based on the 16S rRNA gene) that hybridizes to specific bacteria in the mucosal biofilm. When a treated tissue section is observed under a fluorescent microscope, any bacterium that has hybridized with this probe will illuminate. Computer software can then be used to determine the densities of a bacterium of interest. Probes that can recognize all bacteria (a universal probe) in a given tissue section are also available, allowing the densities of the bacterium/bacterial group of interest to be expressed as a percentage of total intestinal bacteria. This technique has been used to detect the levels of gut microorganisms in stool[39] and mucosal samples.[40]

In probiotic research, FISH has been used to demonstrate that during consumption of *Lactobacillus johnsonii* La1, this probiotic bacterium not only can be detected in the gut, but also alters the densities of other intestinal bacteria such as other *Lactobacillus* species, *Bifidobacterium* species, and *Faecalibacterium prausnitzii*.[41] Additionally, in a clinical trial using VSL#3 in pouchitis patients, FISH demonstrated that a probiotic-induced remission was associated with a high level of the bacterial family Enterobacteriaceae in close contact with the intestinal epithelium.[36] Another interesting study used FISH to illustrate differences in the composition of bacterial communities throughout an intact fecal sample.[42] These studies demonstrate the potential of FISH to display the spatial distribution of probiotic bacteria either on the gut epithelium or within a fecal sample.

PROBIOTIC EFFECTS ON THE INTESTINAL MICROBIOTA

Genetic Fingerprinting of the Gut Microbiota

Genetic fingerprinting of probiotic organisms within the gut microbiota has focused on 2 techniques, namely denaturing gradient gel electrophoresis (DGGE) and terminal-restriction fragment length polymorphism (T-RFLP). These PCR-based techniques provide detailed qualitative information regarding the most abundant bacterial communities encompassed within a sample. In both techniques, the 16S rRNA genes from all bacteria or a group of bacteria (eg, a specific genus) are amplified, but from this point, the manner in which a genetic fingerprint is obtained from a 16S rRNA PCR product differs considerably between both techniques.

Denaturing Gradient Gel Electrophoresis

For DGGE, the complex mixture of 16S rRNA sequences contained within a PCR product is fractionated through a denaturing agarose gel. In this technique, the PCR product that passes through the gel encounters increasing levels of a denaturing agent. PCR products that have weaker bonds (eg, more adenine and tyrosine nucleotides) denature quickly and therefore migrate slower through the gel, while PCR products with stronger bonds (eg, more guanine and cytosine nucleotides) will migrate faster and further down the agarose gel. Ultimately, the differing 16S rRNA genes are separated on an agarose gel, stained with ethidium bromide, and visualized under an ultraviolet light to yield a genetic fingerprint. Using the appropriate conditions, sequences that differ by as little as one nucleotide can be separated. In addition, because the DGGE technique is based on the 16S rRNA gene, a specific band within a genetic fingerprint can be excised from the gel and sequenced, thus allowing the identification of that particular bacterium.

DGGE fingerprinting has been employed in several probiotic clinical studies to determine the presence and persistence of probiotic bacteria following intervention. For example, this technique has been applied to salivary and fecal samples from subjects consuming a probiotic mix of *L. acidophilus* and *B. animalis* ssp. *lactis* BB-12 to demonstrate the effect of their consumption on the stability of the oral and fecal microbiota.[43] DGGE fingerprinting has also been used to detect changes in the gut mucosal microbiota following probiotic consumption. A recent study using DGGE in patients with UC treated with VSL#3 demonstrated that 2 of the 8 probiotic bacteria of the VSL#3 mixture were found in the intestinal mucosa of those patients who responded with remission to the probiotic intervention.[44] This study demonstrates the ability of DGGE to detect changes in the mucosal microbiota. It also suggests that specific probiotics can, at least temporarily, adhere to the intestinal wall and that this adherence may be associated with remission of UC. Another recent study used DGGE fingerprinting to determine the effect of yogurt bacteria in the human intestinal tract.[45] This study showed no qualitative differences in the composition of the intestinal microbiota during probiotic consumption using DGGE fingerprinting. However, quantitative changes were detected in *Bacteroides* species and the LAB group using qPCR.

Terminal-Restriction Fragment Length Polymorphism

With terminal-restriction fragment length polymorphism (T-RFLP)-PCR, a complex mixture of 16S rRNA genes are amplified from an intestinal DNA sample using fluorescently labeled primers. Each amplified 16S rRNA gene will contain a fluorescent probe as a result of the labeled primers. These 16S rRNA genes are then digested with a restriction enzyme. As all restriction enzymes recognize a specific nucleotide sequence, and bacterial species differ on the basis of their 16S rRNA sequence, each 16S rRNA gene amplified from a sample containing a complex community of bacteria will be digested differently and result in a mixture of digested fragments of the 16S rRNA genes. These digested fragments are representative of the bacterial composition in the original sample. The digested 16S rRNA genes of each sample are then separated by capillary or polyacrylamide electrophoresis in a DNA sequencer, and a genetic fingerprint is obtained by reading the fluorescently labeled fragments of each sample. The T-RFLP patterns of numerous bacteria have been determined and entered in an available reference database.[46] Thus, a unique trait of the T-RFLP technique is that the bacteria encompassed within a complex microbiology ecosystem can be predicted by comparing the genetic fingerprints of a sample to the restriction patterns stored within this reference database.

Similarly to DGGE fingerprinting, T-RFLP has been used to identify probiotic organisms and their effect of the gut microbiota in clinical probiotic studies.[47,48] Additionally, T-RFLP has been used to monitor the changes in the gut microbiota during probiotic and antibiotic treatment.[49] A recent mouse model study used DGGE and T-RFLP fingerprinting to investigate the effects of *L. casei* and *L. plantarum* on the gut microbiota.[50] DGGE and T-RFLP were carried out on fecal and mucosal samples. Both techniques demonstrated that probiotic consumption had a greater effect on the microbiota adherent to the intestinal mucosa than the fecal microbiota. Additionally, DGGE demonstrated that fecal and intestinal samples could be separated on the basis of treatment groups, when *Lactobacillus* species primers were used. Sequence analysis of new or more intense bands within DGGE fingerprints from mice that received a probiotic mix identified the presence of *Lactobacillus helveticus*, *L. johnsonii*, and *Lactobacillus gasseri*. T-RFLP demonstrated that out of the *Lactobacillus* species, *L. johnsonii* was the most abundant.

The genetic fingerprints generated using DGGE and T-RFLP to analyze the gut microbiota can also be compared on a phylogenetic level using novel available software (Figure 5-3). These programs enable the comparison of the fingerprint patterns generated from different samples containing a microbial community and determining how similar they are based on the common banding patterns in their fingerprints. This approach allows the comparison of the overall microbial structure between different samples and between individuals with differing disorders/diseases. For example, Figure 5-3A demonstrates the use of T-RFLP to compare the gut microbiota between patients with diarrhea-predominant irritable bowel syndrome (D-IBS) and healthy controls. This figure shows that the T-RFLP fingerprints of the majority of D-IBS samples are similar and cluster separately from healthy controls.

Genetic fingerprinting of the gut microbiota using DGGE and T-RFLP has several limitations. Fingerprinting will generally yield information regarding the most predominant members of a complex microbiota. This is as a result of a PCR bias for the predominant bacteria in a sample, and digested sequences that are present at low concentrations are difficult to visualize or detect. Also, comparisons of T-RFLP patterns to a database are not always accurate as experimental conditions (such as the restriction of 16S rRNA sequences) and apparatuses (such as the model of DNA sequencer used) can vary between laboratories, resulting in slightly different profiles for the same bacterium. The main advantages of these fingerprinting techniques is that, first, the amplified or restricted fragment can be separated from all other genetic bands and sequenced, allowing for the identification of bacterium within a fingerprint. Second, these techniques are cost- and time-effective, and provide a broad view of the intestinal microbiota.

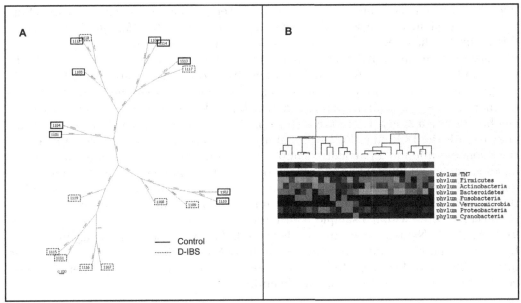

Figure 5-3. Molecular techniques. (A) Phylogenetic clustering of T-RFLP fingerprints from D-IBS patients and healthy controls. (B) Representative heat map generated from 16S rRNA sequences obtained by pyrosequencing. Sequence data are clustered at the phylum level.

SEQUENCING THE 16S RRNA GENE

The techniques discussed so far yield considerable information relating to the structure of the gut microbiota. However, many assumptions are made regarding the bacteria/bacterial species that are going to be investigated. Indeed, alterations that occur in the gut microbiota may occur via bacterial species that have not been taken into account. In order to comprehensively investigate the gut microbiota with respect to a disease state or probiotic intervention, a broad and unbiased technique that details the content of the gut microbiota is needed. To achieve this, PCR and gene sequencing technology of the 16S rRNA gene has been developed. In these technologies, a complex mixture of 16S rRNA genes from a DNA sample is amplified by PCR using primers that recognize all relevant (eg, intestinal) bacteria. The 16S rRNA fragments in this PCR product are then randomly cloned into plasmids and transformed into an appropriate host (usually *E. coli*). Each transformed *E. coli* colony will contain a 16S rRNA sequence that originated from the original PCR product. By randomly choosing transformed *E. coli* colonies, extracting the plasmids they harbor, and sequencing the cloned 16S rRNA fragments from these plasmids, the identities of the different bacteria in the original DNA sample can be determined. The identity of each bacterium within a sample is determined using computer software that compares the 16S rRNA sequences found in a sample with those stored in a database, such as the RDP II. Increasing the number of sequence reactions carried out increases the characteristic detail of the sample of interest. In addition to identification, this technique can be used to estimate the concentration of a bacteria/bacterial group in a sample by determining the percentage of sequences within a sample that share an identity to an organism of interest.

Identification and characterization of microorganisms by sequencing the 16S rRNA gene is advantageous if the composition of the microbiota in certain environments of disease conditions or the effect of particular probiotics are unknown. For example, sequencing techniques were used to detect indigenous probiotic bacteria in the breast milk of healthy women using 16S rRNA clone libraries.[51] This study also demonstrated that the breast milk from each mother harbored a unique microbial composition, and that breast milk was a source of commensal bacteria for the infant gut. Additionally, this technique has been used to investigate the effects of probiotics (*L. casei* and *L. plantarum*) on the intestinal microbiota of mice. This study demonstrated that administration of these probiotics increased the diversity of *Lactobacillus* species in the gut.[50]

There are, however, some caveats to this technique. A researcher is limited by the number of genes that can be sequenced, which is a direct result of how much expense can be put into a study. There are also steps that may create a bias in this technique. First is with the PCR step. PCR will amplify the levels of sequences with respect to their concentration in a particular sample; thus, sequences that are in a majority will be adequately amplified while sequences that are in a minority may undergo a limited amplification or not be amplified at all. Second, sequences that are not recognized by the primers will also not be amplified, resulting in an inaccurate representation of the bacteria harbored within a sample. Third, the cloning process may also allow for some bias as not all DNA sequences are evenly cloned; thus, some sequences may be missed. Regardless of these limitations, sequencing 16S rRNA libraries has become an accepted method that is widely used to describe alterations in microbiota in several disease conditions and following probiotic interventions.[36,50,51]

Novel Sequencing Methods

With the conventional sequencing method of 16S rRNA clone libraries, the detail of characterization of the gut microbiota is determined by the number of clones that are sequenced. For example, in a study of the relationship between the intestinal microbiota and obesity, 18,348 16S rRNA sequences were generated from 12 obese and 2 lean subjects over 4 time periods (approximately 350 base pair sequences per subject).[52] A novel type of nucleotide-sequencing technique termed "pyrosequencing" is a high-throughput nucleotide-sequencing method that can generate up to 100 million nucleotide sequences in a single run. This method is based on the emission of light when a nucleotide is added to a synthesized DNA strand.[53-55] Briefly, the PCR product of a sample containing a complex mixture of 16S rRNA is converted to single strands and embedded onto minute beads. Each bead contains one single-stranded sequence that is amplified on the bead. A complementary strand is then synthesized on these amplified sequences one base pair at a time. When a nucleotide is added to a strand, light is emitted through a chemiluminescent enzymatic reaction, and the type of nucleotide added to each strand is recorded. Using a bead matrix, "bar-coded" technology, and several runs of enzymatic addition of nucleotides, a computer program is able to compile the data of multiple different samples simultaneously. The major advantage of pyrosequencing is the number of sequences that are generated, allowing for deep characterization of complex microbial samples. Traditional sequencing can read approximately 800 base pairs of 100 DNA molecules, whereas the 454's GS FLX pyrosequencing machine can read 250 base pairs from 400,000 DNA molecules. Pyrosequencing has been used to characterize the gut microbiota in animal models[56-58] and in human studies investigating the effects of antibiotics[59] and obesity on the intestinal microbiota[55,60] (see Figure 5-3B). Although the potential for this technique is apparent, there are currently no data available regarding the use of this technique in relation to the characterization or identification of bacteria/bacterial groups in different disease conditions or the effect of probiotic intervention.

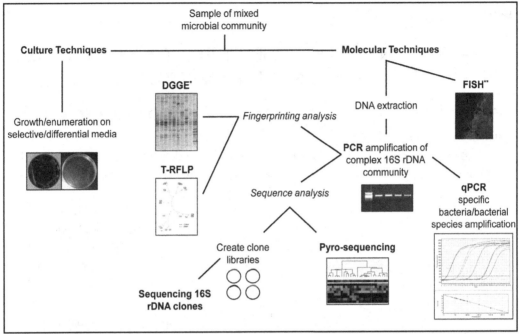

Figure 5-4. Schematic diagram of methods to characterize and identify probiotics in clinical samples. *Photograph used with permission from Bibiloni R, Fedorak RN, Tannock GW, et al. VSL#3 probiotic-mixture induces remission in patients with active UC. *Am J Gastroenterol.* 2005;100(7):1539-1546. **Photograph used with permission from Kim SC, Tonkonogy SL, Jarvis W, et al. Escherichia coli strains differentially induce colitis in IL-10 gene deficient mice. *Gastroenterology.* 2008;134(4):A-650.

CONCLUSION

The emerging data on the important role of the intestinal microbiota in maintaining and promoting human health, and the contribution of dysbiosis in this ecosystem to the development of disease and illness, have led to the realization and acceptance of the intestinal microbiota as an important functional organ and possible terget for intervention.[61] This, together with the increase in the use of probiotics in various clinical conditions, has led to the recent interest in research related to probiotics aiming to provide the rationale for their use, the evidence for their benefits, and the possible mechanisms of their effect(s).

The advent of new molecular methods over the last few years has made the accurate characterization and quantification of complex microbial environments quicker and easier to carry out. The currently available microbiology techniques (Figure 5-4) enable researchers to perform detailed microbiology analyses to confirm the association between the expected/observed effect(s) and the specific probiotic intervention as well as examination of the effect of probiotic intervention on the overall host-harbored microbial communities. However, because all the available methodologies have inherent limitations, no technique can be regarded as a "gold standard" for these purposes, and currently a combination of different techniques is recommended. Greater knowledge and familiarity of investigators with the details, advantages, limitations, and pitfalls of each technique (summarized in Table 5-1) will increase their ability to choose the technique(s) that are likely to provide the comprehensive information in each study, and to appropriately and cautiously interpret and evaluate the meaning and importance of their results.

TABLE 5-1

ADVANTAGES AND DISADVANTAGES OF THE TECHNIQUES USED FOR QUANTIFYING AND IDENTIFYING PROBIOTICS

TECHNIQUE	ADVANTAGES	DISADVANTAGES
Culture techniques:		
Nonselective, Selective, Differential	Identification and quantification of viable/live bacteria	Difficult to grow and identify all bacteria in complex community
		Labor intensive
		Difficult to differentiate probiotics from indigenous bacteria
		Somewhat difficult to reproduce due to varying lab conditions
		Subjective and need skilled personnel
		Subject to contamination
Molecular techniques:		
qPCR	Accurate	Doesn't differentiate between live and dead bacteria
	Sensitive	
	Specific	Groups of bacteria difficult to enumerate
		Difficult to design primers for the selective amplification of a group of bacteria
FISH	Specific	Doesn't differentiate between live and dead bacteria.
	Localization of bacteria within sample	Semi-quantitative
DGGE/T-RFLP fingerprinting	Global representation of gut microbiota	Doesn't differentiate between live and dead bacteria
	Determine effect of probiotic on other members of gut microbiota	Not quantitative
		Mostly represents the predominant members of the gut microbiota
	Can determine the identity of the bacteria within the fingerprint	Variability between laboratories
	Cost effective	

(continued)

TABLE 5-1 *(continued)*

ADVANTAGES AND DISADVANTAGES OF THE TECHNIQUES USED FOR QUANTIFYING AND IDENTIFYING PROBIOTICS

TECHNIQUE	ADVANTAGES	DISADVANTAGES
Sequence analysis • 16S clone libraries • Pyro-sequencing	Quantitative Qualitative Detailed representation of the gut microbiota	Doesn't differentiate between live and dead bacteria Expensive For clone libraries: • Limited by the number of clones sequenced • PCR and cloning bias For pyro-sequencing: • PCR bias

Acknowledgment

The authors would like to thank Andrea M. Azcarate-Peril, PhD and Ajay S. Gulati, MD, for their review and helpful comments.

REFERENCES

1. Floch MH, Walker WA, Guandalini S, et al. Recommendations for probiotic use—2008. *J Clin Gastroenterol.* 2008;42(suppl 2):S104-S108.
2. Turnbaugh PJ, Ley RE, Hamady M, Fraser-Liggett CM, Knight R, Gordon JI. The human microbiome project. *Nature.* 2007;449(7164):804-810.
3. Mohamadzadeh M, Klaenhammer TR. Specific *Lactobacillus* species differentially activate Toll-like receptors and downstream signals in dendritic cells. *Expert Rev Vaccines.* 2008;7(8):1155-1164.
4. Azcarate-Peril MA, Altermann E, Goh YJ, et al. Analysis of the genome sequence of *Lactobacillus gasseri* ATCC 33323 reveals the molecular basis of an autochthonous intestinal organism. *Appl Environ Microbiol.* 2008;74(15):4610-4625.
5. Mohamadzadeh M, Duong T, Hoover T, Klaenhammer TR. Targeting mucosal dendritic cells with microbial antigens from probiotic lactic acid bacteria. *Expert Rev Vaccines.* 2008;7(2):163-174.
6. Conway PL, Henriksson A. Strategies for the isolation and characterization of functional probiotics. In: Gibson SAW, ed. *Human Health: The Contribution of Microorganisms.* Vol 1. New York: Springer-Verlag; 1994:75-94.
7. Strahinic I, Busarcevic M, Pavlica D, Milasin J, Golic N, Topisirovic L. Molecular and biochemical characterizations of human oral lactobacilli as putative probiotic candidates. *Oral Microbiol Immunol.* 2007;22(2):111-117.
8. Reid G, Charbonneau D, Erb J, et al. Oral use of *Lactobacillus rhamnosus* GR-1 and *L. fermentum* RC-14 significantly alters vaginal flora: randomized, placebo-controlled trial in 64 healthy women. *FEMS Immunol Med Microbiol.* 2003;35(2):131-134.
9. Robins-Browne RM, Levine MM. The fate of ingested lactobacilli in the proximal small intestine. *Am J Clin Nutr.* 1981;34(4):514-519.
10. Bouhnik Y, Pochart P, Marteau P, Arlet G, Goderel I, Rambaud JC. Fecal recovery in humans of viable *Bifidobacterium* sp ingested in fermented milk. *Gastroenterology.* 1992;102(3):875-878.

11. Rogosa M, Mitchell JA, Wiseman RF. A selective medium for the isolation and enumeration of oral and fecal lactobacilli. *J Bacteriol.* 1951;62(1):132-133.
12. De Man JC, Rogosa M, Sharpe ME. A medium for the cultivation of Lactobacilli. *J Appl Bacteriol.* 1960;23(1):130-135.
13. Hartemink R, Van Laere KM, Rombouts FM. Growth of enterobacteria on fructo-oligosaccharides. *J Appl Microbiol.* 1997;83(3):367-374.
14. Champagne CP, Gardner NJ. The growth and recovery of an exopolysaccharide-producing *Lactobacillus rhamnosus* culture on growth media containing apple juice or molasses. *J Gen Appl Microbiol.* 2008;54(4):237-241.
15. Mirlohi M, Soleimanian-Zad S, Sheikh-Zeiondin M, Fazeli H. Enumeration of lactobacilli in the fecal flora of infant using two different modified de-Man Rogosa Sharpe media under aerobic and anaerobic incubation. *Pak J Biol Sci.* 2008;11(6):876-881.
16. Tharmaraj N, Shah NP. Selective enumeration of *Lactobacillus delbrueckii* ssp. *bulgaricus, Streptococcus thermophilus, Lactobacillus acidophilus*, bifidobacteria, *Lactobacillus casei, Lactobacillus rhamnosus*, and propionibacteria. *J Dairy Sci.* 2003;86(7):2288-2296.
17. Bujalance C, Jimenez-Valera M, Moreno E, Ruiz-Bravo A. A selective differential medium for *Lactobacillus plantarum. J Microbiol Meth.* 2006;66(3):572-575.
18. Jackson MS, Bird AR, McOrist AL. Comparison of two selective media for the detection and enumeration of lactobacilli in human faeces. *J Microbiol Meth.* 2002;51(3):313-321.
19. Elmer GW, McFarland LV, Surawicz CM, Danko L, Greenberg RN. Behaviour of *Saccharomyces boulardii* in recurrent *Clostridium difficile* disease patients. *Aliment Pharmacol Ther.* 1999;13(12):1663-1668.
20. Pochart P, Marteau P, Bouhnik Y, Goderel I, Bourlioux P, Rambaud JC. Survival of bifidobacteria ingested via fermented milk during their passage through the human small intestine: an in vivo study using intestinal perfusion. *Am J Clin Nutr.* 1992;55(1):78-80.
21. Fujiwara S, Hashiba H, Hirota T, Forstner JF. Proteinaceous factor(s) in culture supernatant fluids of bifidobacteria which prevents the binding of enterotoxigenic *Escherichia coli* to gangliotetraosylceramide. *Appl Environ Microbiol.* 1997;63(2):506-512.
22. Goldin BR, Gorbach SL, Saxelin M, Barakat S, Gualtieri L, Salminen S. Survival of *Lactobacillus* species (strain GG) in human gastrointestinal tract. *Dig Dis Sci.* 1992;37(1):121-128.
23. Millar MR, Bacon C, Smith SL, Walker V, Hall MA. Enteral feeding of premature infants with *Lactobacillus* GG. *Arch Dis Child.* 1993;69(5 Spec No):483-487.
24. Cole JR, Wang Q, Cardenas E, et al. The Ribosomal Database Project: improved alignments and new tools for rRNA analysis. *Nucleic Acids Res.* 2009;37(Database issue):D141-D145.
25. Ludwig W, Strunk O, Westram R, et al. ARB: a software environment for sequence data. *Nucleic Acids Res.* 2004;32(4):1363-1371.
26. Ashelford KE, Weightman AJ, Fry JC. PRIMROSE: a computer program for generating and estimating the phylogenetic range of 16S rRNA oligonucleotide probes and primers in conjunction with the RDP-II database. *Nucleic Acids Res.* 2002;30(15):3481-3489.
27. DeSantis TZ, Hugenholtz P, Larsen N, et al. Greengenes, a chimera-checked 16S rRNA gene database and workbench compatible with ARB. *Appl Environ Microbiol.* 2006;72(7):5069-5072.
28. Hallin PF, Ussery DW. CBS Genome Atlas Database: a dynamic storage for bioinformatic results and sequence data. *Bioinformatics.* 2004;20(18):3682-3686.
29. Peterson DA, Frank DN, Pace NR, Gordon JI. Metagenomic approaches for defining the pathogenesis of inflammatory bowel diseases. *Cell Host Microbe.* 2008;3(6):417-427.
30. Baker GC, Smith JJ, Cowan DA. Review and re-analysis of domain-specific 16S primers. *J Microbiol Meth.* 2003;55(3):541-555.
31. Horz HP, Vianna ME, Gomes BP, Conrads G. Evaluation of universal probes and primer sets for assessing total bacterial load in clinical samples: general implications and practical use in endodontic antimicrobial therapy. *J Clin Microbiol.* 2005;43(10):5332-5337.
32. Collado MC, Donat E, Ribes-Koninckx C, Calabuig M, Sanz Y. Specific duodenal and faecal bacterial groups are associated with paediatric celiac disease. *J Clin Pathol.* 2009;62(3):264-269.
33. Bibiloni R, Mangold M, Madsen KL, Fedorak RN, Tannock GW. The bacteriology of biopsies differs between newly diagnosed, untreated, Crohn's disease and UC patients. *J Med Microbiol.* 2006;55(pt 8):1141-1149.
34. Willing B, Halfvarson J, Dicksved J, et al. Twin studies reveal specific imbalances in the mucosa-associated microbiota of patients with ileal Crohn's disease. *Inflamm Bowel Dis.* 2009;15(5):653-660.
35. Bartosch S, Woodmansey EJ, Paterson JC, McMurdo ME, Macfarlane GT. Microbiological effects of consuming a synbiotic containing *Bifidobacterium bifidum, Bifidobacterium lactis*, and oligofructose in elderly persons, determined by real-time polymerase chain reaction and counting of viable bacteria. *Clin Infect Dis.* 2005;40(1):28-37.

36. Kuhbacher T, Ott SJ, Helwig U, et al. Bacterial and fungal microbiota in relation to probiotic therapy (VSL#3) in pouchitis. *Gut.* 2006;55(6):833-841.

37. Rochet V, Rigottier-Gois L, Sutren M, et al. Effects of orally administered *Lactobacillus casei* DN-114 001 on the composition or activities of the dominant faecal microbiota in healthy humans. *Br J Nutr.* 2006;95(2):421-429.

38. Haarman M, Knol J. Quantitative real-time PCR analysis of fecal *Lactobacillus* species in infants receiving a prebiotic infant formula. *Appl Environ Microbiol.* 2006;72(4):2359-2365.

39. Kalliomaki M, Collado MC, Salminen S, Isolauri E. Early differences in fecal microbiota composition in children may predict overweight. *Am J Clin Nutr.* 2008;87(3):534-538.

40. Janeczko S, Atwater D, Bogel E, et al. The relationship of mucosal bacteria to duodenal histopathology, cytokine mRNA, and clinical disease activity in cats with inflammatory bowel disease. *Vet Microbiol.* 2008;128(1-2):178-193.

41. Garrido D, Suau A, Pochart P, Cruchet S, Gotteland M. Modulation of the fecal microbiota by the intake of a *Lactobacillus johnsonii* La1-containing product in human volunteers. *FEMS Microbiol Lett.* 2005;248(2):249-256.

42. Swidsinski A, Loening-Baucke V, Verstraelen H, Osowska S, Doerffel Y. Biostructure of fecal microbiota in healthy subjects and patients with chronic idiopathic diarrhea. *Gastroenterology.* 2008;135(2): 568-579.

43. Maukonen J, Matto J, Suihko ML, Saarela M. Intra-individual diversity and similarity of salivary and faecal microbiota. *J Med Microbiol.* 2008;57(pt 12):1560-1568.

44. Bibiloni R, Fedorak RN, Tannock GW, et al. VSL#3 probiotic-mixture induces remission in patients with active UC. *Am J Gastroenterol.* 2005;100(7):1539-1546.

45. Garcia-Albiach R, Jose M, de Felipe P, et al. Molecular analysis of yogurt containing *Lactobacillus delbrueckii* subsp. *bulgaricus* and *Streptococcus thermophilus* in human intestinal microbiota. *Am J Clin Nutr.* 2008;87(1):91-96.

46. Shyu C, Soule T, Bent SJ, Foster JA, Forney LJ. MiCA: a web-based tool for the analysis of microbial communities based on terminal-restriction fragment length polymorphisms of 16S and 18S rRNA genes. *Microb Ecol.* 2007;53(4):562-570.

47. Odamaki T, Xiao JZ, Iwabuchi N, et al. Influence of *Bifidobacterium longum* BB536 intake on faecal microbiota in individuals with Japanese cedar pollinosis during the pollen season. *J Med Microbiol.* 2007;56(pt 10):1301-1308.

48. Tsuda Y, Yoshimatsu Y, Aoki H, et al. Clinical effectiveness of probiotics therapy (BIO-THREE) in patients with UC refractory to conventional therapy. *Scand J Gastroenterol.* 2007;42(11): 1306-1311.

49. Jernberg C, Sullivan A, Edlund C, Jansson JK. Monitoring of antibiotic-induced alterations in the human intestinal microflora and detection of probiotic strains by use of terminal restriction fragment length polymorphism. *Appl Environ Microbiol.* 2005;71(1):501-506.

50. Fuentes S, Egert M, Jimenez-Valera M, et al. Administration of *Lactobacillus casei* and *Lactobacillus plantarum* affects the diversity of murine intestinal lactobacilli, but not the overall bacterial community structure. *Res Microbiol.* 2008;159(4):237-243.

51. Martin R, Heilig HG, Zoetendal EG, et al. Cultivation-independent assessment of the bacterial diversity of breast milk among healthy women. *Res Microbiol.* 2007;158(1):31-37.

52. Ley RE, Turnbaugh PJ, Klein S, Gordon JI. Microbial ecology: human gut microbes associated with obesity. *Nature.* 2006;444(7122):1022-1023.

53. Andersson AF, Lindberg M, Jakobsson H, Backhed F, Nyren P, Engstrand L. Comparative analysis of human gut microbiota by barcoded pyrosequencing. *PLoS ONE.* 2008;3(7):e2836.

54. Ronaghi M. Pyrosequencing sheds light on DNA sequencing. *Genome Res.* 2001;11(1):3-11.

55. Turnbaugh PJ, Hamady M, Yatsunenko T, et al. A core gut microbiome in obese and lean twins. *Nature.* 2009;457(7228):480-484.

56. McKenna P, Hoffmann C, Minkah N, et al. The macaque gut microbiome in health, lentiviral infection, and chronic enterocolitis. *PLoS Pathog.* 2008;4(2):e20.

57. Dowd SE, Sun Y, Wolcott RD, Domingo A, Carroll JA. Bacterial tag-encoded FLX amplicon pyrosequencing (bTEFAP) for microbiome studies: bacterial diversity in the ileum of newly weaned Salmonella-infected pigs. *Foodborne Pathog Dis.* 2008;5(4):459-472.

58. Dowd SE, Callaway TR, Wolcott RD, et al. Evaluation of the bacterial diversity in the feces of cattle using 16S rDNA bacterial tag-encoded FLX amplicon pyrosequencing (bTEFAP). *BMC Microbiol.* 2008;8:125.

59. Dethlefsen L, Huse S, Sogin ML, Relman DA. The pervasive effects of an antibiotic on the human gut microbiota, as revealed by deep 16S rRNA sequencing. *PLoS Biol.* 2008;6(11):e280.

60. Armougom F, Raoult D. Use of pyrosequencing and DNA barcodes to monitor variations in Firmicutes and Bacteroidetes communities in the gut microbiota of obese humans. *BMC Genomics.* 2008;9(1):576.

61. Ringel Y, Carroll IM. Alterations in the intestinal microbiota and functional bowel symptoms. *Gastrointest Endosc Clin N Am.* 2009;19(1):141-150, vii.

6

Nutrients to Nourish the Organisms: Prebiotics and Fiber

Harry J. Flint, BSc, PhD and Sylvia H. Duncan, BSc, PhD

A significant proportion of dietary intake remains undigested during passage through the stomach and small intestine, and becomes available as a source of energy and nutrients to the microbiota that colonize the large intestine. While many microorganisms can also be supported by energy sources of endogenous origin (host secretions, especially mucin, and sloughed epithelial cells), the species composition and density of the colonic community is profoundly influenced by the energy supply from dietary residue.[1,2] Research has only recently started to reveal exactly how different dietary components influence the intestinal microbial community. A priori, we might expect that a complex substrate such as plant fiber should promote multiple species, whereas a defined oligosaccharide preparation used as a prebiotic might be more targeted in its effects, but experimental evidence is currently limited. Most important, of course, is to be able to predict the consequences of dietary manipulation of the gut microbial community upon health. Although most major gut pathogens have a long history of research, we are only just beginning to understand the roles of different groups of commensal gut microorganisms that colonize the gut in health and disease. Such understanding is, however, of fundamental importance in predicting the health impact of dietary prebiotics and fiber.

GUT MICROBIOTA

The human intestine harbors many different communities of microorganisms whose composition varies with the anatomical site, environmental and nutritional conditions, and host factors including genotype, immunological status, age, and state of health or disease.[3-5] The most densely colonized region is the large intestine where microbial densities can exceed 10^{11}/g contents and total microbial numbers exceed host cells in the body by a factor of 10. Colonizing microbes include representatives of 3 kingdoms—eukaryotes (protozoa and fungi), bacteria, and archaea. Protozoa found in the gut include many well-known agents of infection (eg, *Cryptosporidium* and *Entamoeba*), but rather less is known about the contribution of eukaryotic microorganisms to the commensal microbiota of healthy subjects. We will focus here

Floch MH, Kim AS, eds.
Probiotics: A Clinical Guide (pp 71-82)
© 2010 Taylor & Francis Group

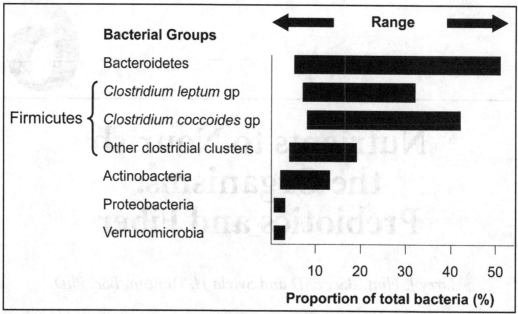

Figure 6-1. Abundance of the major bacterial groups in human fecal samples as determined by molecular methods. The approximate range of abundance (as percentage of total bacterial cells detected by the method used) is shown for healthy adult individuals. Estimates are based largely on studies using fluorescent in situ hybridization.

largely on the bacteria, which are the most numerous microbial inhabitants of the gut and the main targets for prebiotic and probiotic treatments.

Over the past 10 years, the composition of the bacterial community colonizing the large intestine has been documented largely through surveys of ribosomal 16S rRNA sequences, following culture-independent direct PCR amplification.[6] A few studies have examined the intestinal wall[7,8] although the total number of individuals surveyed by these approaches remains small. This sequence information has given rise to enumeration techniques such as FISH and quantitative real-time PCR that can be applied to larger numbers of individuals and that estimate the abundance of specific groups.[9-13] With regard to the fecal and colonic microbiota, there is general agreement that 3 bacterial phyla are dominant: low % G + C Gram-positive firmicutes, high % G + C Gram-positive actinobacteria, and Gram-negative bacteria belonging to bacteroidetes.[6-8,14] Also commonly found, but in lower abundance, are proteobacteria and verrucomicrobia (Figure 6-1).

Initial 16S rRNA-based surveys concluded that some 75% of sequences did not conform to known cultured species of bacteria, and this has been taken to imply that the majority of gut bacteria might be unculturable. More likely, however, is that the culturing effort has simply not kept pace with the ease of characterization by sequencing. Recent isolation studies focusing on butyrate-producers, for example, have yielded many new species that are readily cultured under anaerobic conditions despite being extremely sensitive to oxygen.[1,5,15] For certain groups of firmicutes bacteria such as *Eubacterium rectale/Roseburia*, for example, the available cultured isolates now appear to populate most of the branches of phylogenetic trees that are constructed from directly amplified 16S rRNA sequences.[16] Nevertheless, a very significant proportion of the numerically most abundant bacteria within the human intestinal community remain unstudied, in many cases unnamed, and in some cases uncultured. This should be an important consideration when trying to predict the consequences, for example, of a novel prebiotic.

It should be emphasized that we do not yet have sufficient detailed understanding for any simplistic division of the gut community into "good" and "bad" bacteria. Most pathogenic bacteria are of course well known and well studied, but this has left the great majority of bacteria that colonize the healthy intestine to be classified by default as "harmless commensals." There is good evidence that the numerically predominant commensal bacteria collectively help to create a gut environment that is hostile to many pathogens through competition for nutrients and binding sites, and through the production of fermentation acids and antimicrobial compounds. As we gain more understanding of individual groups, however, it should become apparent that some commensals have more favorable effects on the host, while others may be deleterious, even acting as opportunistic pathogens.

While the major phyla of gut bacteria appear generally well conserved between different individuals, at the level of species, phylotypes, and strains, there is remarkable interindividual variation. This was first revealed by rapid profiling methods such as DGGE analysis,[17] but it has also been confirmed by sequencing approaches.[18,19] As populations of individual bacterial groups are expected to fluctuate constantly with time and dietary intake, it is impossible to conclude from examination of a single sample that a given bacterial clone is absent from that individual's microbiota. Nevertheless, profiling studies do suggest that there is normally a degree of stability in an individual's fecal microbiota over time.[17] A central, unresolved question is whether there is a common "core" human gut microbiota. A small number of species (or phylotypes) appear to be detected among the most abundant organisms present in most individuals, but no single species appears to be universally present at high levels in everyone.[20] Attempts are also being made to define a core "microbiome" in terms of sequences, using metagenomics.[21]

DIETARY FIBER AND NONDIGESTIBLE CARBOHYDRATES

The colonic microbiota are assumed to depend for their energy and nutrient requirements in part on endogenous secretions, such as mucin, and on sloughed epithelial host cells. Under normal dietary conditions, however, the largest source of energy for microbial growth and metabolism comes from dietary residue that has survived passage through the gut to the large intestine.[22] The main components of dietary origin are variously referred to as dietary fiber and nondigestible or "low-digestible" carbohydrates.

As there is no universally agreed definition of dietary fiber, it is necessary to start by considering the range of nondigestible food components more generally. A significant fraction of the digesta escapes absorption in the upper gut (taken to mean the gut as far as the end of the ileum). This is mainly because certain food components resist the battery of digestive enzymes that are produced in salivary, gastric, and pancreatic secretions. Some resistant components are soluble, and these include many oligosaccharides of plant origin in which the constituent sugars are linked by bonds that are not hydrolyzable by the digestive enzymes (eg, β-glycosides, β-fructosides, and β-xylosides). Many resistant components are, however, part of solid or semisolid food particles. Any ingested plant foodstuff comprises a significant quantity of plant cell wall material, whose composition is dominated by the nonstarch polysaccharides cellulose, hemicellulose (xylans, mannans, etc), pectins, and lignins, which are nondigestible fibers. These different polymers are closely associated with each other and with other polymers including lignin and structural proteins within the plant cell wall, and their resistance to degradation can also represent a barrier to the release of other molecules that are held within the plant cell. Other sources of carbohydrates that are essentially undegradable by mammalian digestive enzymes include natural gums and storage carbohydrates such as inulin and fructooligosaccharides (FOS).

Some other polysaccharides found in abundance in foodstuffs contain bonds that are normally degradable by digestive enzymes, but are not always fully digested. This applies to starch, most of which is readily digestible apart from a significant fraction of resistant starch that survives digestion in the small intestine to reach the colon.[23] Resistant starch is classified into 4 types, RS1, RSII, RSIII, and RSIV, that differ in the explanations for their nondigestibility. RS1 is resistant starch that is found in legumes and unprocessed whole grains and therefore is physically inaccessible, while RS2 is the natural granular form found, for example, in uncooked potatoes. RS3 is formed when foods such as potatoes are cooked and cooled, and RS4 is not a natural product but is chemically modified to resist digestion.

Some definitions of dietary fiber are limited to those insoluble nonstarch polysaccharides that are recovered by the Englyst procedure while others include soluble oligosaccharides and resistant starch. A recent review proposed to term all nondigestible carbohydrates as "resistant carbohydrates."[24] Dietary residue can also contain noncarbohydrate material, including dietary protein, that has escaped digestion because of either intrinsic resistance to gut proteases or perhaps incomplete digestion under conditions of high protein intake.[25]

A high proportion of nondigestible residue entering the colon arrives in the form of insoluble particles. Particulate material in feces is assumed to consist of a mixture of incompletely degraded dietary substrate, mainly plant cell wall material rich in cellulose and lignin, together with mucin and cell fragments of microbial and host origin. Fractionation of fecal samples into washed fiber and liquid, followed by 16S rRNA clone library analysis, has however shown that certain firmicute bacteria, especially *Ruminococcus* spp, are detected at significantly higher relative abundance in the fiber-attached community.[19] Related cluster IV ruminococci are important in fiber breakdown in the rumen, and isolates have now been obtained from human feces.[26] In vitro fermentor systems are being adapted to study the colonization of insoluble substrates by human colonic bacteria.[27,28] In a recent study, substrate-attached bacteria surveyed by 16S rRNA sequence analysis were found to be highly specific for the substrate used (mucin, wheat bran, or porcine mucin) with 80% of sequences detected on starch particles being accounted for by 3 groups of bacteria—*Ruminococcus bromii, E. rectale,* and *Bifidobacterium* spp.[29]

IMPACT OF PREBIOTICS ON THE INTESTINAL MICROBIOTA

Prebiotics have been defined as "a selectively fermented ingredient that allows specific changes, both in the composition and/or activity in the gastrointestinal microflora that confers benefits upon host well-being and health."[30] Prebiotics currently in use, or proposed for use, are mainly carbohydrates of low digestibility that are found naturally in foodstuffs, although novel prebiotics are also being produced on the basis of synthetic oligosaccharides.[31] Candidate prebiotics include mannooligosaccharides, pectic oligosaccharides, xylooligosaccharides, galactooligosaccharides (GOS),[32] transgalactosylated oligosaccharides, and chitooligosaccharides, but most studies have focused on the use of inulin and FOS.[2]

While most of the above-mentioned prebiotics are derived from plant material, oligosaccharides of low digestibility are also produced by mammalian cells. In particular, oligosaccharides comprising the sugars L-fucose, D-glucose, or D-galactose are the third largest component of human milk where they occur at concentrations of around 10 g/L.

Breastfed infants have an intestinal microbiota that is dominated by bifidobacteria, which differs from the intestinal microbiota of formula-fed infants that tends to harbor a greater diversity of organisms, including more enterococci[33] with concomitant higher levels of ammonia, amines, and phenols.[34] The high numbers of bifids in the feces of breastfed babies is thought to result from their abilities to utilize oligosaccharides in breast milk, including GOS.

Until recently, prebiotics were assessed mainly by their ability to promote specific groups of bacteria regarded as beneficial, in particular bifidobacteria, and on evidence that they deliver health benefits.[35,36] It would be surprising, however, if their effects on the microbial community were limited to a single group of bacteria.[5] In studies where a wide range of gut bacterial variation has been surveyed, it has been shown that inulin and FOS, for example, promote one or more groups of bacteria in addition to their effects on bifidobacteria.[37-39] In some cases, it is reasonable to suppose that these other groups might contribute to the mode of action of the prebiotic. There is recent evidence that *Faecalibacterium prausnitzii*, for example, has a beneficial anti-inflammatory effect in patients suffering from CD,[40] and this group was shown to be stimulated by inulin in a recent human dietary study.[38]

We know relatively little about the selective effects of prebiotics at the species/strain level. Subtle variations in the ability to utilize carbohydrates undoubtedly occur within most groups of bacteria; consequently, prebiotics may promote only certain species within a given genus such as bifidobacteria.[38] As there is extensive inter-individual variation in gut microbiota composition, this suggests that there should be inter-individual variation in the response of the microbial community to prebiotics.

Extensive metabolic cross-feeding occurs between the primary degraders of complex substrates and other bacterial species that depend on their products in the large intestine.[5] This involves utilization of fermentation products as well as cross-feeding of partial degradation products from dietary substrates. FOS and GOS have been shown to increase acetate and butyrate formation in model fermentor systems with transient accumulation of lactate.[41] Lactate is formed by many species, including bifidobacteria, and is metabolized by other bacteria, including the butyrate producers *E. hallii* and *Anaerostipes caccae*.[42,43] Thus, direct stimulation of lactate producers may lead indirectly to increased butyrate formation. In addition, butyrate-producing species that are unable to utilize lactate or grow on complex carbohydrates can benefit from the cross-feeding of partial breakdown products released by other species from polysaccharides.[43,44] This is one documented example out of many potential cross-feeding interactions, and it seems likely, therefore, that the effects of prebiotics will often extend to different groups of microorganism.

METABOLIC IMPACT OF PREBIOTICS AND DIETARY FIBER

Active fermentation of carbohydrates in the colon results in the formation of SCFA,[45] mainly acetate, propionate, and butyrate together with gases, mainly H_2, CO_2, and methane. The total concentration of SCFA in the large intestine may reach upwards of 100 mM.[46] Dietary shifts can result in changes in SCFA production rates and in the molar proportions of different SCFA detected in feces. Weight loss diets that are high in protein but low in carbohydrates, for example, were recently shown to reduce fecal butyrate by up to fourfold.[1] Meanwhile higher proportions of propionate and butyrate and lower acetate have been reported to result from increasing prebiotic or fiber intake.[47]

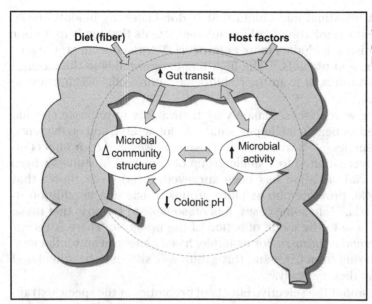

Figure 6-2. Diagrammatic representation of the interactions between diet, gut pH, and the gut microbial community in the human large intestine.

(Figure labels: Diet (fiber); Host factors; ↑ Gut transit; Microbial Δ community structure; ↑ Microbial activity; ↓ Colonic pH)

SCFA have a variety of likely effects upon health. Butyrate is considered beneficial for gut health, because it serves as the major energy source for the colonocytes and has a role in preventing colorectal cancer.[48,49] Propionate is metabolized in the liver and is gluconeogenic. Activation of the gut receptors GPR 41 and GPR 43 by SCFA influences gut motility and reduces inflammatory responses.[50,51] Acetate is metabolized in the peripheral tissues and is a precursor for cholesterol metabolism and lipid formation. A shift in fermentation products away from acetate (normally present at the highest concentration) towards propionate and butyrate may therefore be beneficial and may help to explain the decrease in cholesterol levels in volunteers consuming fiber.[52]

In general, high fiber diets increase fecal bulking, SCFA production, and transit rates through the large intestine.[53-56] These mild laxative effects can be particularly beneficial in elderly individuals suffering from constipation.[57] Active fermentation of fiber and prebiotics also tends to decrease the pH in the proximal large intestine (Figure 6-2).[58] There is evidence that such shifts in pH can have a major effect on the gut microbial community, with a slightly acidic pH, for example, promoting butyrate formation, and lower pHs resulting in lactate accumulation.[59,60]

The potential impact of prebiotics and fiber extends beyond gut health to include cardiovascular and metabolic health, including type 2 diabetes.[61] This is because of the systemic consequences of changes in bacterial populations that affect inflammation and the immune system and because of changes in microbially produced metabolites. In a study on healthy humans, a 4-weekly supplementation with resistant starch (30 g/day) produced a significant improvement in insulin sensitivity that might be linked to changes in SCFA formation.[62] There is recent evidence that FOS may help in improving insulin sensitivity by stimulating bifidobacteria in a mouse model under conditions of high fat intake.[61] In this case, the mechanism was suggested to involve an improvement in barrier function, reducing bacterial endotoxin-mediated inflammation. Inulin-type fructans have the potential to modulate lipid and glucose metabolism.[63]

There has been much interest in the potential role of nondigestible dietary carbohydrates for body weight control and obesity.[64] Colonic fermentation provides an additional source of energy to the host via absorption of SCFA, which is estimated to contribute around 10% of dietary calorific intake.[65] It has been suggested that bacterial fermentative activity in the colon may contribute to fat deposition.[66,67] The energy recovered from a mole of ingested sugar by this route is, however, less than for a mole of sugar directly absorbed in the small intestine.[68] The net effect must, therefore, depend largely on how alternative sources of dietary carbohydrate influence satiety. High intakes of the monosaccharides such as glucose and fructose present in soft drinks appear to increase serum ghrelin, activating hunger signals and decreasing satiety.[62,69] It has been suggested that FOS intake, on the other hand, results in decreased ghrelin levels that may help in the control of food intake.[70] Drastic reduction in total dietary carbohydrate intake in weight loss diets alters the composition of the colonic microbial community as well as fecal metabolite profiles.[71]

Increased SCFA concentrations may also increase the solubility of certain minerals, such as calcium, and enhance the absorption and expression of calcium-binding proteins.[72] Consuming inulin fructans has also been shown to improve bone health by increasing calcium absorption while β-glucans may lower total cholesterol levels.[73]

Microbial degradation of dietary plant fiber that reaches the colon results in the release of a variety of phenolic compounds, such as ferulic acid, that exist bound within plant cell wall structures.[74-76] Many of these released plant metabolites are subject to further metabolism by the microbial community. A number of these plant phenolic compounds and their metabolites have significant bioactivity in cell culture assays designed to test antioxidant capacity and anti-inflammatory and/or anticancer activities.[77]

CONCLUSION

Prebiotics provide a convenient and effective approach for modifying the composition of the intestinal microbial community and its metabolic products. We still have a long way to go, however, before we can claim any detailed understanding of the effects of prebiotics, including how reproducible these are across different individuals. Each new prebiotic preparation needs to be rigorously tested to establish that its effects are neutral or beneficial and that it does not stimulate the "wrong" groups of microorganism. As we have shown, prebiotics are likely to have complex effects upon the composition and metabolism of the gut microbiota that will inevitably include nontarget organisms. Consuming excessive amounts of prebiotics, or fiber, may have negative consequences, leading to excess gas formation, bloating, and osmotic diarrhea,[31] and these effects may be more pronounced in some individuals than others. These effects are less likely with more slowly fermentable products such as acacia gum.[78] Natural sources of dietary fiber are chemically more complex than prebiotic oligosaccharides and are the source of a wide array of phytochemicals, many of which are considered to confer health benefits. For this reason, it can be argued that prebiotics should not be used to replace natural sources of fiber in the diet, but only as supplements to a balanced diet. Fiber may indeed have effects similar to prebiotics in stimulating the growth of potentially beneficial gut microorganisms such as bifidobacteria.[79]

Acknowledgment
The authors are grateful to the Scottish Government Rural Environment Research and Analysis Directorate for support.

REFERENCES

1. Duncan SH, Belenguer A, Holtrop G, Johnstone AM, Flint HJ, Lobley GE. Reduced dietary intake of car-bohydrates by obese subjects results in decreased concentrations of butyrate and butyrate-producing bacteria in feces. *Appl Environ Microbiol.* 2007;73(4):1073-1078.
2. Macfarlane S, Macfarlane GT, Cummings JH. Review article: prebiotics in the gastrointestinal tract. *Aliment Pharmacol Ther.* 2006;24:701-714.
3. Hopkins MJ, Sharp R, Macfarlane GT. Age and disease related changes in intestinal bacterial popu-lations assessed by cell culture, 16S rRNA abundance and community cellular fatty acid profiles. *Gut.* 2001;48:198-205.
4. Zoetendal EG, Collier CT, Koike S, Mackie RI, Gaskins HR. Molecular ecological analysis of the gastro-intestinal microbiota: a review. *J Nutr.* 2004;34:465-472.
5. Flint HJ, Duncan SH, Scott KP, Louis P. Interactions and competition within the microbial community of the human colon: links between diet and health. *Environ Microbiol.* 2007;9:1101-1111.
6. Suau A, Bonnet R, Sutren M, et al. Direct analysis of genes encoding 16S rRNA from complex communi-ties reveals many novel molecular species within the human gut. *Appl Environ Microbiol.* 1999;24: 4799-4807.
7. Hold GL, Pryde SE, Russell VJ, Furrie E, Flint HJ. Assessment of microbial diversity in human colonic samples by 16S rDNA sequence analysis. *FEMS Microbiol Ecol.* 2002;39:33-39.
8. Eckburg PB, Bernstein CN, Purdom E, et al. Diversity of the human intestinal microbial flora. *Science.* 2005;308:1635-1638.
9. Franks AH, Harmsen HJM, Raangs GC, Jansen GJ, Schut F, Welling GW. Variations of bacterial popula-tions in human feces measured by fluorescent in situ hybridisation with group-specific 16S rRNA-targeted oligonucleotide probes. *Appl Environ Microbiol.* 1998;64:3336-3345.
10. Lay C, Rigottier-Gois L, Holmstrom Rjilic M, et al. Colonic microbiota signatures across five northern European countries. *Appl Environ Microbiol.* 2005;7:933-946.
11. Mueller S, Saunier K, Hanisch C, et al. Differences in fecal microbiota in different European study populations in relation to age, gender, and country: a cross-sectional study. *Appl Environ Microbiol.* 2006;72:1027-1033.
12. Harmsen HJM, Raangs GC, He T, Degener JE, Welling GW. Extensive set of rRNA-based probes for detec-tion of bacteria in human faeces. *Appl Environ Microbiol.* 2002;68:2982-2990.
13. Matsuki T, Watanabe K, Fujimoto J, et al. Development of 16S rRNA-gene-targeted group-specific prim-ers for the detection and identification of predominant bacteria in human feces. *Appl Environ Microbiol.* 2002;68:5445-5451.
14. Duncan SH, Louis P, Flint HJ. Cultivable bacterial diversity from the human colon. *Lett Appl Microbiol.* 2007;44:343-359.
15. Barcenilla A, Pryde SE, Martin JC, Duncan SH, Stewart CS, Flint HJ. Phylogenetic relationships of domi-nant butyrate producing bacteria from the human gut. *Appl Environ Microbiol.* 2002;66:1654-1661.
16. Aminov RI, Walker AW, Duncan SH, Harmsen HJM, Welling GW, Flint HJ. Molecular diversity, cultiva-tion, and improved FISH detection of a dominant group of human gut bacteria related to *Roseburia* and *Eubacterium rectale. Appl Environ Microbiol.* 2006;72:6371-6376.
17. Zoetendal EG, Akkermans ADL, de Vos WM. Temperature gradient gel electrophoresis analysis of 16S rRNA from human fecal samples reveals stable and host-specific communities of active bacteria. *Appl Environ Microbiol.* 1998;64:3854-3859.
18. Ley RE, Turnbaugh PJ, Klein S, Gordon JI. Microbial ecology: human gut microbes associated with obesity. *Nature.* 2006;444:1022-1023.
19. Walker AW, Duncan SH, Harmsen HJM, Holtrop G, Welling GW, Flint HJ. The species composition of the human intestinal microbiota differs between particle-associated and liquid phase communities. *Environ Microbiol.* 2008;10:3275-3283.
20. Tap J, Mondot S, Levenez F, et al. Towards the human intestinal microbiota phylogenetic core. *Environ Microbiol.* 2009;11(10):2574-2584.
21. Turnbaugh PJ, Backhed F, Fulton L, Gordon JI. Diet-induced obesity is linked to marked but reversible alterations in the mouse distal gut microbiome. *Cell Host Microbe.* 2008;3:213-223.
22. Cummings JH, Macfarlane GT. The control and consequences of bacterial fermentation in the human colon. *J Appl Bacteriol.* 1991;70:443-459.
23. Topping DL, Clifton PM. Short-chain fatty acids and human colonic function: roles of resistant starch and non-starch polysaccharides. *Physiol Rev.* 2001;81:1031-1064.
24. Englyst KN, Liu S, Englyst HN. Nutritional characterization and measurement of carbohydrates. *Eur J Clin Nutr.* 2007;61:S19-S39.

25. Magee EA, Richardson CJ, Hughes R, Cummings JH. Contribution of dietary protein to sulphide production in the large intestine: an in vitro and a controlled feeding trial in humans. *Am J Clin Nutr.* 2000;72:1488-1494.
26. Robert C, Bernalier-Donadille A. The cellulolytic microflora of the human colon: evidence of microcrystalline cellulose-degrading bacteria in methane excreting subjects. *FEMS Microbiol Ecol.* 2003;46:81-89.
27. Probert HM, Apajalathti JHA, Rautonen N, Stowell J, Gibson GR. Polydextrose, lactitol, and fructooligosaccharide fermentation by colonic bacteria in a three-stage continuous culture system. *Appl Environ Microbiol.* 2004;70:4505-4511.
28. Macfarlane S, Woodmansey EJ, Macfarlane GT. Colonization of mucin by human intestinal bacteria and establishment of biofilm communities in a two-stage continuous culture system. *Appl Environ Microbiol.* 2005;71:7483-7492.
29. Leitch ECM, Walker AW, Duncan SH, Holtrop G, Flint HJ. Selective colonization of insoluble substrates by human colonic bacteria. *Environ Microbiol.* 2007;72:667-679.
30. Gibson GR, Roberfroid MB. Dietary modulation of the human colonic microbiota: introducing the concept of prebiosis. *J Nutr.* 1995;125:1401-1412.
31. Gibson GR, Rastall RA, Roberfroid MB. Prebiotics. In: Gibson GR, Roberfroid MB, eds. *The Colonic Microbiota: Nutrition and Health.* London: Kluwer Academic Publishers; 1999:101-124.
32. Macfarlane GT, Steed H, Macfarlane S. Bacterial metabolism and health related effects of galactooligosaccharides and other prebiotics. *J Appl Microbiol.* 2007;104:305-344.
33. Harmsen HJM, Wildeboer-Veloo ACM, Raangs GC, et al. Analysis of intestinal flora development in breast-fed and formula-fed infants by using molecular identification and detection methods. *J Pediatr Gastroneterol Nutr.* 2000;30:61-67.
34. Heavey PM, Savage SAH, Parrett A, Cecchini C, Edwards CA, Rowland IR. Protein-degradation products and bacterial enzyme activities in faeces of breast-fed and formula-fed infants. *Br J Nutr.* 2003;89:509-515.
35. Fuller R, Gibson GR. Probiotics and prebiotics: microflora management for improved gut health. *Clin Microbiol Infect.* 1998;4:477-480.
36. Bouhnik Y, Raskine L, Simoneau G, et al. The capacity of nondigestible carbohydrates to stimulate fecal bifidobacteria in healthy humans: a double-blind, randomized, placebo-controlled, parallel-group, dose-response relation study. *Am J Clin Nutr.* 2004;80:1658-1664.
37. Kruse H-P, Kleessen B, Blaut M. Effects of inulin on fecal bifidobacteria in human subjects. *Br J Nutr.* 1999;82:375-382.
38. Ramirez-Farias C, Slezak K, Fuller K, et al. Effect of inulin on the human gut microbiota: stimulation of *Bifidobacterium adolescentis* and *Faecalibacterium prausnitzii. Br J Nutr.* 2009;101:541-550.
39. Apalajahti JH, Kettunen H, Kettunen A, et al. Culture-independent microbial community analysis reveals that inulin in the diet primarily affects previously unknown bacteria in the mouse cecum. *Appl Environ Microbiol.* 2002;68:4986-4995.
40. Sokol H, Pigneur B, Watterlot L, et al. *Faecalibacterium prausnitzii* is an anti-inflammatory commensal bacterium identified by gut microbiota analysis of Crohn disease patients. *PNAS USA.* 2008;105:16731-16736.
41. Hopkins MJ, Macfarlane GT. Nondigestible oligosaccharides enhance bacterial colonization resistance against *Clostridium difficile* in vitro. *Appl Environ Microbiol.* 2003;69:1920-1927.
42. Duncan SH, Louis P, Flint HJ. Lactate-utilizing bacteria, isolated from human faeces, that produce butyrate as a major fermentation product. *Appl Environ Microbiol.* 2004;70:5810-5817.
43. Belenguer A, Duncan SH, Calder AG, et al. Two routes of metabolic cross-feeding between *Bifidobacterium adolescentis* and butyrate-producing anaerobes from the human gut. *Appl Environ Microbiol.* 2006;72:3593-3599.
44. Falony G, Viachou A, Verbrugge K, de Vuyst L. Cross-feeding between *Bifidobacterium longum* BB536 and acetate converting, butyrate-producing colon bacteria during growth on oligofructose. *Appl Env Microbiol.* 2006;72:7835-7841.
45. Macfarlane GT, Gibson GR. Microbiological aspects of the production of short-chain fatty acids in the large bowel. In: Cummings JH, Rombeau JL, Sakata S, eds. *Physiological and Clinical Aspects of Short-Chain Fatty Acids.* Cambridge: Cambridge University Press; 1995.
46. Macfarlane GT, Gibson GR, Cummings JH. Comparison of fermentation reactions in different regions of the human colon. *J Appl Bacteriol.* 1992;72:57-64.
47. Queenan KM, Stewart ML, Smith KN, Thomas W, Fulcher RG, Slavin JL. Concentrated oat beta-glucan, a fermentable fiber, lowers serum cholesterol in hypercholesterolemic adults in a randomized trial. *Nutr J.* 2007;6:6.
48. Pryde SE, Duncan SH, Hold GL, Stewart CS, Flint HJ. The microbiology of butyrate formation in the human colon. *FEMS Microbiol Lett.* 2002;217:133-139.

49. McIntyre AP, Gibson P, Young GP. Butyrate production from dietary fiber and protection against large bowel cancer in a gut model. *Gut.* 1993;34:386-391.

50. Brown AJ, Goldsworthy SM, Barnes AA, et al. The orphan G protein coupled receptors GPR41 and GPR43 are activated by propionate and other short chain fatty acids. *J Biol Chem.* 2003;2778:11312-11319.

51. Tazoe H, Otomob Y, Kaji I, Tanaka R, et al. Roles of short chain fatty acid receptors, GPR41 and GPR43 on colonic functions. *J Physiol Pharmacol.* 2008;59:251-262.

52. Brown L, Rosner B, Willett WW, Sacks FM. Cholesterol-lowering effects of dietary fiber: a meta-analysis. *Am J Clin Nutr.* 1999;69:30-42.

53. Lewis SJ, Heaton KW. Increasing butyrate concentration in the distal colon by accelerating intestinal transit. *Gut.* 1997;41:245-251.

54. Richardson A, Delbridge AT, Brown NJ, Rumsey RDE, Read NW. Short chain fatty acids in the terminal ileum accelerate stomach to caecum transit time in the rat. *Gut.* 1991;32:266-269.

55. Knusden KEB, Laerke HN. Whole grain cereals and gut health. *Agro-Food Ind Hi Tec.* 2008;19:6-8.

56. Lampe JW, Slavin JL, Melcher EA, Potter JD. Effects of cereal and vegetable fiber feeding on potential risk-factors for colon cancer. *Cancer Epidemiol Biomarkers and Prevent.* 1992;1:207-211.

57. Woodmansey EJ. Intestinal bacteria and ageing. *J Appl Microbiol.* 2007;102:1178-1186.

58. Bown RL, Gibson JA, Sladen GE, Hicks B, Dawson A. Effects of lactulose and other laxatives on ileal and colonic pH as measured by a radiotelemetry device. *Gut.* 1974;15:999-1004.

59. Walker AW, Duncan SH, Leitch ECM, Child MW, Flint HJ. pH and peptide supply can radically alter bacterial populations and short-chain fatty acid ratios within microbial communities from the human colon. *Appl Environ Microbiol.* 2005;71:3692-3700.

60. Belenguer A, Duncan SH, Holtrop G, Anderson SE, Lobley GE, Flint HJ. Impact of pH on lactate formation and utilization by human fecal microbial communities. *Appl Environ Microbiol.* 2007;73:6526-6533.

61. Cani PD, Neyrinck M, Fava F, et al. Selective increases of bifidobacteria in gut microflora improve high-fat-diet-induced diabetes in mice through a mechanism associated with endotoxaemia. *Diabetologia.* 2007;50:2374-2383.

62. Robertson MD, Bickerton AS, Dennis AL, Vidal H, Frayn KN. Insulin-sensitizing effects of dietary resistant starch and effects on skeletal muscle and adipose tissue metabolism. *Am J Clin Nutr.* 2005;82:559-567.

63. Delzenne NM, Cani PD, Daubioul C, Neyrinck AM. Impact of inulin and oligofructose on gastrointestinal peptides. *Br J Nutr.* 2005;93:S157-S161.

64. Nilsson AC, Ostman EM, Holst JJ, Bjorck IME. Including indigestible carbohydrates in the evening meal of healthy subjects improves glucose tolerance, lowers inflammatory markers, and increases satiety after a subsequent standardized breakfast. *J Nutr.* 2008;138:732-739.

65. Bergman EN. Energy contributions of volatile fatty acids from the gastrointestinal tract in various species. *Physiol Rev.* 1990;70:567-590.

66. Backhed F, Ding H, Wang T, et al. The gut microbiota as an environmental factor that regulates fat storage. *Proc Nat Acad Sci U S A.* 2004;101:15718-15723.

67. Turnbaugh PJ, Ley RE, Mahowald MA, Magrini V, Mardis ER, Gordon JI. An obesity-associated gut microbiome with increased capacity for energy harvest. *Nature.* 2006;444:1027-1031.

68. Roberfroid MB. Calorific value of inulin and oligofructose. *J Nutr.* 1999;129:1436S-1437S.

69. Lindqvist A, Baelemans A, Erlanson-Albertsson C. Effects of sucrose, glucose and fructose on peripheral and central appetite signals. *Regul Pept.* 2008;150:26-32.

70. Delzenne NM, Cani PD, Neyrinck AM. Modulation of glucagon-like peptide 1 and energy metabolism by inulin and oligofructose: experimental data. *J Nutr.* 2007;137:2547S-2551S.

71. Duncan SH, Lobley GE, Holtrop G, Ince J, Johnstone AM, Flint HJ. Human colonic microbiota associated with diet, obesity and weight loss. *Int J Obesity.* 2008;32:1720-1724.

72. Scholz-Aherns KE, Ade P, Marten B, et al. Prebiotics, probiotics and synbiotics affect mineral absorption, bone mineral content, and bone structure. *J Nutr.* 2007;137:838S-846S.

73. Smith KN, Queenan KM, Thomas W, Fulcher RG, Slavin JL. Physiological effects of concentrated barley beta-glucan in mildly hypercholesterolemic adults. *J Am College Nutr.* 2008;27:434-440.

74. Manach C, Scalbert A, Morand C, Remesy C, Jimenez L. Polyphenols: food sources and bioavailability. *Am J Clin Nutr.* 2004;79:727-747.

75. Russell WR, Labat A, Scobbie L, Duncan SH. Availability of blueberry phenolics for microbial metabolism in the colon and the potential inflammatory implications. *Mol Nutr Food.* 2007;51:726-731.

76. Costabile A, Klinder A, Fava F, et al. Wholegrain wheat breakfast cereal has a prebiotic effect on the human gut microbiota: a double-blind, placebo-controlled, crossover study. *Br J Nutr.* 2008;99:110-120.

77. Russell WR, Scobbie L, Chesson A, et al. Anti-inflammatory implications of the dietary phenolic compounds. *Nutr Cancer Int J.* 2008;60:636-642.

78. Goetze O, Fruehauf H, Pohl D. Effect of a prebiotic mixture on intestinal comfort and general wellbeing in health. *Br J Nutr.* 2008;100:1077-1085.
79. Scott KP, Duncan SH, Flint HJ. Dietary fiber and the gut microbiota. *Nutr Bull.* 2008;33:201-211.

7

Fermentation and the Effects of Probiotics on Host Metabolism

George T. Macfarlane, BSc, PhD; Sandra Macfarlane, BSc, PhD; and Katie L. Blackett, BSc, PhD

FERMENTATION AND THE PHYSIOLOGIC SIGNIFICANCE OF THE COLONIC MICROBIOTA

The large intestinal microbiota interacts with the human host in multiple ways and plays a key role in many physiologic processes, such as vitamin formation, protection from invading pathogens, bile acid and steroid transformations, metabolism of xenobiotic compounds, mineral absorption, and immune system development and function. The microbiota also participates in the activation and destruction of toxins, genotoxins, and mutagens. The metabolic activities of intestinal microorganisms therefore play a key role in host physiology in both health and disease.[1] Colonic bacteria are responsible, in part, for stimulating colonic motility through fecal bulking, while they also carry out the final stages of the digestive process. Measurements made using materials taken from human sudden death victims have shown that substrate availability, bacterial populations, and the metabolism of the microbiota vary along the length of the gut,[2,3] and this is strongly affected by intestinal transit time.[4] The nutritional and environmental determinants, together with the anatomic, physiologic, and microbiologic factors that affect metabolic processes in the large gut, are complex and interdependent. In particular, the chemical composition of the fermentable substrate, the amount of substrate available, its physical form (eg, particle size, solubility, and association with indigestible complexes such as tannins, lignin, and silica), the bacterial species composition of the microbiota, ecological factors (eg, competitive and cooperative interactions between different groups of bacteria), and the availability of inorganic electron acceptors such as NO_3^- and SO_4^{2-} all affect the way substrates are digested and fermentation products are formed.

The principal sources of carbon and energy for bacteria growing in the large bowel are resistant starches, plant cell wall polysaccharides, and host mucopolysaccharides, as well as various proteins, peptides, and other lower-molecular-weight carbohydrates that escape digestion and absorption in the upper gut.[1,5] While many different types of carbohydrates are used as fermentation substrates in the colon, these substances are

Floch MH, Kim AS, eds.
Probiotics: A Clinical Guide (pp 83-94)
© 2010 Taylor & Francis Group

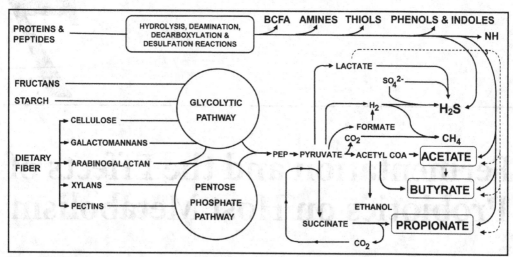

Figure 7-1. General scheme showing the major fermentation pathways in the human large intestine.

metabolized in a relatively small number of biochemical pathways (Figure 7-1), and there is considerable metabolic redundancy in the ecosystem. Complex polymers are first broken down by a wide range of bacterial polysaccharidases, glycosidases, proteases, and peptidases to smaller oligomers and their component sugars and amino acids, which then serve as substrates in various fermentation processes. Carbohydrate metabolism is quantitatively more important than amino acid fermentation in the human large intestine, particularly in the cecum and proximal colon, where substrate availability is greatest.

As illustrated in Figure 7-1, acetate, propionate, and butyrate are the main products of both carbohydrate and protein breakdown in the large gut. A variety of other fermentation products are also formed, including hydroxy and dicarboxylic acids, particularly lactate and succinate, the gases hydrogen and carbon dioxide, and other neutral, acidic, and basic end products. Minor metabolic products such as ethanol, lactate, and succinate are essentially fermentation intermediates that, under normal circumstances, are metabolized by cross-feeding species and generally do not accumulate to a significant degree in the gut (discussed further in the text). A vast majority of SCFA (95% to 99%) formed by intestinal microorganisms are absorbed and metabolized by the host, and they constitute a major source of energy reclamation from the large gut. Theoretical calculations show that up to 540 kcal/day might be obtained from colonic fermentation, possibly contributing to as much as 10% of the host's daily energy requirements.[1,5] SCFA interact with a wide range of physiologic functions in the body, including colonocyte metabolism, epithelial cell growth and differentiation,[6] cellular transport processes,[7] the metabolism of lipids and carbohydrates in the liver,[8] and gut motility,[9] as well as energy generation in muscle, kidney, heart, and brain.[10] SCFA also inhibit phagocytic cell function.[11,12] Butyrate is thought to be protective against colorectal cancer and has been shown to arrest cell growth early in G1 and induce cell differentiation, while stimulating cytoskeletal organization and alterations in gene expression.[13-16] The arrest of cell growth by butyrate is associated with differentiation, which occurs in many human cell lines. Butyrate modulates the expression of many different genes and differentiation in tumor cells, and is linked to changes in their cytoskeletal architecture and adhesion properties.[17]

PUTREFACTION IN THE LARGE INTESTINE AND THE EFFECTS OF FERMENTABLE CARBOHYDRATE ON THESE PROCESSES

Apart from the chemical and physical nature of the substrate, host physiology plays an important role in determining how substrates are broken down and the types of fermentation products that can be formed. For example, it has been shown that long colonic transits affect the breakdown of carbohydrates, proteins, and xenobiotic substances and have been associated with the occurrence of large bowel cancer.[4,18-21] For more than 100 years, it has been understood that the absorption of toxic substances from the large intestine can lead to autointoxication, increased body temperature, depression, sleeplessness, fetid breath, vomiting, skin diseases, and headaches. More recent studies have shown that protein breakdown and amino acid fermentation are quantitatively most important in the distal gut, where there are usually low levels of readily fermentable carbohydrate.[2] As a consequence, concentrations of putrefactive substances such as phenols and indoles are considerably higher in this region of the bowel. Many products of dissimilatory amino acid metabolism are toxic to the host—eg, high levels of ammonia for neoplastic growth—and can also be responsible for hepatic coma. Some indoles and phenols are believed to act as cocarcinogens, while secondary amines can become involved in N-nitrosation reactions. However, carbohydrate and acid pH strongly affect amino acid and peptide fermentations. In vitro fermentation studies[20,21] have demonstrated that the microbiota ferments peptides more rapidly than free amino acids, and that at acidic pH values characteristic of those found in the proximal large bowel, ammonia formation was reduced by 60% and 35%, respectively, during growth at pH 5.5, compared to control cultures maintained at pH 6.8. Moreover, when starch was included in the cultures at pH 6.8, net ammonia formation was reduced by 43% and 37%, respectively. The reduction in ammonia accumulation can be explained not only by the greater requirement for nitrogen for biosynthetic purposes by carbohydrate-utilizing species in the starch cultures, but also by direct effects of pH on amino acid and peptide transport systems in the bacteria.[22]

CONTROL OF CARBOHYDRATE ASSIMILATION IN MAJOR GROUPS OF SACCHAROLYTIC BACTERIA IN THE LARGE GUT

Many different types of carbohydrates are available for fermentation for bacteria growing in the proximal large bowel. However, concentrations of individual substrates are continually changing as they are broken down, replenished, or replaced. For the most part, saccharolytic bacteria exist in a multisubstrate-limited environment in the large gut, particularly in the distal bowel, where they must be able to adapt to changing nutritional circumstances, as dietary carbohydrate becomes depleted. Many gut species are able to regulate the assimilation and metabolism of polysaccharides and oligosaccharides by controlling the synthesis and activities of polysaccharide/oligosaccharide depolymerizers, and substrate uptake systems, as well as by more responsive and rapid-acting mechanisms that operate at the level of substrate transport into the cells.[23] These catabolite regulatory processes are determined to a large degree by the types and relative amounts of fermentable substrate in the ecosystem, and are of ecologic significance to the microbiota and, ultimately, are of physiologic importance to the host. Because individual species and groups of bacteria form different types of fermentation products, catabolite regulatory mechanisms ultimately affect

TABLE 7-1

EXAMPLES OF CARBOHYDRATE SUBSTRATE PREFERENCES IN HUMAN BIFIDOBACTERIAL ISOLATES*

ORGANISMS

B. pseudolongum	Sequential uptake of galactose, followed by glucose and xylose
B. adolescentis	Glucose and galactose coutilized; mannose and arabinose uptake repressed
B. catenulatum	Only utilized glucose and galactose. Galactose taken up after glucose depletion
B. angulatum	Glucose and galactose coutilized; xylose uptake repressed
B. infantis	Glucose repressed mannose and galactose utilization
B. bifidum	Sequential uptake of glucose > galactose > mannose
B. breve	Glucose and arabinose coutilized; mannose and galactose uptake repressed
B. longum	Glucose and xylose coutilized; galactose uptake repressed

Data from Degnan BA, Macfarlane GT. Comparison of carbohydrate substrate preferences in eight species of bifidobacteria. *FEMS Microbiol Lett.* 1991;68(2):151-156.

*The bacteria were grown on mixtures of glucose, galactose, mannose, xylose, and arabinose.

the way these metabolites are produced from individual substrates. Catabolite regulatory activities in the colon should in principle allow bacteria to selectively use certain substrates to the exclusion of others. This may enable some species to compete more effectively for a limited range of preferred substrates in specialized metabolic niches, thereby ensuring survival. A characteristic feature of catabolite regulation in many bacteria is the manifestation of substrate preferences during growth in the presence of different carbon sources.

Distinct substrate preferences have been demonstrated in bifidobacteria in a study by Degnan and Macfarlane,[24] in which 8 different species were investigated for their abilities to utilize a mixture of 5 different sugars (glucose, galactose, mannose, xylose, and arabinose). The results are shown in Table 7-1. The experiment showed that while individual bifidobacteria adopted specific strategies with respect to the way in which they acquired these growth substrates, with the exception of *Bifidobacterium pseudolongum*, glucose was a preferred carbon source in all of the species tested and that hexoses were generally utilized in preference to pentoses.

In other experiments on carbohydrate uptake strategies, other important saccharolytic gut anaerobes, including *Bacteroides ovatus*, were shown to be able to simultaneously assimilate glucose, galactose, mannose, and xylose, while arabinose uptake was repressed.[25] In carbohydrate-limited chemostats, however, starch and arabinogalactan were coutilized.[26] Similarly, in *Bacteroides thetaiotaomicron*, arabinose, xylose, glucose, and galactose were simultaneously taken up; however, if mannose was also present, utilization of glucose and galactose was strongly inhibited. This effect was less marked with the pentoses arabinose and xylose.[27] The strong regulatory role of mannose in sugar transport indicates that this bacterium may occupy a specialized metabolic niche in the colon. While the control of carbohydrate assimilation in *Bact. thetaiotaomicron* can be attributed either to catabolite repression of the synthesis of sugar transport systems or to a more rapid-acting mechanism (catabolite inhibition/ inducer exclusion), the immediate inhibitory effects of mannose observed in these studies suggested the latter.

These investigations showed that carbohydrate uptake was more strictly controlled in bifidobacteria compared to the bacteroides tested. However, as with the bacteroides, each bifidobacterial species adopted specific strategies for regulating sugar uptake. The sequential utilization of sugars in these organisms indicates the existence of catabolite regulatory mechanisms; however, these control processes have not been characterized in great detail.

To assess other aspects of catabolite regulation of carbohydrate metabolism in gut microorganisms, experiments were carried out using pure cultures of bacteroides and bifidobacteria. Synthesis of polysaccharide-degrading enzymes was shown to be tightly controlled in *Bact. ovatus* and generally required induction by polymerized carbon sources.[28] The importance of carbohydrate concentration in catabolite regulation in the human colon was evident in the studies with *Bact. ovatus*, indicating that in the large gut, these regulatory mechanisms will be of greatest significance in the cecum and proximal colon. Similar studies with bifidobacteria have shown that while the formation of arabinogalactan-degrading enzymes is catabolite regulated in *B. longum*, this was not the case for starch-degrading enzymes in *B. angulatum* and *B. pseudolongum*. These results suggest that catabolite repression of polysaccharide- and oligosaccharide-hydrolyzing enzymes may be less important in bifidobacteria than in bacteroides.[25,29]

CONTROL OF FERMENTATION REACTIONS IN PROBIOTIC ORGANISMS

The principal probiotics used in humans include various LAB, particularly species belonging to the genus *Lactobacillus* and bifidobacteria, which have an actinobacterial lineage. In some individuals, bifidobacteria can occur in high numbers and can constitute a significant component of the microbiota; however, LAB cell population densities are generally orders of magnitude lower, even in people who regularly consume probiotics. As a consequence of this disparity in numbers, bifidobacteria are likely to be considerably more important in nutrient metabolism in the colonic ecosystem. LAB, and bifidobacteria in particular, are primarily saccharolytic organisms; however, it is worth noting that both groups can produce significant amounts of putrefactive substances such as amines, phenols, and indoles under certain circumstances.[19-21] As in all fermentative bacteria, primary metabolism is predicated by the requirement to maintain redox balance, mainly through controlling the reduction and oxidation of flavins and pyridine nucleotides. This regulates carbon flow through the bacteria, the energy and cell growth yields that can be obtained from any given substrate, and the fermentation products that are formed. As a general principle, while the formation of reduced end products of metabolism such as lactate, succinate, butyrate, ethanol, and hydrogen is used to maintain redox balance in colonic microorganisms, the generation of more oxidized metabolites such as acetate is linked to ATP synthesis. As a consequence, bacteria that form more reduced fermentation products are able to achieve comparatively lower ATP yields. Many gut species exhibit metabolic flexibility by employing branched fermentation pathways because this enables them to control the thermodynamic efficiency of substrate catabolism through regulating ATP formation and redox balance. In this respect, pyruvate and acetyl-CoA are key points of control in both LAB and bifidobacterial metabolism.

In both LAB and bifidobacteria, lactate and, to a lesser extent, ethanol variously function as electron acceptors in fermentation reactions, which serve to oxidize reduced coenzymes generated in the early stages of substrate catabolism. The recycled oxidized forms enable fermentation processes to be maintained in operation. Cummings and colleagues[30] have shown that, in normal circumstances, most of the lactate in the large bowel accumulates in the cecum, reflecting the high levels of fermentable substrate available in this part of the gut. In some bacteria, lactate formation is pH dependent,[31] while investigations have shown that its production in the large bowel is particularly associated with starch fermentation.[32-34]

The majority of lactate-producing bacteria in the human large intestine form the L-isomer, although some indigenous and probiotic lactobacilli (eg, *L. bulgaricus, L. acidophilus, L. johnsonii, L. delbrueckii* ssp. *lactis*) also produce the D-isomer, which, in some circumstances, is not well metabolized by humans. For example, excessive D-lactate formation has been reported to occur in patients with short bowel syndrome, due to high substrate levels and bacterial overgrowth. D-Lactic acidosis resulting in encephalopathy has been linked with antibiotic use, as well as the consumption of dairy products and lactobacillus probiotics.[35,36] In one patient, metabolic acidosis was linked to high levels of antibiotic-resistant *L. acidophilus* in stools. D-Lactic acidosis can also be a concern in some young children; however, in a double-blinded, randomized, controlled trial involving 71 infants aged between 4 and 5 months, consumption of *L. johnsonii* in those receiving formula feeding showed no increase in urinary lactate excretion, leading the authors to conclude that lactobacillus supplementation was not a risk with respect to lactic acidosis.[37]

A number of intestinal bacteria form ethanol as a major end product of metabolism in mixed fermentations. Ethanol is a highly reduced metabolite, which, in bacteria, consumes 2 moles of NADH per mole of alcohol produced. In contrast to ethanol fermentation in yeasts, which oxidizes only one molecule of NADH, and where the alcohol is formed from pyruvate by pyruvate decarboxylase and alcohol dehydrogenase, the vast majority of bacteria make ethanol from acetyl-CoA, via acetaldehyde dehydrogenase and alcohol dehydrogenase. In ethanol-producing organisms that metabolize carbohydrates using the Embden-Meyerhof-Parnas (EMP) pathway, acetate must be produced to maintain redox balance, because this mechanism can only supply half of the NADH that would be needed if ethanol was the sole fermentation product.

Lactic Acid Bacteria Fermentations

As discussed previously, the loose association of organisms grouped together as LAB produces lactate as a major end product of fermentation, and with respect to the human large bowel and probiotic use, these organisms can include enterococci, streptococci, pediococci, and leuconostocs, as well as lactobacilli. The genera *Enterococcus* and *Lactobacillus* include species that undertake homolactic-type fermentations, as well as those that are heterofermentative. Homolactic species convert glucose into 2 lactates through the EMP pathway, with the formation of 2 moles of ATP per mole of hexose consumed. The reduction of pyruvate to lactate maintains redox balance. However, lactate need not be the only fermentation metabolite produced by homofer-

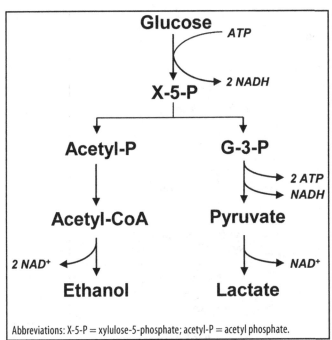

Figure 7-2. Outline of heterolactic fermentation in LAB.

Abbreviations: X-5-P = xylulose-5-phosphate; acetyl-P = acetyl phosphate.

mentative LAB. Modeling studies show that when some lactobacilli are grown under nutrient-limited conditions, the bacteria metabolize sugars to acetate, formate, and ethanol, whereas only trace amounts of these fermentation products are formed if carbon availability is increased, when lactate becomes the principal product of metabolism.[38,39] Heterofermentative lactobacilli form lactate, ethanol, and carbon dioxide by the hexose monophosphate shunt, in which the oxidation of one hexose molecule generates one ATP during substrate-level phosphorylation. This corresponds to 50% of the energy yield that is achieved during homolactic fermentations. An outline of the heterolactic fermentation pathway in lactobacilli is summarized in Figure 7-2. The key enzyme in these reactions is a phosphoketolase that hydrolyzes xylulose-5-phosphate to acetyl-CoA and glyceraldehyde-3-phosphate (G-3-P). Both lactate and ethanol serve as electron sinks, while ATP is generated during the conversion of G-3-P to pyruvate. Heterofermentative LAB are able to ferment pentoses in the phosphoketolase pathway, which is an inducible system; however, many homofermentative species are unable to ferment pentoses or are facultatively heterofermentative with respect to pentose catabolism.[40] A number of LAB are aerotolerant and can oxidize NADH with oxygen using superoxide dismutase and peroxidases, which enables pyruvate to be converted to acetyl-CoA instead of lactate, thereby leading to the generation of more acetate and ATP.[41]

Bifidobacterial Metabolism

Bifidobacteria can constitute a significant component of the gut microbiota in some people.[42] Consequently, like other numerically important saccharolytic species, such as bacteroides, they are likely to play an important role in carbohydrate fermentation in the large bowel. The principal products of bifidobacterial metabolism were initially thought to be acetate and lactate in a 3:2 ratio.[43] Hexoses are fermented by the fructose-6-phosphate shunt, which involves a series of cleavage and isomerization reactions that yield pentose phosphates. They are converted to acetyl phosphate and G-3-P. ATP is produced from acetyl phosphate, while G-3-P is metabolized to pyru-

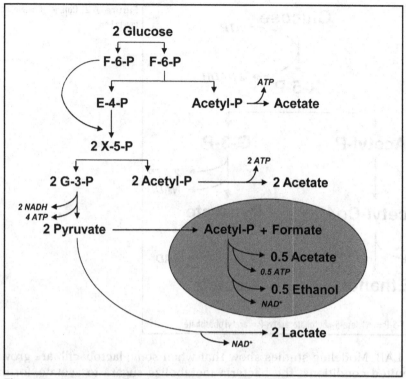

Figure 7-3. Routes of carbon dissimilation in bifidobacteria. The shaded area shows how these bacteria can obtain extra ATP under carbon-limiting conditions.

vate.[44] However, as shown in Figure 7-3, in energy-limiting environments, bifidobacteria can also produce ethanol and formate.[45] This is because either pyruvate can be reduced by NADH to produce lactate as an electron sink product under nutrient-rich conditions or, alternatively, it can undergo phosphoroclastic cleavage to formate and acetyl phosphate. Half of the resulting acetyl phosphate is reduced to ethanol to facilitate NADH oxidation, while the remainder is available to make extra ATP through the formation of acetate.[45] Furthermore, ATP can also be generated through end-product efflux-type mechanisms.[46]

As shown in Table 7-2, continuous culture experiments with *Bifidobacterium breve* demonstrate that carbon availability has a major effect on fermentation product formation.[47] These studies show that acetate and formate are the main fermentation products in carbon-limited chemostats, whereas under nitrogen limitation, acetate and lactate predominate. These investigations showed that the metabolic fate of pyruvate is dependent on carbon availability. Under carbon limitation, pyruvate was preferentially cleaved to acetate and formate instead of being reduced to lactate, enabling the bacterium to generate extra ATP. In contrast, the increase in availability of fermentable carbohydrate in nitrogen-limited chemostats provided sufficient ATP for growth, and under these circumstances, the reduction of pyruvate to lactate served as an uncoupling mechanism, which facilitated carbon flow through the cells without concomitant generation of energy in substrate-level phosphorylation reactions.

TABLE 7-2

EFFECT OF CARBON AVAILABILITY AND GROWTH RATE ON FERMENTATION PRODUCT FORMATION IN CONTINUOUS CULTURES OF B. BREVE

MOLAR RATIOS OF PRINCIPAL FERMENTATION PRODUCTS

GROWTH CONDITIONS	D*	ACETATE	LACTATE	ETHANOL	FORMATE
Glucose limited	0.10	59	0	8	32
Glucose excess	0.09	70	25	3	0

Data from Degnan BA, Macfarlane GT. Effect of dilution rate and carbon availability on *Bifidobacterium breve* fermentation. *Appl Microbiol Biotechnol.* 1994;40:800-805.

*Dilution rate per hour.

ECOLOGIC SIGNIFICANCE OF CROSS-FEEDING OF PROBIOTIC METABOLITES IN THE LARGE GUT

Considerable work has been done aimed at developing new nondigestible carbohydrates with a view to stimulating the growth of specific groups of beneficial organisms such as bifidobacteria and lactobacilli in the large bowel.[48] Other important objectives are to increase carbohydrate fermentation and SCFA formation in the distal colon using slowly digestible carbohydrates and to identify preferential substrates for the new groups of butyrate-producing anaerobes that have recently been characterized in the gut, such as eubacteria and roseburias.[49,50] Ecologic and physiologic studies on gut bacteria[51,52] have shown how metabolic cross-feeding of lactate and acetate is important in propionate butyrate formation in the microbiota. Results suggest that many low G+C Gram-positive species can be selected against in in vitro incubations, giving an incomplete picture of substrate catabolism in comparative fermentation tests. However, as summarized in Figure 7-4, coculture studies have shown how cross-feeding occurs between bifidobacteria, which do not form butyrate, and butyrate-producing *Roseburia* sp, *Anaerostipes caccae*, and *Eubacterium hallii*. Two different cross-feeding processes were demonstrated in this work, involving the utilization of bifidobacterial metabolites such as lactate and acetate by *A. caccae* and *E. hallii* and the uptake of hydrolysis products formed by bifidobacteria growing on FOS by the *Roseburia* and *E. hallii*. These studies demonstrated for the first time how large amounts of butyrate can be produced during the breakdown of FOS and inulins by probiotic bacteria in the colonic microbiota.

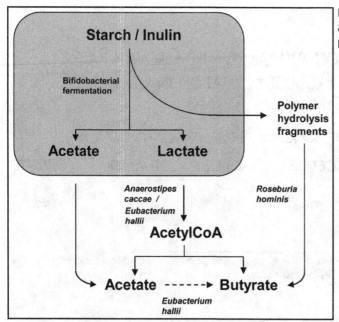

Figure 7-4. Cross-feeding of bifidobacterial and LAB polymer hydrolysis and fermentation products to produce butyrate in the large gut.

REFERENCES

1. Macfarlane GT, Cummings JH. The colonic flora, fermentation and large bowel digestive function. In: Phillips SF, Pemberton JH, Shorter RG, eds. *The Large Intestine: Physiology, Pathophysiology and Disease.* New York: Raven Press; 1991:51-92.
2. Macfarlane GT, Gibson GR, Cummings JH. Comparison of fermentation reactions in different regions of the human colon. *J Appl Bacteriol.* 1992;72(1):57-64.
3. Macfarlane GT, Macfarlane S, Gibson GR. Validation of a three-stage compound continuous culture system for investigating the effect of retention time on the ecology and metabolism of bacteria in the human colon. *Microbiol Ecol.* 1998;35:180-187.
4. Cummings JH, Hill MJ, Bone ES, Branch WJ, Jenkins DJA. The effect of meat protein and dietary fiber on colonic function and metabolism. Part II. Bacterial metabolites in feces and urine. *Am J Clin Nutr.* 1979;32(10):2094-2101.
5. Cummings JH, Macfarlane GT. The control and consequences of bacterial fermentation in the human colon. *J Appl Bacteriol.* 1991;70(6):443-459.
6. deFazio A, Chiew Y-E, Donoghue C, Lee CS, Sutherland RL. Effect of sodium butyrate on estrogen receptor and epidermal growth factor receptor gene expression in human breast cancer cell lines. *J Biol Chem.* 1992;267(25):18008-18012.
7. del Castillo JR, Muniz R, Sulbaran-Carrasco MC, Pekerar S. Cellular metabolism of colonocytes. In: Binder HJ, Cummings JH, Soergel KH, eds. *Short Chain Fatty Acids.* London, UK: Kluwer Academic; 1994:180-191.
8. Demigne C, Remesey C. Short chain fatty acids and hepatic metabolism. In: Binder HJ, Cummings JH, Soergel KH, eds. *Short Chain Fatty Acids.* London, UK: Kluwer Academic; 1994:272-282.
9. Cherbut C, Blottiere H, Kaeffer B, Galmiche JP. Short-chain fatty acids: a luminal modulatory signal for gastrointestinal motility. In: Malkki Y, Cummings JH, eds. *Dietary Fibre and Fermentation in the Colon.* Brussels: European Commission; 1996:203-208.
10. Cummings JH. Short chain fatty acids. In: Gibson GR, Macfarlane GT, eds. *Human Colonic Bacteria: Role in Nutrition, Physiology, and Health.* Boca Raton, FL: CRC Press; 1995:101-130.
11. Eftimiadi C, Tonetti M, Cavallero A, Sacco O, Rossi GA. Short-chain fatty acids produced by anaerobic bacteria inhibit phagocytosis by human lung macrophages. *J Infect Dis.* 1990;161(1):138-142.
12. Tonetti M, Cavallero A, Botta GA, Niederman R, Eftimiadi C. Intracellular pH regulates the production of different oxygen metabolites in neutrophils: effects of organic acids produced by anaerobic bacteria. *J Leukoc Biol.* 1991;49(2):180-188.
13. Prasad KN, Sinha PK. Effect of sodium butyrate on mammalian cells in culture: a review. *In Vitro.* 1976;12(2):125-132.

14. Kruh J. Effects of sodium butyrate, a new pharmacological agent, on cells in culture. *Mol Cell Biochem.* 1982;42(2):65-82.

15. Fregeau CJ, Helgason CD, Bleackley RC. Two cytotoxic cell proteinase genes are differentially sensitive to sodium butyrate. *Nucleic Acids Res.* 1992;20(12):3113-3119.

16. Hague A, Elder DJE, Hicks DJ, Paraskeva C. Apoptosis in colorectal tumour cells: induction by the short chain fatty acids butyrate, propionate and acetate and by the bile salt deoxycholate. *Int J Cancer.* 1995;60(3):400-406.

17. Wilson JR, Weiser MM. Colonic cancer cell (HT29) adhesion to laminin is altered by differentiation: adhesion may involve galactosyltransferase. *Exp Cell Res.* 1992;201(2):330-334.

18. Cummings JH, Bingham SA, Heaton KW, Eastwood MA. Fecal weight, colon cancer risk, and dietary intake of nonstarch polysaccharides (dietary fiber). *Gastroenterology.* 1992;103(6):1783-1789.

19. Smith EA, Macfarlane GT. Formation of phenolic and indolic compounds by anaerobic bacteria in the human large intestine. *Microb Ecol.* 1997;33:180-188.

20. Smith EA, Macfarlane GT. Enumeration of human colonic bacteria producing phenolic and indolic compounds: effects of pH, carbohydrate availability and retention time on dissimilatory aromatic amino acid metabolism. *J Appl Bacteriol.* 1996;81:288-302.

21. Smith EA, Macfarlane GT. Studies on amine production in the human colon: enumeration of amine forming bacteria and physiological effects of carbohydrate and pH. *Anaerobe.* 1996;2:285-297.

22. Smith EA, Macfarlane GT. Enumeration of amino acid fermenting bacteria in the human large intestine: effects of pH and starch on peptide metabolism and dissimilation of amino acids. *FEMS Microbiol Ecol.* 1998;25(4):355-368.

23. Macfarlane GT, Degnan BA. Catabolite regulatory mechanisms in relation to polysaccharide breakdown and carbohydrate utilization. In: Malkki Y, Cummings JH, eds. *Dietary Fibre and the Human Colon.* Luxembourg: Office for Official Publications of the European Communities; 1996:117-129.

24. Degnan BA, Macfarlane GT. Comparison of carbohydrate substrate preferences in eight species of bifidobacteria. *FEMS Microbiol Lett.* 1991;68(2):151-156.

25. Degnan BA. *Transport and Metabolism of Carbohydrates by Anaerobic Gut Bacteria* [PhD Thesis]. Cambridge, UK: University of Cambridge; 1992.

26. Macfarlane GT, Gibson GR. Co-utilization of polymerized carbon sources by *Bacteroides ovatus* grown in a two-stage continuous culture system. *Appl Environ Microbiol.* 1991;57(1):1-6.

27. Degnan BA, Macfarlane GT. Carbohydrate utilization patterns and substrate preferences in *Bacteroides thetaiotaomicron. Anaerobe.* 1995;1(1):25-33.

28. Macfarlane GT, Hay S, Macfarlane S, Gibson GR. Effect of different carbohydrates on growth, polysaccharidase and glycosidase production by *Bacteroides ovatus*, in batch and continuous culture. *J Appl Bacteriol.* 1990;68(2):179-187.

29. Degnan BA, Macfarlane GT. Arabinogalactan utilization in continuous cultures of *Bifidobacterium longum*: effect of co-culture with *Bacteroides thetaiotaomicron. Anaerobe.* 1995;1:103-112.

30. Cummings JH, Pomare EW, Branch WJ, Naylor CPE, Macfarlane GT. Short chain fatty acids in human large intestine, portal, hepatic and venous blood. *Gut.* 1987;28:1221-1227.

31. Macfarlane GT, Gibson GR. Metabolic activities of the normal colonic flora. In: Gibson SAW, ed. *Human Health: The Contribution of Microorganisms.* London, UK: Springer Verlag; 1994:17-52.

32. Macfarlane GT, Englyst HE. Starch utilization by the human large intestinal microflora. *J Appl Bacteriol.* 1986;60:195-201.

33. Englyst HN, Hay S, Macfarlane GT. Polysaccharide breakdown by mixed populations of human faecal bacteria. *FEMS Microbiol Ecol.* 1987;95:163-171.

34. Etterlin C, McKeowen A, Bingham SA, Elia M, Macfarlane GT, Cummings JH. D-Lactate and acetate as markers of fermentation in man. *Gastroenterology.* 1992;102:A551.

35. Coronado BE, Opal SM, Yoburn DC. Antibiotic-induced D-lactic acidosis. *Ann Intern Med.* 1995;122(11): 839-842.

36. Uchida H, Yamamoto H, Kisaki Y, Fujino J, Ishimaru Y, Ikeda H. D-Lactic acidosis in short-bowel syndrome managed with antibiotics and probiotics. *J Ped Surg.* 2009;39(4):634-636.

37. Haschke-Becher E, Brunser O, Cruchet S, Gotteland M, Haschke F, Bachmann C. Urinary D-lactate excretion in infants receiving *Lactobacillus johnsonii* with formula. *Ann Nutr Metab.* 2008;53:240-244.

38. DeVries W, Gerbrandy SJ, Stouthamer AH. Carbohydrate metabolism in *Bifidobacterium bifidum. Biochim Biophys Acta.* 1967;136:415-425.

39. DeVries W, Kapteijn WMC, Van der Beek EG, Stouthamer AH. Molar growth yields and fermentation balances of *Lactobacillus casei* L3 in batch cultures and in continuous cultures. *J Gen Microbiol.* 1970;63:333-345.

40. Kandler O. Carbohydrate metabolism in lactic acid bacteria. *Antonie van Leeuwenhoek.* 1983;49: 209-224.

41. Hamilton WA. Energy transduction in anaerobic bacteria. In: Anthony C, ed. *Bacterial Energy Transduction.* London, UK: Academic Press; 1988:83-149.

42. Macfarlane S, Macfarlane GT. Bacterial diversity in the large intestine. *Advan Appl Microbiol.* 2004;54:261-289.

43. Rasic JL. The role of dairy foods containing bifido- and acidophilus bacteria in nutrition and health? *North Eur Dairy J.* 1983;48:80.

44. Modler HW, McKellar RC, Yaguchi M. Bifidobacteria and bifidogenic factors. *Can Inst Food Sci Technol J.* 1990;23:29-41.

45. DeVries W, Stouthamer AH. Fermentation of glucose, lactose, galactose, mannitol and xylose by bifidobacteria. *J Bacteriol.* 1968;96:472-478.

46. Bezkorovainy A. Nutrition and metabolism of bifidobacteria. In: Bezkorovainy A, Miller-Catchpole R, eds. *Biochemistry and Physiology of Bifidobacteria.* Boca Raton, FL: CRC Press; 1989.

47. Degnan BA, Macfarlane GT. Effect of dilution rate and carbon availability on *Bifidobacterium breve* fermentation. *Appl Microbiol Biotechnol.* 1994;40:800-805.

48. Rastall RA, Gibson GR, Gill HS, et al. Modulation of the microbial ecology of the human colon by probiotics, prebiotics and synbiotics to enhance human health: an overview of enabling science and potential applications. *FEMS Microbial Ecol.* 2005;52:145-152.

49. Hold GL, Schwiertz A, Aminov RI, Blaut M, Flint HJ. Oligonucleotide probes detect quantitatively significant groups of butyrate producing bacteria in human feces. *Appl Environ Microbiol.* 2003;69:4320-4324.

50. Aminov RI, Walker AW, Duncan SH, Harmsen HJM, Welling GW, Flint HJ. Molecular diversity, cultivation, and improved detection by fluorescent in situ hybridization of a dominant group of human gut bacteria related to *Roseburia* spp. or *Eubacterium rectale. Appl Environ Microbiol.* 2006;72:6371-6376.

51. Belenguer A, Duncan SH, Calder A, et al. Two routes of metabolic cross-feeding between *Bifidobacterium adolescentis* and butyrate-producing anaerobes from the human gut. *Appl Environ Microbiol.* 2006;72:3593-3599.

52. Bourriaud C, Robins RJ, Martin L, et al. Lactate is mainly fermented to butyrate by human intestinal microfloras but inter-individual variation is evident. *J Appl Microbiol.* 2005;99:201-212.

8

Use of Probiotic Yogurts in Health and Disease

Mary Ellen Sanders, PhD and Daniel Merenstein, MD

Live active cultures have been delivered in fermented dairy foods for thousands of years. Contamination of milk with lactic acid bacteria from the environment resulted in acidified foods more resistant to spoilage and pathogen growth. Refinements of the fermentation process have led to a range of modern products with a staggering array of diversity with regard to the microbiological and compositional uniqueness, often signatures of local traditions. Products such as cheese, yogurt, kefir, and buttermilk are important components of the diets of many countries worldwide. The contribution of such products to global nutrition is well accepted; however, the unique benefit of the live microbes delivered in these products has become an active topic for research in recent years. To the extent live microbes can provide a health benefit underlies the concept of probiotics. These live microbes have long been thought to contribute to health, but it has only been in the past couple of decades that possible health effects have been tested using well-controlled human studies.

There is often a lack of appreciation for the role of foods as delivery agents for bioactive components. Pill forms of probiotics are often viewed as more medicinal or effective. However, the only categories of products in the United States that contain probiotics are foods and dietary supplements. Currently, there are no probiotic drugs. The only types of claims that can be made for foods and dietary supplements are FDA-approved health claims or structure-function claims that do not require premarket regulatory approval. Although regulatory requirements preclude use of therapeutic claims on food products, many studies have been conducted on yogurt with such clinical endpoints. No claims that relate to curing, treating, mitigating, or preventing disease can be legally made for foods or supplements. Therefore, both foods and dietary supplements are similar in the functions they perform (beyond providing nutrition) and the claims that can be made.

The aim of this chapter is to review the evidence that yogurt can deliver benefits beyond nutrition for both healthy and diseased individuals. This chapter will address the available literature on health effects of yogurt on human subjects. In many cases, the evidence reviewed deals with "live active culture" yogurts to which additional

Floch MH, Kim AS, eds.
Probiotics: A Clinical Guide (pp 95-120)
© 2010 Taylor & Francis Group

probiotic bacteria have been added—ie, probiotic yogurts. It is worth noting that not all yogurts contain added probiotic bacteria, and therefore not all yogurts should be considered functionally equivalent. Furthermore, this chapter will explore the possible role of the dairy matrix in delivering these benefits beyond what can be delivered by dietary supplements or dried forms of probiotics.

YOGURT

Conventional yogurt is a fermented dairy product derived from the fermentation of milk with 2 specific species of bacteria: *Streptococcus thermophilus* (*S. thermophilus*) and *Lactobacillus delbrueckii* spp. *bulgaricus* (*L. bulgaricus*). Legal standards of identity for yogurt exist (which must be met to call a product "yogurt") that specify the required composition of the product with regard to macronutrients, acidity, and other added ingredients, including additional, nonstarter microbes (Codex Standard for Fermented Milks, Codex standard 243-2003). But yogurts can vary with regard to the minimum level of acidity, the numbers of each of the starter bacterial strains, the presence of added functional ingredients (eg, fiber and prebiotics), and whether or not there are added probiotic bacteria, such as additional species of *Lactobacillus* or *Bifidobacterium*. With regard to levels of live bacteria in yogurt, the Codex standard stipulates that the total starter bacteria must be 10^7 CFU/g and any added probiotic bacteria must be present at 10^6 CFU/g. However, if the product is heat treated after fermentation, there is no Codex requirement for viable microorganisms. Such products must be labeled as heat treated; however, it should be recognized that not all products labeled as "yogurt" necessarily are a source of live, active cultures.

Although probiotic effects are considered to be strain specific, it is common that the *S. thermophilus* and *L. bulgaricus* strains used in manufacturing yogurt are not specifically identified. Unlike the probiotic components of a particular brand of yogurt that are consistent over time, the starter strains of *S. thermophilus* and *L. bulgaricus* may change. This generally occurs because of technological issues such as bacteriophage buildup against the starter strains (resulting in a failed fermentation), requiring the substitution of phage-unrelated strains for production. In general, the contribution of the *S. thermophilus* and *L. bulgaricus* strains to health effects is considered to be secondary to those mediated by the added probiotic bacteria, with one exception. The yogurt starter bacteria seem to be best suited for aiding digestion of lactose in lactose maldigesters (see "Lactose Digestion" section).

This chapter will specifically address the evidence for health benefits attributed to the live microbial components of yogurt. This chapter is not meant to be a comprehensive review of efficacy evidence for probiotics, but instead focuses specifically on the value of yogurt as a delivery vehicle.

DESCRIPTION OF LITERATURE SEARCH

Eligibility Criteria

Studies were included if they met the following criteria: (1) conducted with human subjects; (2) the product studied was referred to as a yogurt or would be recognized by the general public as a yogurt-like product; (3) an intervention was conducted; (4) a clinical trial was conducted; (5) published in English through the end of 2008. Furthermore, studies were evaluated using the Strength of Recommendation Taxonomy (SORT), an approach developed by the American Academy of Family Physicians to aid evaluation of efficacy of human studies.[1] This strategy is based on a combination of previous evidence taxonomies. The SORT approach provides grades of A, B, or C to human studies on the basis of meeting quality criteria. The focus of this review is on A-rated studies, as these studies provide consistent and good-quality patient-oriented evidence. However, so as not to exclude a large body of research on yogurt effects on microbiota and immune biomarkers, these nonpatient-oriented studies were included in these sections.

The following discussion focuses on the clinical endpoints that have been addressed by yogurt intervention studies. Studies focused on blood pressure, cancer risk, hepatic encephalopathy, and vancomycin-resistant *Enterococcus* have been published, but we deemed that there were insufficient data on these endpoints to include.

Search Strategy

Literature searches were conducted using the following electronic databases: PubMed, Cochrane Review of Databases, EMBASE, and Web of Science. Search terms included *yogurt, yoghurt, dairy products, cultured milk, kefir,* and *probiotics.*

ALLERGIES

Our review found 2 studies that met our entry criteria. One study used in-house volunteers and appeared not to be properly blinded.[2] The other study was well conducted but the placebo was not a matching yogurt-like drink but instead included fermented milk. In this study, fermented milk (*L. casei* DN-114 001, *L. bulgaricus, S. thermophilus*) was evaluated in children 2 to 5 years old who suffered from allergies or asthma.[3] They consumed the product or fermented milk for 12 months. There was a 33% lower incidence of allergic rhinitis in the fermented milk group but no differences in asthma control or medication usage.

On the basis of the available data, there is insufficient evidence to recommend yogurt or probiotic-supplemented, yogurt-like drinks for treating or preventing allergies. However, more studies with *L. casei* DN-114 001 should be conducted as there appears to be some benefit in children previously diagnosed with allergies, but more studies using better matched controls are needed.

GASTROINTESTINAL DISEASES

Radiation-Induced Diarrhea

Diarrhea is one of the most common and debilitating adverse events of radiation therapy. One study was conducted in women undergoing radiation for pelvic cancer.[4] The study enrolled patients undergoing pelvic radiotherapy and randomized them to receive 10^8 CFU/g fermented milk (*L. casei* DN-114 001, *L. bulgaricus, S. thermophilus*) in addition to *S. thermophilus* and *L. bulgaricus,* or the same amount of sterilized matching placebo. The intervention did not prevent radiation-induced diarrhea.

Diarrhea

Consistent with other probiotic research, the abundance of yogurt research has been on gastrointestinal illnesses, most specifically diarrhea (Table 8-1) and *Helicobacter*

 (text continued on page 101)

TABLE 8-1

STUDIES ON THE EFFECT OF CONVENTIONAL YOGURT (CONTAINING *L. BULGARICUS* AND *S. THERMOPHILUS*) AND PROBIOTIC YOGURT (CONTAINING ADDITIONAL PROBIOTIC STRAINS INDICATED PARENTHETICALLY) ON DIARRHEA

REFERENCE	INTERVENTION	PLACEBO	STUDY POPULATION	PRIMARY OUTCOME	RESULTS
5	Probiotic yogurt (*L. rhamnosus*, GR-1 and *L. reuteri* RC-14)	Conventional yogurt	HIV-positive adult women with moderate diarrhea	Resolution of diarrhea	12/12 supplemented group had resolution of diarrhea at day 2 compared to 2/12 in the conventional yogurt at day 15
6	Fermented probiotic milk (LGG, *L. acidophilus* La-5, and *Bifidobacterium* Bb-12)	Milk drink with heat-killed bacteria	Adult hospitalized patients on antibiotics	Prevention of antibiotic-associated diarrhea	2/34 (6%) in the active group versus 8/29 (28%) in the placebo group experienced diarrhea
7	Probiotic yogurt (*S. thermophilus*, *L. acidophilus*, *B. lactis*) or conventional yogurt with *S. thermophilus* and *L. bulgaricus*	No yogurt	Over age 1 receiving antibiotics	Prevention of antibiotic-associated diarrhea	Total patients, 407; no statistical differences in the three arms ($P = .20$): 7% in the bio-yogurt group, 11% in the commercial-yogurt group, and 14% in the no-yogurt group
8	*Lactobacillus* fermented milk	Placebo with no organisms	Hospitalized adults on antibiotics	Prevention of antibiotic-associated diarrhea	Total patients, 89; 7 of 44 patients (16%) in the lactobacilli group had diarrhea compared to 16 of 45 patients (36%) in the placebo group

(continued)

TABLE 8-1 (continued)

REFERENCE	INTERVENTION	PLACEBO	STUDY POPULATION	PRIMARY OUTCOME	RESULTS
9	Commercial yogurt	No treatment	Hospitalized adults on antibiotics	Prevention of antibiotic-associated diarrhea	Yogurt group had 105 participants versus 97 in the control. Yogurt group had 12% diarrhea rate versus 24% in the no-yogurt group
10	Fermented milk (*L. casei* DN-114 001, *L. bulgaricus, S. thermophilus*) or dahi (*L. lactis, L. lactis cremoris, Leuconostoc mesenteroides cremoris*)	Ultra PY with no cultures	Hospitalized children with acute diarrhea	Resolution of diarrhea	Total participants, 75; mean days of diarrhea were PY = 2.1; Dahi = 1.8; Fermented milk = 1.5
11	Fermented milk (*L. casei* DN-114 001, *L. bulgaricus, S. thermophilus*) or dahi (*L. lactis, L. lactis cremoris, Leuconostoc mesenteroides cremoris*)	Ultra PY with no cultures	Community children in India with acute diarrhea	Resolution of community diarrhea	Total participants, 75; mean days of diarrhea were PY = 2.4; Dahi = 2.2; Fermented milk = 1.9
12	Commercially manufactured product containing *L. casei* DN-114 001	Conventional yogurt used in the control group did not contain live bacteria	Healthy military recruits	Incidence and duration of diarrhea	No differences: probiotic yogurt group had 254 participants, 12% acquired diarrhea that lasted a mean of 3 days; conventional yogurt group had 248 participants; 16% acquired diarrhea for 2.6 days

TABLE 8-1 *(continued)*

STUDIES ON THE EFFECT OF CONVENTIONAL YOGURT (CONTAINING *L. BULGARICUS* AND *S. THERMOPHILUS*) AND PROBIOTIC YOGURT (CONTAINING ADDITIONAL PROBIOTIC STRAINS INDICATED PARENTHETICALLY) ON DIARRHEA

REFERENCE	INTERVENTION	PLACEBO	STUDY POPULATION	PRIMARY OUTCOME	RESULTS
13	Fermented milk (*L. casei* DN-114 001, *L. bulgaricus, S. thermophilus*)	Conventional yogurt	Healthy children in daycare	Frequency and duration of diarrhea	Fermented milk group had 384 participants; conventional yogurt had 395. Duration of diarrhea was similar but 16% in the fermented milk group had diarrhea compared to 22% in the yogurt group
14	Formula with yogurt starter cultures	Formula	Hospitalized children with acute diarrhea	Resolution of diarrhea	Both groups had 56 children. Two days after admission, 62% of the milk group had diarrhea compared to 35% in the yogurt starter culture group
15	Fermented milk (*L. casei* DN-114 001, *L. bulgaricus, S. thermophilus* or conventional yogurt	Jellied milk	Healthy children in daycare	Incidence of diarrhea	No differences in diarrhea incidence

pylori infections (Table 8-2). Similar to other disease categories, there are a variety of different interventions and placebos used in the clinical trials. It is difficult to craft an overall conclusion due to the heterogeneity in the studies. For example, of the 12 studies that met our inclusion criteria, 5 examined the role of yogurt in treating individuals who suffered from acute diarrhea, 4 examined the role in preventing antibiotic-associated diarrhea (AAD), and 3 looked at preventing diarrhea in a healthy population. Definitions of diarrhea varied within the studies. In addition to differences in the primary outcome, studies varied with regard to different products studied, controls used, and study settings. In addition, methodological problems existed with many of the studies, such as very small patient populations,[5] questionable placebo,[7] and emphasizing per-protocol analysis rather than intention-to-treat analysis.[5,7,13] However, even considering study limitations, some success and rationale in preventing and treating diarrhea with yogurt or yogurt-like products was observed in 8 of the studies.[5,6,8-11,13,16]

H. pylori

Studies on *H. pylori* were more homogeneous than those with diarrhea endpoints, due to consistency of the primary outcome among studies. Studies tracked impact on *H. pylori* colonization, and standard medical treatments were part of the intervention (see Table 8-2). Of the 6 studies that met the inclusion criteria, 3 had positive outcomes, 2 of which were conducted by the same research team with the same probiotic-fortified yogurt.[17-19] Neither of these studies used a placebo; comparison was with a control group receiving only standard medical treatments. Standard treatment of *H. pylori* is generally an intensive 2-week treatment of at least 2 different antibiotics. The *H. pylori* results, taken in conjunction with the previously discussed AAD studies, suggest some role for probiotic-fortified yogurt in eradicating *H. pylori*.

LIPIDS

In the literature, the primary outcome on the impact of yogurt on lipid profiles was reduction of cholesterol levels. However, the 10 studies that met the inclusion criteria used many different interventions and placebos (Table 8-3). Unfortunately, as in the field as a whole, the studies gave mixed results, with many different strains and groups examined. However, there are some promising studies that suggest there may be a role of probiotic-supplemented yogurt in positively impacting lipid levels, either lowering LDL or raising HDL cholesterol.

VAGINAL INFECTIONS

Three studies have examined the role of yogurts in vaginal infections.[20-22] Two of these studies included evaluations of the ability of the probiotic strains in the yogurt to colonize the healthy vaginal epithelium. Interestingly, LGG at 10^9 CFU/g was administered for 1 month to postmenopausal women and was found not to adhere to the epithelium.[20] However, yogurt with 10^8 CFU/g of *L. acidophilus* (strain not reported) was found to colonize both the rectum and vagina in women with a history of vaginal infections who consumed the yogurt for 2 consecutive months.[21] A similar study examined the role of consuming 10^8 CFU/g of *L. acidophilus* for 6 months in women with chronic vaginal *Candida* infections.[22] In the per-protocol analysis of the 13 women who finished the study, the mean number of infections was 2.54 in the control group compared to

    (text continued on page 105)

TABLE 8-2

STUDIES ON THE EFFECT OF CONVENTIONAL YOGURT AND PROBIOTIC YOGURT ON *H. PYLORI**

REFERENCE	INTERVENTION	PLACEBO	STUDY POPULATION	RESULTS
23	Routine therapy plus probiotic yogurt (*L. acidophilus* HY2177, *L. casei* HY2743, *B. longum* HY8001, and *S. thermophilus* B-1)	Routine therapy	+ *H. pylori*	No differences
24	Routine therapy plus probiotic yogurt (*B. animalis* and *L. casei*)	Routine therapy plus milk	Children + *H. pylori*	No differences
19	Enhanced medical therapy plus probiotic yogurt (*L. acidophilus* La5, *B. lactis* Bb12, *L. bulgaricus*, and *S. thermophilus*)	Enhanced medical therapy	Adults with *H. pylori* who failed routine therapy	Yogurt group had 59 patients versus 49 in control. Statistically significant differences were found; 85% in yogurt versus 71% in control
18	Routine therapy plus fermented milk (*L. casei* DN-114 001, *L. bulgaricus*, *S. thermophilus*)	Routine therapy plus unfermented pasteurized milk	Adults with *H. pylori*	Fermented milk group had 39 patients and milk had 47 patients; statistically significant differences were found; 85% versus 58% in milk
17	Routine therapy plus probiotic yogurt (*L. acidophilus* La5, *B. lactis* Bb12, *L. bulgaricus*, and *S. thermophilus*)	Routine therapy	Adults with *H. pylori*	Each group had 11 participants; statistically significant differences; 91% versus 78% in the control group
25	One intervention that included *L. casei* 03, *L. acidophilus* 2412, *L. acidophilus* ACD1 with a commercial starter containing *L. bulgaricus*, *S. thermophilus*, and *L. acidophilus*	Only one group	Adult women with asymptomatic *H. pylori*	In 26 of 27 subjects, the urea breath test values remained positive

*Primary outcome is eradication of *H. pylori*.

TABLE 8-3

STUDIES ON THE EFFECT OF CONVENTIONAL YOGURT AND PROBIOTIC YOGURT ON SERUM LIPIDS*

REFERENCE	INTERVENTION	PLACEBO	STUDY POPULATION	RESULTS
26	Yogurt supplemented with *L. casei* ssp. *casei*	Conventional yogurt	Normocholesterolemic women	Significant improvement in the ratio of LDL/HDL and total/HDL cholesterol in both groups, but no differences among groups
27	Yogurt supplemented with *B. longum* strain BL1	Conventional yogurt	Hypercholesterolemic adults	Some decreases in the supplemented group of individuals with moderate hypercholesterolemia compared to conventional yogurt
28	Yogurt supplemented with *L. acidophilus* 145 and *B. longum* 913	Conventional yogurt	Normo- and hypercholesterolemic women	Supplemented group had an increase in HDL compared to conventional yogurt
29	Kefir	Milk	Hypercholesterolemic men	No changes in cholesterol levels
30	Group 1: probiotic yogurt (2 strains of *S. thermophilus* and 2 strains of *L. acidophilus*, (Stla)). Group 2: placebo yogurt, acidified with delta-acid-lactone. Group 3: probiotic yogurt (2 strains of *S. thermophilus* and *L. rhamnosus*, Stlr). Group 4: probiotic yogurt (*E. faecium* and 2 strains of *S. thermophilus*).	Group 5 was given 2 placebo pills daily	Overweight adults	No significant changes among groups

(continued)

TABLE 8-3 (continued)

STUDIES ON THE EFFECT OF CONVENTIONAL YOGURT AND PROBIOTIC YOGURT ON SERUM LIPIDS*

REFERENCE	INTERVENTION	PLACEBO	STUDY POPULATION	RESULTS
31	Fermented milk (L. casei TMC0409 and S. thermophilus TMC1543)	Milk	Hypercholesterolemic men	Each group had 10 participants, and the supplemented group had a statistically significant increase in HDL and decrease in triglycerides
32	Probiotic yogurt (L. acidophilus L1)	Conventional yogurt	Hypercholesterolemic adults	No changes in cholesterol levels
33	Probiotic yogurt (L. acidophilus L1 and S. thermophilus MUH34)	Conventional yogurt	Hypercholesterolemic adults	Seventy-eight subjects; the supplemented group had a 3.5% decrease in total cholesterol
34	Conventional yogurt or whole milk	Skimmed milk	Males 16 to 18 years	No significant differences, but skimmed milk was the only intervention that lowered total cholesterol
35	PY or conventional yogurt	2% butter fat milk	Healthy adults	Twenty-one subjects in both yogurt groups; mean decrease in total cholesterol was 7.5% in both yogurt groups

* All primary outcomes are based on changes in cholesterol.

0.38 in the intervention. This study has several important limitations. The control group was instructed not to eat any yogurt, but had no other interventions. Additionally, the study started with 33 women but analyzed only 13 participants who properly followed the intervention. The 3 studies together evaluated a total of only 109 women consuming yogurt, so although they provide some suggestion that probiotic yogurts may treat or prevent vaginal infections, much more research with larger studies, targeted probiotics, and defined patient groups is needed for a definitive conclusion.

LACTOSE DIGESTION

The ability of lactose-intolerant subjects to tolerate a lactose load when delivered in yogurt with live starter cultures, compared to milk, is the focus of several human studies (Table 8-4). These studies have typically used breath hydrogen excretion (BH_2) as the biomarker of lactose maldigestion; some studies have also recorded the impact on symptoms. Studies have typically not been blinded and in some cases have included pasteurized yogurt (PY) (with no viable cultures) for comparison. Studies differ with regard to subject inclusion criteria due to different definitions of lactose maldigestion, which is generally defined as increase in BH_2 >20 ppm after ingestion of 440 mL milk with 18 to 50 g lactose delivered in milk or water. However, these studies have yielded consistent results: Subjects consuming yogurt excrete lower levels of BH_2 than subjects consuming milk or PY. Most studies were conducted in healthy subjects, but other subjects included children on chemotherapy and adults with short-bowel syndrome. Interestingly, although studies show that the live cultures are important for this effect, the level of BH_2 for PYs was between those for yogurt and milk, possibly due to reduced oro-fecal transit time observed with yogurt and PY compared to milk.[36-40] It was also observed that yogurt does not help with additional lactose load beyond the lactose in yogurt, and meals do not interfere with the ability of yogurt to suppress BH_2.[41] Effects are due to intraluminal bacterial lactase activity, as no changes in mucosal lactase were observed after 1 week of yogurt consumption.[40] Although clear differences in BH_2 results were observed between PY and yogurt with live active cultures, results with symptoms were more equivocal among studies.[35,39,42,43] In total, these studies indicate that yogurt with live cultures is tolerated better than milk containing the same amount of lactose.

NUTRITIONAL STATUS

The role of yogurt in improving nutritional status has been reported in a few studies (Table 8-5). These studies are diverse in objectives and design. Some studies document the nutritional value of adding yogurt to the diet but offer no insight into unique properties of yogurt (such as live cultures) beyond its nutritional value. Studies were conducted on different populations: Chinese children,[44] Egyptian children,[45] and healthy women.[46] Parra and Martinez[47] found that short-term assimilation of leucine was improved for both lactose-intolerant and lactose-tolerant subjects consuming yogurt compared to PY, suggesting a role of live cultures in this effect. In a study by Elmadfa et al,[48] no effect was observed on vitamin B status when healthy subjects consumed either yogurt or PY compared to baseline, but in a study by Fabian et al,[46] consumption of yogurt improved vitamin B status. Also, no impact of a probiotic yogurt was seen on isoflavone bioavailability when combined with a diet high in soy.[49] In sum, the effects of yogurt with live cultures compared to yogurt without live cultures on nutritional status has not been sufficiently evaluated.

     (text continued on page 109)

TABLE 8-4

Studies on the Effect of Conventional Yogurt and Probiotic Yogurt on Lactose Digestion

REFERENCE	INTERVENTIONS	STUDY POPULATION	PRIMARY OUTCOME	RESULTS
36	12 g lactose consumed in milk or yogurt	Twelve children (2.4 to 13.5 years) with malignancies and chemotherapy-induced lactose intolerance	BH_2	Yogurt reduced BH_2 compared to milk and was well tolerated by subjects
38	20 g lactose in 440 mL milk or 442 mL yogurt	Seventeen LM patients with short-bowel syndrome (mean small bowel length 67 cm) with either a terminal jejunostomy (group A, $n = 6$) or a jejunocolic anastomosis (group B, $n = 11$)	Fecal weight, symptoms, lactose and hexose flow rates in stomal effluents (group A), and breath-hydrogen excretion (group B)	Patients with short-bowel syndrome were able to tolerate lactose (no symptoms, no effect on fecal weight) from both milk and yogurt, although less lactose was recovered from stomal effluent with yogurt feeding. No difference in BH_2 between yogurt and milk
37	11 g lactose consumed in milk, yogurt, or PY	Fifty-three healthy, institutionalized Caucasian elderly (67 to 95 years)	BH_2	19/53 were LM***; yogurt reduced BH_2 in 19 LM tested; some intermediate benefit from PY
41	20 g lactose in milk, yogurt, yogurt + meal or meal with no lactose, fed in random order	Twelve healthy LM* adults	BH_2	Yogurt reduced BH_2 compared to milk; consumption of the meal with yogurt did not affect yogurt's ability to reduce BH_2
41	Milk (20 g lactose) or 5 servings of yogurt with 10, 15, 20, 25 or 30 g lactose/serving	Ten healthy LM* adults	BH_2	Yogurt reduced BH_2 compared to milk; yogurt did not impact BH_2 if additional lactose was added

(continued)

TABLE 8-4 (continued)

REFERENCE	INTERVENTIONS	STUDY POPULATION	PRIMARY OUTCOME	RESULTS
42	Comparison of 5 products, including yogurt, with milk, 18 g lactose	Ten LM* black subjects	BH_2	Yogurt reduced BH_2 and symptoms compared to milk; correlation between symptoms reported and mean peak BH_2; yogurt (454 U lactase) outperformed lactase tablets (756 U lactase)
40	125 g yogurt or PY, tid for 7 days; 16 subjects divided equally in yogurt and PY groups; Double-blind, placebo-controlled design	Sixteen healthy Cameroon-born, LM adults (18 to 26 years)	BH_2 compared to baseline milk BH_2 and between yogurt and PY; mucosal lactase levels (via endoscopic duodenal biopsies)	Yogurt reduced BH_2 compared to milk baseline and PY; results on day 1 were the same as day 8; no alteration in mucosal lactase activity was observed. No reported symptoms in yogurt or PY group
39	20 g lactose in milk, yogurt, PY, buttermilk, sweet and acidophilus milk	Nine healthy LM* adults (20 to 28 years)	BH_2 and symptoms	Yogurt reduced BH_2 compared to milk and PY; no symptoms for subjects consuming yogurt or PY, but buttermilk nor sweet acidophilus milk did not improve symptoms compared to milk
50	25 g lactose in yogurt or PY	Twenty-two healthy LM***** adults (20 to 24 years)	BH_2, symptoms, gastric emptying and oro-fecal transit time	Yogurt reduced BH_2 and gastrointestinal symptoms compared to milk and PY; no differences in gastric emptying or oro-fecal transit time (although results approached significance, $P = .0524$, with PY slower oro-fecal transit time than conventional yogurt)
51	25 g lactose in milk, conventional yogurt, PY and yogurt with reduced starter bacteria (10^6 or 10^5 CFU/g compared to 10^8 CFU/g in conventional yogurt)	Twenty-four healthy LM**** men (21 to 35 years)	BH_2 and symptoms	Yogurt reduced BH_2 compared to milk, PY or yogurt with reduced numbers of starter bacteria; results with PY or yogurt with reduced numbers of starter bacteria fell in between results with milk and conventional yogurt; results on symptoms paralleled BH_2 results

LM (lactose maldigester) defined by increase in BH_2 >20 ppm after ingestion of 440 mL milk with 18 g lactose; LM*, 20 g lactose in milk; LM**, 50 g lactose in 250 mL water; LM***, 11 g lactose in 250 mL milk; LM****, increase in BH_2 >30 ppm with 25 g lactose in 250 mL tap water; LM*****, increase in BH_2 >20 ppm after ingestion of water with 25 g lactose.

TABLE 8-5

STUDIES ON THE EFFECT OF CONVENTIONAL YOGURT AND PROBIOTIC YOGURT ON NUTRITIONAL STATUS

REFERENCE	INTERVENTION	PLACEBO	STUDY POPULATION	PRIMARY OUTCOME	RESULTS
47	Yogurt administered in a single-blinded, sequential administration study	PY (administration to all subjects following yogurt administration period)	Thirty-three healthy subjects with mild lactose intolerance (>20 ppm increase in BH_2 after ingestion of 25 g lactose in 250 mL water) or lactose-tolerant	Leucine uptake	Short-term assimilation of leucine was improved in yogurt compared to PY; no difference between lactose-intolerant and lactose-tolerant subjects
49	Yogurt with LGG, L. acidophilus, and B. bifidus (strain designations not provided)	Two-arm study with yogurt compared to resistant starch	Thirty-one healthy women on soy diet	Isoflavone bioavailability	Yogurt had no effect on isoflavone bioavailability
45	Yogurt; control group received no intervention	None	Children, $n = 402$ (3 to 5 years) with low height/weight	Vitamin and mineral update; incidence and duration of infections; weight and height	Yogurt added to the diet improved intake of calcium, zinc, and vitamin B2, reduced incidence and duration of upper-respiratory infection and diarrhea of children, increased height and weight gain
48	"Mild" yogurt made with S. thermophilus, L. acidophilus, and LGG	PY (sequential feeding study, administration of PY for 2 weeks followed by yogurt for 2 weeks)	Twelve healthy adults (25 to 36 years)	Impact of live cultures in yogurt on B vitamin (B1, B2, B6) status of the healthy adult	No difference in vitamin B1, B2, and B6 status of healthy subjects was observed when yogurt with live cultures (S. thermophilus, L. acidophilus, and LGG) was compared to PY
46	Yogurt containing S. thermophilus, L. bulgaricus, and L. casei DN-114 001	Two-arm study with yogurt compared to yogurt + added probiotic	Thirty-three healthy women	Plasma and urine concentrations vitamin B1, B2, and B6	200 g of both yogurts increased total intake of vitamin B1 and B2 compared to periods without yogurt intake

EFFECTS OF YOGURT ON COMMENSAL MICROBIOTA BIOCHEMISTRY AND INTESTINAL FUNCTION

The ability of yogurt to impact the populations or activities of microbes associated with the human body is not well understood. Although it is conventionally understood that one substantial value of fermented dairy products with live active cultures is its ability to "balance" our colonizing microbes, evidence is insufficient. This is due in part to the need for studies using modern methods that detect the impact of yogurt on dominant microbial communities including noncultured microbes, methods that have become established only in recent years.[52] When considering the studies published to date, some general conclusions can be made about the effects of yogurt on fecal microbiota (Table 8-6). Transient increases in the levels of genus, species, or strain that was fed (depending on specificity of methods used) are often observed, most typically when *Bifidobacterium* or intestinal *Lactobacillus* species are also included in the yogurt. Some studies show changes in populations of other colonizing microbes, but groups that change are not consistent among studies (Table 8-6). Changes in the microbiota are transient and return to baseline within weeks after feeding has stopped. Changes are sometimes observed in fecal biochemical parameters (such as SCFA, ammonia, amines, pH, phenols, ρ-cresol, and enzymatic activities).

The studies evaluating microbiological effects of yogurt are summarized in Table 8-6 and below. Studies have predominantly been conducted on fecal samples, which serve as surrogates of intestinal microbiota; however, nasal and oral microbiology has also been evaluated. In interpreting these results, it is important to recognize that the clinical significance of any effects on normal colonizing microbiota populations is largely unknown. The ability to alter levels of pathogens may be important from the perspectives of both reducing the risk of infectious disease for the host and pathogen transmission. But the health advantages of altering normal colonizing bacteria have yet to be demonstrated. Recent advances in molecular techniques that target the DNA of colonizing microbes rather than the ability to culture them are beginning to provide a deeper understanding of microbial colonization patterns associated with compromised health, such as IBD and obesity.[53,54] Such observations provide the basis for the hypothesis that direct manipulation of colonizing microbes with administration of exogenous microbes such as those contained in yogurt might lead to improved health. This mechanistic hypothesis has yet to be proven.

When considering how yogurt, and the live cultures contained within, can impact microbiological endpoints in human studies, perhaps the most obvious assessment is isolating the fed strain(s) from feces or mucosal tissues after consumption of the yogurt. The strength of the data documenting such recovery of yogurt strains varies with the microbiological composition of the yogurt, and specifically if the yogurt is conventional yogurt with only yogurt starters, or yogurt containing added probiotic bacteria. The starter bacteria in yogurt (*S. thermophilus* and *L. bulgaricus*) are not as well suited to survive intestinal transit as some other species sometimes added to yogurt. Reports on isolation[55-57] or failed isolation[58] of yogurt starters from feces after yogurt consumption have been published. Low numbers (up to ~10^5 CFU/g) of viable *L. bulgaricus*, but not *S. thermophilus* (except in one case), were recovered from healthy subjects consuming 6×10^9 and 5×10^{10} CFU/d of *L. bulgaricus* and *S. thermophilus* in yogurt, respectively.[55] Culture-based recovery was followed by DNA-based confirmation of species in this study. Brigidi et al[56] reported successful isolation of *S. thermophilus* from feces, but the primers used were not tested for the ability to distinguish between *S. salivarius* and *S. thermophilus*, and therefore may not have been sufficiently specific, as suggested by Elli,

 (text continued on page 113)

Table 8-6

STUDIES ON THE EFFECT OF CONVENTIONAL YOGURT AND PROBIOTIC YOGURT ON FECAL MICROBIOTA AND BIOCHEMISTRY

REFERENCE	INTERVENTION/ PLACEBO	STUDY POPULATION	PRIMARY OUTCOME	RESULTS
59	Conventional yogurt, probiotic yogurt (L. casei), or second probiotic yogurt (L. acidophilus); strains not reported	Fifteen healthy adults	Fecal microbiota (Lactobacillus, Bifidobacterium, and 4 other taxonomic groups) using DNA-based methods	Neither probiotic yogurt significantly altered fecal levels of the 6 taxonomic groups; conventional yogurt increased relative % of C. coccoides/E. rectale and decreased bacteroides and prevotella groups
44	Subjects consumed both capsule with B. longum (strain not reported) and probiotic yogurt (B. animalis DN-173 010); no control	Eleven healthy, lactose-intolerant subjects	Composition of the fecal microbiota using fluorescent in situ hybridization; fecal β-galactosidase and symptoms after yogurt feeding and lactose challenge were measured	In addition to increasing total bacteria, C. coccoides/E. rectale increased during product consumption compared to baseline; increased β-galactosidase activity in feces and decreased total symptom score after lactose challenge
60	This was not an intervention study, but subjects selected from a larger dietary cohort study	Thirty yogurt consumers and 21 non-consumers; a single fecal sample was obtained from all 51 subjects	Feces evaluated for composition of microbiota (DNA-based identification of 8 taxonomic groups) and 9 metabolic bacterial enzyme activities	Enteric bacteria lower in yogurt consumers; proportion of bifidobacteria positively correlated with yogurt consumption; β-galactosidase higher in yogurt consumers; no difference in bile acids or SCFA
61	Conventional yogurt or probiotic yogurt (B. longum BB536)	Forty adults with Japanese cedar pollinosis (fecal samples from a subset: only 10 of these)	Terminal restriction fragment length polymorphism used to characterize the bacterial communities of the feces of the subjects	Bifidobacterium increased in BB536 group compared to placebo. B. fragilis group increased in placebo group but not BB536 group

(continued)

TABLE 8-6 (continued)

REFERENCE	INTERVENTION/ PLACEBO	STUDY POPULATION	PRIMARY OUTCOME	RESULTS
62	Conventional yogurt or probiotic yogurt (without L. bulgaricus but with L. coryniformis CECT5711 and L. gasseri CECT5714)	Thirty healthy adults	Blood and fecal parameters	Probiotic yogurt consumption compared to conventional yogurt resulted in higher fecal lactic acid bacteria and increased SCFA; no differences in cytotoxicity, fecal pH, ammonium concentration, or enzymatic activities; fed probiotic strains were isolated from feces
63	Probiotic yogurt (B. lactis LKM512)	Six elderly patients in hospital for long term	Fecal biochemistry	Increased spermine, decreased haptoglobin, and reduced mutagenicity of feces
64	Conventional yogurt, gelled milk (no live cultures) and probiotic yogurt (L. casei DN-114 001)	Thirty-nine healthy infants (10 to 18 months)	Fecal microbiota, bacterial enzyme activity and SCFA	Compared to baseline, no changes in number of anaerobes, bifidobacteria, bacteroides, or enterobacteria; yogurt + L. casei group showed increased Lactobacillus and decreased activity of β-glucuronidase and β-glucosidase; yogurt group showed increased Enterococcus and decreased branched chain and long-chain fatty acids
65	Conventional yogurt and probiotic yogurt (L. acidophilus NCFB 1748, B. lactis Bb12, and L. paracasei ssp. paracasei F19)	Twenty-four healthy adults (21 to 48 years)	Impact of yogurt or probiotic yogurt on antibiotic-induced disturbances of fecal microbiota	Compared to conventional yogurt, yogurt with added probiotics prevented antibiotic-induced reductions in lactobacilli and bacteroides; other microbiological changes occurred compared to baseline, but did not differ between groups
66	PY and probiotic yogurt (L. paracasei A)	Twenty-six healthy infants (12 to 14 months)	Fecal microbiology and strain-specific fecal isolation of L. paracasei A (culture and DNA-based methods)	Isolation of probiotic strain from feces; increased levels of lactobacilli; minimal other effects on microbiota

(continued)

Table 8-6 (continued)

STUDIES ON THE EFFECT OF CONVENTIONAL YOGURT AND PROBIOTIC YOGURT ON FECAL MICROBIOTA AND BIOCHEMISTRY

REFERENCE	INTERVENTION/ PLACEBO	STUDY POPULATION	PRIMARY OUTCOME	RESULTS
67	Conventional yogurt or probiotic yogurt (*B. lactis* LKM512)	Seven healthy adults	Fecal biochemistry	Probiotic yogurt increased spermidine and reduced mutagenicity of feces compared to conventional yogurt
68	Conventional yogurt or probiotic yogurt (*B. lactis* LKM512)	Ten adults with moderate atopic dermatitis	Fecal microbiology assessed by terminal restriction fragment length polymorphism	Many fecal microbiology changes observed after both conventional and probiotic yogurt consumption, depending on individuals; increased spermidine

et al,[55] del Campo et al[58] administered yogurt or PY for 15 days to 114 healthy subjects in a double-blind, crossover study. PCR testing with species-specific primers of presumptive isolates grown from feces failed to identify any colonies of *L. bulgaricus* or *S. thermophilus* from any fecal sample. In addition, direct DNA amplification of these species from feces was negative. DNA hybridization experiments did reveal DNA compatible with *L. bulgaricus* in 10% of the subjects consuming yogurt, but this method detects DNA, not viable cells. Different culture media and molecular methods used may account for some of the differences between results by Elli[55] and del Campo.[58] Taken together, these results suggest that *L. bulgaricus*, and perhaps *S. thermophilus*, may survive intestinal transit, but at low efficiency. Other probiotic species more suited to intestinal transit and administered in yogurt at the same levels as *L. bulgaricus* and *S. thermophilus* have been recovered at levels of up to 10^8 CFU/g compared to <10^5 CFU/g.[59]

When considering the impact of yogurt on intestinal function, several studies on yogurt with *B. animalis* DN-173 010 have demonstrated its ability to accelerate colonic transit time. One such study documented this effect compared to conventional yogurt in healthy women in a double-blind, crossover study.[69] However, no impact on fecal bacterial mass or secondary bile acids was detected.

Two studies evaluated the effect of conventional yogurt compared to yogurt containing additional probiotic bacteria on the level of mutans streptococci in saliva, useful as an indicator of caries risk. Caglar et al[70] studied yogurt containing *B. animalis* DN-173 010 in 21 healthy adults (21 to 24 years) in a double-blind, randomized crossover study. After consumption of the yogurt for 2 weeks, no changes in salivary *Lactobacillus* populations were observed, but modest reductions on salivary mutans streptococci were observed with the *Bifidobacterium*-containing yogurt. Nikawa et al[71] conducted a double-blind study of 40 healthy women who consumed yogurt containing *S. thermophilus* and *L. reuteri* ATCC55730 for 2 weeks; half the subjects received placebo yogurt before probiotic yogurt and the other half received probiotic yogurt before placebo yogurt. The group receiving placebo yogurt first showed no difference in mutans streptococci after placebo yogurt consumption, but *L. reuteri* yogurt resulted in reduced levels compared to baseline. The other group showed reductions with both *L. reuteri* yogurt and placebo yogurt, perhaps reflecting a carry-over effect from the *L. reuteri* yogurt. These 2 studies suggest that yogurt containing certain probiotic strains may reduce mutans streptococci, but the clinical significance of the observations have yet to be demonstrated.

Gluck and Gebbers[72] evaluated levels of potentially pathogenic nasal bacteria in 209 healthy subjects who consumed either fermented milk with *S. thermophilus* plus 3 additional probiotic bacteria or conventional yogurt for 3 weeks in an open, prospective trial. Results showed that those consuming probiotic milk, but not conventional yogurt, showed reductions in potentially pathogenic nasal bacteria (eg, *Staphylococcus aureus*, *S. pneumoniae*, and β-hemolytic streptococci) compared to baseline. Therefore, conventional yogurt does not appear to be effective at modulating nasal levels of potential pathogens.

IMMUNE FUNCTION

The gastrointestinal tract is a critical immune organ and serves as a key mucosal interface between the environment (lumen) and the host. Numerous animal, ex vivo, and human studies have documented the ability of yogurt, and the live cultures contained in yogurt, to impact immune system function.[73] Although many of these studies have tracked movement in markers of immune function (populations and activity of immune cells such phagocytes and lymphocytes, and blood-borne factors, including complement, antibodies, and cytokines), the most important expression of improved immune function is improved health, such as resistance to infectious disease or cancer, lack of allergic responses, or appropriateness of the inflammatory response.

Thirteen human clinical studies were retrieved from our literature search that concerned yogurt and immune function. Two additional ones[74,75] were conducted on fermented milks, not yogurt, and were therefore not included in this review. Some characteristics of these studies are shown in Table 8-7. All studies evaluated immune biomarkers, but only 4 studies also looked at some health or clinical parameters.[68,76-78] Although methods and endpoints varied, both conventional yogurt and probiotic yogurts were associated with movement in some immune biomarkers. The health endpoints evaluated in all 4 studies tracking them were allergy symptoms; 3 of 4 studies showed improvement in some measure of allergy symptoms.[76-78] Immune biomarker results are useful for establishing mechanisms of action, but need to be bolstered by patient-oriented health outcomes to understand the significance of the magnitude and type of biomarker movements observed.

YOGURT AS A DELIVERY VEHICLE FOR PROBIOTIC-DERIVED BENEFITS

The evidence for the impact of yogurt containing live microbes on numerous efficacy endpoints have been reviewed. Yogurt is not unique in being able to deliver these benefits; other product formats, including nonyogurt dairy products and dietary supplements, have been documented to show similar types of effects. Currently, there is a lack of human intervention studies comparing different probiotic delivery formats that would lead to conclusions about singular attributes of one format over another. In fact, none of the studies reviewed compared yogurt to other formats for delivery of the same live microbes. Such studies are important to determine the impact of delivery vehicle for functionality of health-promoting microbes.

Hypothetically, yogurt might be advantageous over other formats for several reasons. Yogurt is a popular food choice and, as such, provides a convenient, pleasing way for consumers to regularly add healthful bacteria to their diet. The authors of this chapter have conducted 4 yogurt trials in the past 3 years, and their compliance rates are consistently 90% or greater, much higher than expected in drug or supplement trials. Milk-based products such as yogurt, in addition to a healthful blend of macronutrients, also provide functional micronutrients that may complement the effects of probiotics. For example, dietary calcium has been shown to inhibit enteric infection by enterotoxigenic *Escherichia coli*. Oligosaccharides in milk—nondigestible to humans—likely provide prebiotic substrates to encourage growth of beneficial colonizing bacteria and inhibit pathogen binding to epithelial cell surfaces.[79] Antimicrobial effects of lactoferrin and immunomodulatory, antibacterial, antihypertensive effects of peptides in milk are well documented.[80] Dairy delivery may be especially suitable for probiotic effects on dental caries, because calcium is an important mineral in bones and teeth.

Although data are currently lacking to support additive or synergistic effects of milk delivery and microbial effects, it is a promising area for research.

(text continued on page 117)

TABLE 8-7

STUDIES ON THE EFFECT OF CONVENTIONAL YOGURT AND PROBIOTIC YOGURT ON VARIOUS IMMUNE ENDPOINTS

REFERENCE	PROBIOTIC STRAINS IN ADDITION TO YOGURT STARTERS?	RESULTS	IMMUNE-RELATED HEALTH ENDPOINT	IMMUNE FUNCTION TARGETED
68	Probiotic yogurt (B. lactis LKM512) or conventional yogurt	Increased IFN-γ in both probiotic yogurt and conventional yogurt compared to baseline; no statistically significant improvement in symptoms	Atopic dermatitis, $n = 10$ subjects with moderate atopic dermatitis	Allergy symptoms Cellular immune functions
76	Conventional yogurt, PY or no yogurt	Decrease in allergic symptoms in both age groups consuming yogurt; little effect on IFN-γ and IgE production	Allergic symptoms, $n = 60$ healthy young adults or seniors	Health parameters Vaccine response Cellular immune functions
77	Probiotic yogurt (L. acidophilus and Bifidobacterium, strains not disclosed), milk or no intervention	Yogurt increased IFN (and reduced IL-4) and improved symptoms	Symptoms of rhinopathy, $n = 13$ rhinopathic subjects, 7 healthy controls	Cellular immune functions; allergy symptoms
78	Probiotic yogurt (B. longum BB536) or conventional yogurt	Probiotic yogurt reduced eye symptoms compared to conventional yogurt; decreased IFN levels	Symptoms of Japanese cedar pollinosis, $n = 40$ subjects with pollinosis	Cellular immune functions; allergy symptoms
81	Probiotic yogurt (L. casei DN-114 001) or conventional yogurt	Increased % of granulocytes and monocytes showing phagocytic activity by probiotic yogurt consumption; oxidative burst activity and specific immune parameters did not change	None, $n = 26$ healthy adults	Cellular immune functions

(continued)

TABLE 8-7 *(continued)*

Studies on the Effect of Conventional Yogurt and Probiotic Yogurt on Various Immune Endpoints

REFERENCE	PROBIOTIC STRAINS IN ADDITION TO YOGURT STARTERS?	RESULTS	IMMUNE-RELATED HEALTH ENDPOINT	IMMUNE FUNCTION TARGETED
82	Probiotic yogurt (*L. casei* DN-114 001) or conventional yogurt	Increased number of cytotoxic T lymphocytes and CD69 on T lymphocytes compared to baseline	None, n = 33 healthy women	Cellular immune functions
83	Probiotic yogurt (*L. casei* DN-114 001) or conventional yogurt	No significant differences in cytokine responses between conventional and probiotic yogurt	None, n = 33 healthy women	Cytokine responses
84	Probiotic yogurt (*L. rhamnosus* GR-1 and *L. reuteri* RC-14) or conventional yogurt	Modulation of inflammatory cytokines	None, n = 40 (20 IBD, 20 healthy)	Anti-inflammatory
85	Conventional yogurt or skimmed milk	Increased CD4+/CD8+ ratio and production of IFN-c by lymphocytes in anorexia patients consuming yogurt	None, n = 16 anorexia nervosa patients and 16 healthy controls	Cellular immune functions
86	Probiotic yogurt (*L. gasseri* CECT 5714 and *L. coryniformis* CECT 5711) or conventional yogurt	Increased % of some white blood cell subsets and cytokine expression modified in both groups compared to baseline; effects stronger in probiotic yogurt	None, n = 30 healthy adults	Cellular immune functions
87	Conventional yogurt or no yogurt control group	No benefit of yogurt observed	None, n = 25 healthy women	Cellular immune functions
88	Conventional yogurt or milk	No benefit of yogurt observed	None, n = 20 healthy adults with atopic histories	Cellular, humoral, and phagocytic function

(continued from page 114)

CONCLUSION

The numerous studies reviewed in this chapter indicate that yogurt, and the live microbes contained in it, can deliver health benefits beyond its nutritive value. Benefits include improving tolerance to lactose in lactose maldigesters, modulating immune function, managing AAD, and reducing intestinal transit time. These observations suggest that the medical community should consider yogurt for its functional effects. It should be recognized that not all yogurts are functionally equivalent, however, especially with regard to additional live probiotics they might contain. Unless demonstrated otherwise, probiotic effects are considered to be specific to the strain and dose present in the product.[89] Therefore, health care professionals must be mindful of the scientific evidence available to substantiate claims made for specific products.

REFERENCES

1. Ebell MH, Siwek J, Weiss BD, et al. Strength of recommendation taxonomy (SORT): a patient-centered approach to grading evidence in the medical literature. *Am Fam Physician.* 2004;69(3):548-556.
2. Ishida Y, Nakamura F, Kanzato H, et al. Effect of milk fermented with *Lactobacillus acidophilus* strain L-92 on symptoms of Japanese cedar pollen allergy: a randomized placebo-controlled trial. *Biosci Biotechnol Biochem.* 2005;69(9):1652-1660.
3. Giovannini M, Agostoni C, Riva E, et al. A randomized prospective double blind controlled trial on effects of long-term consumption of fermented milk containing *Lactobacillus casei* in pre-school children with allergic asthma and/or rhinitis. *Pediatr Res.* 2007;62(2):215-220.
4. Giralt J, Regadera JP, Verges R, et al. Effects of probiotic *Lactobacillus casei* DN-114 001 in prevention of radiation-induced diarrhea: results from multicenter, randomized, placebo-controlled nutritional trial. *Int J Radiat Oncol Biol Phys.* 2008;71(4):1213-1219.
5. Anukam KC, Osazuwa EO, Osadolor HB, Bruce AW, Reid G. Yogurt containing probiotic *Lactobacillus rhamnosus* GR-1 and *L. reuteri* RC-14 helps resolve moderate diarrhea and increases CD4 count in HIV/AIDS patients. *J Clin Gastroenterol.* 2008;42(3):239-243.
6. Wenus C, Goll R, Loken EB, Biong AS, Halvorsen DS, Florholmen J. Prevention of antibiotic-associated diarrhoea by a fermented probiotic milk drink. *Eur J Clin Nutr.* 2008;62(2):299-301.
7. Conway S, Hart A, Clark A, Harvey I. Does eating yogurt prevent antibiotic-associated diarrhoea? A placebo-controlled randomised controlled trial in general practice. *Br J Gen Pract.* 2007;57(545):953-959.
8. Beausoleil M, Fortier N, Guenette S, et al. Effect of a fermented milk combining *Lactobacillus acidophilus* Cl1285 and *Lactobacillus casei* in the prevention of antibiotic-associated diarrhea: a randomized, double-blind, placebo-controlled trial. *Can J Gastroenterol.* 2007;21(11):732-736.
9. Beniwal RS, Arena VC, Thomas L, et al. A randomized trial of yogurt for prevention of antibiotic-associated diarrhea. *Dig Dis Sci.* 2003;48(10):2077-2082.
10. Agarwal KN, Bhasin SK, Faridi MM, Mathur M, Gupta S. *Lactobacillus casei* in the control of acute diarrhea: a pilot study. *Indian Pediatr.* 2001;38(8):905-910.
11. Agarwal KN, Bhasin SK. Feasibility studies to control acute diarrhoea in children by feeding fermented milk preparations Actimel and Indian dahi. *Eur J Clin Nutr.* 2002;56(suppl 4):S56-S59.
12. Pereg D, Kimhi O, Tirosh A, Orr N, Kayouf R, Lishner M. The effect of fermented yogurt on the prevention of diarrhea in a healthy adult population. *Am J Infect Control.* 2005;33(2):122-125.
13. Pedone CA, Arnaud CC, Postaire ER, Bouley CF, Reinert P. Multicentric study of the effect of milk fermented by *Lactobacillus casei* on the incidence of diarrhoea. *Int J Clin Pract.* 2000;54(9):568-571.
14. Boudraa G, Benbouabdellah M, Hachelaf W, Boisset M, Desjeux JF, Touhami M. Effect of feeding yogurt versus milk in children with acute diarrhea and carbohydrate malabsorption. *J Pediatr Gastroenterol Nutr.* 2001;33(3):307-313.
15. Pedone CA, Bernabeu AO, Postaire ER, Bouley CF, Reinert P. The effect of supplementation with milk fermented by *Lactobacillus casei* (strain DN-114 001) on acute diarrhoea in children attending day care centres. *Int J Clin Pract.* 1999;53(3):179-184.
16. Boudraa G, Touhami M, Pochart P, Soltana R, Mary JY, Desjeux JF. Effect of feeding yogurt versus milk in children with persistent diarrhea. *J Pediatr Gastroenterol Nutr.* 1990;11(4):509-512.

17. Sheu BS, Wu JJ, Lo CY, et al. Impact of supplement with *Lactobacillus*- and *Bifidobacterium*-containing yogurt on triple therapy for *Helicobacter pylori* eradication. *Aliment Pharmacol Ther*. 2002;16(9): 1669-1675.

18. Sykora J, Valeckova K, Amlerova J, et al. Effects of a specially designed fermented milk product containing probiotic *Lactobacillus casei* DN-114 001 and the eradication of *H. pylori* in children: a prospective randomized double-blind study. *J Clin Gastroenterol*. 2005;39(8):692-698.

19. Sheu BS, Cheng HC, Kao AW, et al. Pretreatment with *Lactobacillus*- and *Bifidobacterium*-containing yogurt can improve the efficacy of quadruple therapy in eradicating residual *Helicobacter pylori* infection after failed triple therapy. *Am J Clin Nutr*. 2006;83(4):864-869.

20. Colodner R, Edelstein H, Chazan B, Raz R. Vaginal colonization by orally administered *Lactobacillus rhamnosus* GG. *Isr Med Assoc J*. 2003;5(11):767-769.

21. Shalev E, Battino S, Weiner E, Colodner R, Keness Y. Ingestion of yogurt containing *Lactobacillus acidophilus* compared with pasteurized yogurt as prophylaxis for recurrent candidal vaginitis and bacterial vaginosis. *Arch Fam Med*. 1996;5(10):593-596.

22. Hilton E, Isenberg HD, Alperstein P, France K, Borenstein MT. Ingestion of yogurt containing *Lactobacillus acidophilus* as prophylaxis for candidal vaginitis. *Ann Intern Med*. 1992;116(5):353-357.

23. Kim MN, Kim N, Lee SH, et al. The effects of probiotics on PPI-triple therapy for *Helicobacter pylori* eradication. *Helicobacter*. 2008;13(4):261-268.

24. Goldman CG, Barrado DA, Balcarce N, et al. Effect of a probiotic food as an adjuvant to triple therapy for eradication of *Helicobacter pylori* infection in children. *Nutrition*. 2006;22(10):984-988.

25. Wendakoon CN, Thomson AB, Ozimek L. Lack of therapeutic effect of a specially designed yogurt for the eradication of *Helicobacter pylori* infection. *Digestion*. 2002;65(1):16-20.

26. Fabian E, Elmadfa I. Influence of daily consumption of probiotic and conventional yoghurt on the plasma lipid profile in young healthy women. *Ann Nutr Metab*. 2006;50(4):387-393.

27. Xiao JZ, Kondo S, Takahashi N, et al. Effects of milk products fermented by *Bifidobacterium longum* on blood lipids in rats and healthy adult male volunteers. *J Dairy Sci*. 2003;86(7):2452-2461.

28. Kiessling G, Schneider J, Jahreis G. Long-term consumption of fermented dairy products over 6 months increases HDL cholesterol. *Eur J Clin Nutr*. 2002;56(9):843-849.

29. St-Onge MP, Farnworth ER, Savard T, Chabot D, Mafu A, Jones PJ. Kefir consumption does not alter plasma lipid levels or cholesterol fractional synthesis rates relative to milk in hyperlipidemic men: a randomized controlled trial. *BMC Complement Altern Med*. 2002;2:1.

30. Agerholm-Larsen L, Raben A, Haulrik N, Hansen AS, Manders M, Astrup A. Effect of 8 week intake of probiotic milk products on risk factors for cardiovascular diseases. *Eur J Clin Nutr*. 2000;54(4):288-297.

31. Kawase M, Hashimoto H, Hosoda M, Morita H, Hosono A. Effect of administration of fermented milk containing whey protein concentrate to rats and healthy men on serum lipids and blood pressure. *J Dairy Sci*. 2000;83(2):255-263.

32. de Roos NM, Schouten G, Katan MB. Yoghurt enriched with *Lactobacillus acidophilus* does not lower blood lipids in healthy men and women with normal to borderline high serum cholesterol levels. *Eur J Clin Nutr*. 1999;53(4):277-280.

33. Anderson JW, Gilliland SE. Effect of fermented milk (yogurt) containing *Lactobacillus acidophilus* L1 on serum cholesterol in hypercholesterolemic humans. *J Am Coll Nutr*. 1999;18(1):43-50.

34. Rossouw JE, Burger EM, Van der Vyver P, Ferreira JJ. The effect of skim milk, yoghurt, and full cream milk on human serum lipids. *Am J Clin Nutr*. 1981;34(3):351-356.

35. Hepner G, Fried R, St Jeor S, Fusetti L, Morin R. Hypocholesterolemic effect of yogurt and milk. *Am J Clin Nutr*. 1979;32(1):19-24.

36. Pettoello-Mantovani M, Guandalini S, diMartino L, et al. Prospective study of lactose absorption during cancer chemotherapy: feasibility of a yogurt-supplemented diet in lactose malabsorbers. *J Pediatr Gastroenterol Nutr*. 1995;20(2):189-195.

37. Varela-Moreiras G, Antoine JM, Ruiz-Roso B, Varela G. Effects of yogurt and fermented-then-pasteurized milk on lactose absorption in an institutionalized elderly group. *J Am Coll Nutr*. 1992;11(2):168-171.

38. Arrigoni E, Marteau P, Briet F, Pochart P, Rambaud JC, Messing B. Tolerance and absorption of lactose from milk and yogurt during short-bowel syndrome in humans. *Am J Clin Nutr*. 1994;60(6): 926-929.

39. Savaiano DA, AbouElAnouar A, Smith DE, Levitt MD. Lactose malabsorption from yogurt, pasteurized yogurt, sweet acidophilus milk, and cultured milk in lactase-deficient individuals. *Am J Clin Nutr*. 1984;40(6):1219-1223.

40. Lerebours E, N'Djitoyap Ndam C, Lavoine A, Hellot MF, Antoine JM, Colin R. Yogurt and fermented-then-pasteurized milk: effects of short-term and long-term ingestion on lactose absorption and mucosal lactase activity in lactase-deficient subjects. *Am J Clin Nutr*. 1989;49(5):823-827.

41. Martini MC, Kukielka D, Savaiano DA. Lactose digestion from yogurt: influence of a meal and additional lactose. *Am J Clin Nutr*. 1991;53(5):1253-1258.

42. Onwulata CI, Rao DR, Vankineni P. Relative efficiency of yogurt, sweet acidophilus milk, hydrolyzed-lactose milk, and a commercial lactase tablet in alleviating lactose maldigestion. *Am J Clin Nutr.* 1989;49(6):1233-1237.

43. Marteau P, Pochart P, Flourie B, et al. Effect of chronic ingestion of a fermented dairy product containing *Lactobacillus acidophilus* and *Bifidobacterium bifidum* on metabolic activities of the colonic flora in humans. *Am J Clin Nutr.* 1990;52(4):685-688.

44. He T, Priebe MG, Zhong Y, et al. Effects of yogurt and bifidobacteria supplementation on the colonic microbiota in lactose-intolerant subjects. *J Appl Microbiol.* 2008;104(2):595-604.

45. Mohammad MA, Molloy A, Scott J, Hussein L. Plasma cobalamin and folate and their metabolic markers methylmalonic acid and total homocysteine among Egyptian children before and after nutritional supplementation with the probiotic bacteria *Lactobacillus acidophilus* in yoghurt matrix. *Int J Food Sci Nutr.* 2006;57(7-8):470-480.

46. Fabian E, Majchrzak D, Dieminger B, Meyer E, Elmadfa I. Influence of probiotic and conventional yoghurt on the status of vitamins B1, B2 and B6 in young healthy women. *Ann Nutr Metab.* 2008;52(1):29-36.

47. Parra D, Martinez JA. Amino acid uptake from a probiotic milk in lactose intolerant subjects. *Br J Nutr.* 2007;98(suppl 1):S101-S104.

48. Elmadfa I, Heinzle C, Majchrzak D, Foissy H. Influence of a probiotic yoghurt on the status of vitamins B(1), B(2) and B(6) in the healthy adult human. *Ann Nutr Metab.* 2001;45(1):13-18.

49. Larkin TA, Price WE, Astheimer LB. Increased probiotic yogurt or resistant starch intake does not affect isoflavone bioavailability in subjects consuming a high soy diet. *Nutrition.* 2007;23(10):709-718.

50. Labayen I, Forga L, Gonzalez A, Lenoir-Wijnkoop I, Nutr R, Martinez JA. Relationship between lactose digestion, gastrointestinal transit time and symptoms in lactose malabsorbers after dairy consumption. *Aliment Pharmacol Ther.* 2001;15(4):543-549.

51. Pelletier X, Laure-Boussuge S, Donazzolo Y. Hydrogen excretion upon ingestion of dairy products in lactose-intolerant male subjects: Importance of the live flora. *Eur J Clin Nutr.* 2001;55(6):509-512.

52. Eckburg PB, Bik EM, Bernstein CN, et al. Diversity of the human intestinal microbial flora. *Science.* 2005;308(5728):1635-1638.

53. Frank DN, St Amand AL, Feldman RA, Boedeker EC, Harpaz N, Pace NR. Molecular-phylogenetic characterization of microbial community imbalances in human inflammatory bowel diseases. *Proc Natl Acad Sci U S A.* 2007;104(34):13780-13785.

54. Ley RE, Turnbaugh PJ, Klein S, Gordon JI. Microbial ecology: human gut microbes associated with obesity. *Nature.* 2006;444(7122):1022-1023.

55. Elli M, Callegari ML, Ferrari S, et al. Survival of yogurt bacteria in the human gut. *Appl Environ Microbiol.* 2006;72(7):5113-5117.

56. Brigidi P, Swennen E, Vitali B, Rossi M, Matteuzzi D. PCR detection of *Bifidobacterium* strains and *Streptococcus thermophilus* in feces of human subjects after oral bacteriotherapy and yogurt consumption. *Int J Food Microbiol.* 2003;81(3):203-209.

57. Mater DD, Bretigny L, Firmesse O, et al. *Streptococcus thermophilus* and *Lactobacillus delbrueckii* subsp. *bulgaricus* survive gastrointestinal transit of healthy volunteers consuming yogurt. *FEMS Microbiol Lett.* 2005;250(2):185-187.

58. del Campo R, Bravo D, Canton R, et al. Scarce evidence of yogurt lactic acid bacteria in human feces after daily yogurt consumption by healthy volunteers. *Appl Environ Microbiol.* 2005;71(1):547-549.

59. Uyeno Y, Sekiguchi Y, Kamagata Y. Impact of consumption of probiotic lactobacilli-containing yogurt on microbial composition in human feces. *Int J Food Microbiol.* 2008;122(1-2):16-22.

60. Alvaro E, Andrieux C, Rochet V, et al. Composition and metabolism of the intestinal microbiota in consumers and non-consumers of yogurt. *Br J Nutr.* 2007;97(1):126-133.

61. Odamaki T, Xiao JZ, Iwabuchi N, et al. Fluctuation of fecal microbiota in individuals with Japanese cedar pollinosis during the pollen season and influence of probiotic intake. *J Investig Allergol Clin Immunol.* 2007;17(2):92-100.

62. Olivares M, Diaz-Ropero MA, Gomez N, et al. Oral administration of two probiotic strains, *Lactobacillus gasseri* CECT5714 and *Lactobacillus coryniformis* CECT5711, enhances the intestinal function of healthy adults. *Int J Food Microbiol.* 2006;107(2):104-111.

63. Matsumoto M, Ohishi H, Benno Y. Impact of LKM512 yogurt on improvement of intestinal environment of the elderly. *FEMS Immunol Med Microbiol.* 2001;31(3):181-186.

64. Guerin-Danan C, Chabanet C, Pedone C, et al. Milk fermented with yogurt cultures and *Lactobacillus casei* compared with yogurt and gelled milk: influence on intestinal microflora in healthy infants. *Am J Clin Nutr.* 1998;67(1):111-117.

65. Sullivan A, Barkholt L, Nord CE. *Lactobacillus acidophilus, Bifidobacterium lactis* and *Lactobacillus* F19 prevent antibiotic-associated ecological disturbances of *Bacteroides fragilis* in the intestine. *J Antimicrob Chemother.* 2003;52(2):308-311.

66. Marzotto M, Maffeis C, Paternoster T, et al. *Lactobacillus paracasei* A survives gastrointestinal passage and affects the fecal microbiota of healthy infants. *Res Microbiol.* 2006;157(9):857-866.

67. Matsumoto M, Benno Y. Consumption of *Bifidobacterium lactis* LKM512 yogurt reduces gut mutagenicity by increasing gut polyamine contents in healthy adult subjects. *Mutat Res.* 2004;568(2):147-153.

68. Matsumoto M, Aranami A, Ishige A, Watanabe K, Benno Y. LKM512 yogurt consumption improves the intestinal environment and induces the T-helper type 1 cytokine in adult patients with intractable atopic dermatitis. *Clin Exp Allergy.* 2007;37(3):358-370.

69. Marteau P, Cuillerier E, Meance S, et al. *Bifidobacterium animalis* strain DN-173 010 shortens the colonic transit time in healthy women: a double-blind, randomized, controlled study. *Aliment Pharmacol Ther.* 2002;16(3):587-593.

70. Caglar E, Sandalli N, Twetman S, Kavaloglu S, Ergeneli S, Selvi S. Effect of yogurt with *Bifidobacterium* DN-173 010 on salivary mutans streptococci and lactobacilli in young adults. *Acta Odontol Scand.* 2005;63(6):317-320.

71. Nikawa H, Makihira S, Fukushima H, et al. *Lactobacillus reuteri* in bovine milk fermented decreases the oral carriage of mutans streptococci. *Int J Food Microbiol.* 2004;95(2):219-223.

72. Gluck U, Gebbers JO. Ingested probiotics reduce nasal colonization with pathogenic bacteria (*Staphylococcus aureus, Streptococcus pneumoniae,* and beta-hemolytic streptococci). *Am J Clin Nutr.* 2003;77(2):517-520.

73. Borchers AT, Selmi C, Meyers FJ, Keen CL, Gershwin ME. Probiotics and immunity. *J Gastroenterol.* 2009;44(1):26-46.

74. Parra MD, Martinez de Morentin BE, Cobo JM, Mateos A, Martinez JA. Daily ingestion of fermented milk containing *Lactobacillus casei* DN114001 improves innate-defense capacity in healthy middle-aged people. *J Physiol Biochem.* 2004;60(2):85-91.

75. Marcos A, Warnberg J, Nova E, et al. The effect of milk fermented by yogurt cultures plus *Lactobacillus casei* DN-114001 on the immune response of subjects under academic examination stress. *Eur J Nutr.* 2004;43(6):381-389.

76. Van de Water J, Keen CL, Gershwin ME. The influence of chronic yogurt consumption on immunity. *J Nutr.* 1999;129(suppl 7):1492S-1495S.

77. Aldinucci C, Bellussi L, Monciatti G, et al. Effects of dietary yoghurt on immunological and clinical parameters of rhinopathic patients. *Eur J Clin Nutr.* 2002;56(12):1155-1161.

78. Xiao JZ, Kondo S, Yanagisawa N, et al. Effect of probiotic *Bifidobacterium longum* BB536 [corrected] in relieving clinical symptoms and modulating plasma cytokine levels of japanese cedar pollinosis during the pollen season. A randomized double-blind, placebo-controlled trial. *J Investig Allergol Clin Immunol.* 2006;16(2):86-93.

79. Tao N, DePeters EJ, Freeman S, German JB, Grimm R, Lebrilla CB. Bovine milk glycome. *J Dairy Sci.* 2008;91(10):3768-3778.

80. Legrand D, Pierce A, Elass E, Carpentier M, Mariller C, Mazurier J. Lactoferrin structure and functions. *Adv Exp Med Biol.* 2008;606:163-194.

81. Klein A, Friedrich U, Vogelsang H, Jahreis G. *Lactobacillus acidophilus* 74-2 and *Bifidobacterium animalis* subsp *lactis* DGCC 420 modulate unspecific cellular immune response in healthy adults. *Eur J Clin Nutr.* 2008;62(5):584-593.

82. Meyer AL, Micksche M, Herbacek I, Elmadfa I. Daily intake of probiotic as well as conventional yogurt has a stimulating effect on cellular immunity in young healthy women. *Ann Nutr Metab.* 2006;50(3):282-289.

83. Meyer AL, Elmadfa I, Herbacek I, Micksche M. Probiotic, as well as conventional yogurt, can enhance the stimulated production of proinflammatory cytokines. *J Hum Nutr Diet.* 2007;20(6):590-598.

84. Lorea Baroja M, Kirjavainen PV, Hekmat S, Reid G. Anti-inflammatory effects of probiotic yogurt in inflammatory bowel disease patients. *Clin Exp Immunol.* 2007;149(3):470-479.

85. Nova E, Toro O, Varela P, Lopez-Vidriero I, Morande G, Marcos A. Effects of a nutritional intervention with yogurt on lymphocyte subsets and cytokine production capacity in anorexia nervosa patients. *Eur J Nutr.* 2006;45(4):225-233.

86. Olivares M, Diaz-Ropero MP, Gomez N, et al. The consumption of two new probiotic strains, *Lactobacillus gasseri* CECT 5714 and *Lactobacillus coryniformis* CECT 5711, boosts the immune system of healthy humans. *Int Microbiol.* 2006;9(1):47-52.

87. Campbell CG, Chew BP, Luedecke LO, Shultz TD. Yogurt consumption does not enhance immune function in healthy premenopausal women. *Nutr Cancer.* 2000;37(1):27-35.

88. Wheeler JG, Bogle ML, Shema SJ, et al. Impact of dietary yogurt on immune function. *Am J Med Sci.* 1997;313(2):120-123.

89. Sanders ME. Use of probiotics and yogurts in maintenance of health. *J Clin Gastroenterol.* 2008;42(suppl 2):S71-S74.

9

Single and Multiple Probiotic Organisms in Therapy of Disease

Pramod Gopal, PhD and Gerald W. Tannock, PhD

The probiotic concept has a long history, but progress in the scientific and medical evaluation and validation of these products has been slow. Even today, adequate information by which the consumer and health professional can judge the efficacy and safety of retailed probiotics is often lacking.[1] Murch[2] has pointed out that there are more than 1.25 million Internet pages concerning probiotics, leading to his conclusion that "no other therapeutic modality spans the divide between internet voodoo and cutting edge high tech in this way." As pointed out by Katz,[3] more than half of the "probiotic papers" recorded in the PubMed database (NCBI) are reviews, not reports of the results of experimental science. Despite these concerns, a considerable list of health-promoting activities of probiotics that encompass a wide range of diseases has appeared in the literature (Table 9-1). The mechanistic explanations for these activities are often broad and somewhat vague, encompassing production of antimicrobial agents, blocking adhesion of pathogens and toxins to epithelial cells, and modulating the immune response. Nevertheless, some members of the medical profession, as well as the laity, have greeted with enthusiasm the use of current probiotic products as prophylaxis for atopic diseases (allergies), IBDs (CD, UC), and pouchitis.

Some probiotic products contain single strains of bacteria while others are composed of multiple bacterial strains of different genera and species. Whether there is a scientific rationale for the inclusion of several strains in probiotic products or it is a mere marketing strategy ("more bangs for your buck") is an open question. It is difficult to answer because of the paucity of reports of studies in which the efficacy of single-strain compared to multistrain probiotics was tested. In this chapter, we will consider the rationale for using multistrain probiotics, discuss the difficulties arising in the manufacture of multistrain probiotics, discuss the difficulties posed in evaluating the effects of probiotics and the meta-analysis evidence that some single- and multistrain probiotics are efficacious, discuss examples of multistrain probiotics, and point to the advantages of using probiotic strains singly rather than in combination.

(text continued on page 124)

Floch MH, Kim AS, eds.
Probiotics: A Clinical Guide (pp 121-130)
© 2010 Taylor & Francis Group

TABLE 9-1

PROBIOTIC PRODUCTS AND SUGGESTED HEALTH BENEFITS*†‡

PRODUCT	COMPANY	SUGGESTED HEALTH BENEFIT	BACTERIAL STRAIN
Single-strain probiotics			
BioGaia-ProBiotic Drops	BioGaia	Colic in babies	L. reuteri ATCC 55730
Align	Procter & Gamble	Mild to moderate IBS	B. infantis 35624
BioGaia Chewable Tablets	BioGaia	Antibiotic-associated diarrhea	L. reuteri ATCC 55730
Ultra Bifidus	Metagenics	Benefits defined for strain	B. lactis Bl-01
Culturelle LGG	ConAgra	Enhances body's natural defenses	L. rhamnosus strain GG
Lalflor	Institut Rosell	Clostridium difficile diarrhea	S. cerevisiae (S. boulardii)
HOWARU-Bifidus	Danisco	Immune modulation/protection against infections	B. animalis ssp. lactis HN019
HOWARU-Rhamnosus	Danisco	Enhance natural immunity	L. rhamnosus HN001
HOWARU-Dophilus	Danisco	Immune health and improve intestinal lactose intolerance	L. acidophilus NCFM
Zenflo	Institut Rosell	Irritable bowel syndrome	L. plantarum v299
Multistrain probiotics			
LactoViden ID	Metagenics	Healthy mucosal barrier	L. acidophilus NCFM, L. salivarius Ls-33, L. paracasei Lpc-37, L. plantarum Lp-115, S. thermophilus St-21
BifoViden ID	Metagenics	Minor intestinal irritations	B. lactis Bl-01, B. lactis Bl-07, S. thermophilus St-21

(continued)

TABLE 9-1 (continued)

PRODUCT	COMPANY	SUGGESTED HEALTH BENEFIT	BACTERIAL STRAIN
VSL#3	Sigma Tau Pharmaceutical Inc	Dietary management of UC, IBD, and ileal pouch	L. casei, L. plantarum, L. acidophilus, L. delbrueckii ssp. bulgaricus, B. longum, B. breve, B. infantis, S. thermophilus
ProbioKid	Institut Rosell	Healthy immune system	L. helveticus Rosell-52, B. infantis Rosell-33, B. bifidum Rosell-71
Lacidofil	Institut Rosell	IBS, dysbacteriosis, lactose intolerance	L. acidophilus Rosell-52, L. rhamnosus Rosell-11, B. longum Rosell-175
Protecflor	Institut Rosell	Traveler's diarrhea	S. boulardii, L. acidophilus Rosell-52, L. rhamnosus Rosell-11, B. longum Rosell-175
BioK+ CL1285	BioK	C. difficile diarrhea	L. acidophilus CL 1285, L. casei Lbc80r
Fem-Dophilus	Urexbiotech	Bacterial vaginosis	L. rhamnosus GR-1, L. reuteri RC-14
BLIS Bio Restore	BLIS Technologies	Postantibiotic treatment	S. salivarius K12, L. rhamnosus, B. lactis
Food format probiotics			
Activia	Danone	Gut health/gut transit	B. animalis DN-173010
Actimel	Danone	Immune benefit	L. casei DN114001
Yakult	Yakult-Honsha	Enhances body's natural defenses	L. casei strain Shirota
Gefilus	Valio	Gut health	L. rhamnosus GG

* Examples of some probiotic products.

† Information on the strain composition of each product has been gathered from the Internet and advertising brochures. Manufacturers often change strains used in products, so this list is based on best available information.

‡ Health benefits are listed on the basis of information available on the Internet and may not be proven.

RATIONALE FOR MULTI- VERSUS SINGLE-STRAIN PROBIOTICS

Adaptation and Persistence

It has been postulated that the ingestion of multiple bacterial strains increases the chances of achieving a probiotic effect. The healthy bowel is colonized by biodiverse and numerous microbiota that form a stable, self-regulating microbial community. The intrinsic factors that regulate the types and proportions of bacterial populations in the community act to competitively exclude allochthonous organisms, including probiotic strains that are introduced into the already-colonized bowel ecosystem. There is, however, considerable variation in the composition of the microbiota between human subjects.[4] Therefore, if several bacterial strains are included in a probiotic product, perhaps at least one will be adapted for persistence in the bowel of a particular human.

Synergism

Synergistic interactions between probiotic strains may enhance binding of bacterial cells to mucosal surfaces. This is a somewhat vexed proposition because although the results of in vitro experiments support this hypothesis, the existence of mucosa-associated populations in the human bowel is controversial.[5] Moreover, there is not any evidence from in vivo experiments to validate the claims of enhanced binding seen in vitro.[6-8]

Multivalency

Particular probiotics are claimed to have specific beneficial effects (see Table 9-1). One probiotic strain may target, for example, competition with pathogens. Another may produce an immunomodulatory effect.[9] Therefore, probiotic products containing several bacterial strains could benefit the consumer in several ways, rather like a multivalent vaccine promotes immunity to several pathogens.

DIFFICULTIES IN MANUFACTURING MULTISTRAIN PROBIOTICS

Commercial manufacture of probiotics involves the following general steps: fermentation, concentration using centrifugation or ultrafiltration, addition of matrix material, drying, milling, and packaging. Freeze drying is one of the most commonly used methods of drying, but some manufacturers use spray drying. Freeze drying is a "gentler" process and generally results in a higher proportion of viable cells in the preparation. Spray drying, on the other hand, is a more economical process. The choice of drying method is dependent on the characteristics of the probiotic strain to be included in the product.

For the manufacture of single strains, the manufacturing process is relatively straightforward. The main challenges involve optimization of the fermentation step (to achieve maximum biomass) and the drying conditions. The selection of appropriate stabilizers (cryoprotectants, lyoprotectants) has a huge effect on the shelf stability of the final product. It is, therefore, extremely important to pay attention to the composition of the matrix during the developmental process. Factors such as glass transition temperature (T_g) and water activity (a_w) of excipients (inactive substances used as carriers for the active ingredients) need to be taken into account. Optimization of freeze-drying parameters is another crucial step that affects viability (final yield) and survivability (shelf life) of the strain. It is important to note that each strain has specific requirements, hence the process needs to be customized.

The manufacture of probiotics containing multiple strains offers additional challenges compared to single-strain manufacture. There are many strains that can be cocultured. This cost-effective method is usually suitable for strains of the same genus. A notable exception, however, is coculturing in the manufacture of probiotics that contain strains of lactobacilli whose growth is compatible with that of strains of *Bifidobacterium* or *Leuconostoc*. The main problem with coculture is the lack of control of the composition of the final product. Adjustment of the proportions of strains in the innoculum does not always result in a consistent final product. Another issue associated with coculturing is the variable susceptibility of the strains to stabilizing and freeze-drying conditions. Often, one strain survives the process much better than others.

The most common method for the manufacture of probiotics containing multiple strains is back-blending of individual strains—ie, preparations of individual strains are manufactured and then milled and mixed in appropriate proportions to give the required final multistrain product. There are losses in yield associated with back-blending and milling. It is also important to ensure the compatibility of individual matrices before back-blending is carried out.

Another major issue associated with the manufacture of multistrain probiotics is ensuring that the correct cell numbers of each strain are present in the product and that they have appropriate shelf stability. There has been loss of credibility of probiotic products due to industrial failings on both aspects. Products said to contain multiple strains have often been found to contain less than what is claimed on labels. Temmerman et al[10] evaluated 55 European probiotics and found that live bacteria could not be detected in 40%. Forty-seven percent of the bacterial identifications were inaccurate. Using a culture-independent approach, Temmerman et al[11] also analyzed 10 European probiotic products, including dairy products, fruit juices, and freeze-dried powders. Many products were incorrectly labelled as to bacteriological content.

DIFFICULTIES IN INTERPRETING HEALTH BENEFITS ASSOCIATED WITH PROBIOTICS

Subjectivity

In the self-care health arena, there have been limited randomized, blind, and placebo-controlled trials, and there is a lingering impression that subjective benefits recorded by consumers may be heavily influenced by the "placebo effect." Controlled human trials that use objective measurements of efficacy (eg, measurement of blood chemistries or immunological factors) are more reliable, but often these trials do not utilize actual probiotic products but instead use experimental preparations. Therefore, direct application of experimental trials to real life may not always be possible.[1]

Lack of Valid Comparisons

Care must be taken in the interpretation of studies where both probiotics and prebiotics were administered to subjects. For example, Kukkonen and colleagues[12] administered a mixture of bacterial strains (*Lactobacillus rhamnosus* GG, *L. rhamnosus* LC705, *B. breve* Bb99, *Propionibacterium freudenreichii* ssp. *shermanii* JS) and galac-tooligosaccharides (prebiotic) to babies in a large trial concerned with the prevention of allergies. The placebo group received neither bacteria nor galactooligosaccharides. In the absence of groups that were administered either probiotic or prebiotic alone, it is impossible to conclude whether the observed reduction in eczema and atopic eczema in the treated group was due to the administration of probiotic, prebiotic, or synbiotic.

Variable Outcomes Between Trials

Where a probiotic has been tested in several independent trials, variation in outcomes may occur.[13] In other words, some trials may indicate a beneficial effect, another may not. For example, Kopp et al[14] found that administration of *L. rhamnosus* GG during pregnancy and to newborn offspring neither reduced the incidence of atopic eczema nor altered its severity. In contrast, Kalliomaki et al[15] showed a preventative effect of *L. rhamnosus* GG with regard to atopic eczema in at-risk children in a similar trial. Therefore, the results of meta-analysis, which supply a statistical overview of a number of trials, may be the best indicators of probiotic efficacy under these circumstances.

META-ANALYSIS EVIDENCE THAT SINGLE- AND MULTISTRAIN PROBIOTICS ARE EFFECTIVE

The efficacy of probiotics in the prevention and treatment of diarrhea associated with the use of antibiotics has been subjected to meta-analysis.[16] The outcomes of 9 randomized, double-blind, placebo-controlled trials were analyzed. Antibiotics were administered together with the probiotics or placebo. The odds ratio in favor of probiotic over placebo in preventing diarrhea was 0.39 (95% confidence interval [CI] 0.25 to 0.62; $P < .001$) for *S. boulardii* and 0.34 (0.19 to 0.61; $P < .01$) for lactobacilli. The authors of the report concluded that the results of the analysis suggested that probiotics could be used to prevent the occurrence of AAD. Similarly, Johnston and colleagues[17] concluded from a meta-analysis of 6 studies of AAD in children that there was significant benefit in the use of probiotics over placebo (relative risk 0.43, 95% CI 0.25 to 0.75; $I^2 = 70.1\%$). Neither study found evidence that probiotics could be used to treat AAD. Sazawal et al[18] reached similar conclusions with regard to the use of probiotics to prevent diarrhea. They analyzed the results of 34 trials. The authors pointed out that most of the trials had been conducted in developed countries in health-care environments; however, the greatest need to prevent diarrhea was in communities in developing countries. The probiotic effect did not differ to any extent between microbial strains (*S. boulardii*, *L. rhamnosus* GG, *L. acidophilus*, *L. bulgaricus*, *L. fermentum*, *B. longum*, *B. bifidum*, *Enterococcus* SF68) used alone or in combination. In contrast, meta-analysis of 7 studies that tested the effect of maintenance treatment with probiotics (*L. rhamnosus* GG, *E. coli* Nissle 1917, VSL#3, *S. boulardii*) among patients with CD in remission did not demonstrate any benefit of probiotic treatment.[19]

PROBIOTIC EFFECTS OF MULTISTRAIN PROBIOTICS

Alleviation of Symptoms of Irritable Bowel Syndrome

A multistrain (*L. rhamnosus* GG, *L. rhamnosus* LC705, *B. breve* Bb99, *P. freudenreichii* ssp. *shermanii* JS) probiotic was tested in a randomized, double-blind, placebo-controlled trial.[20] One hundred and three subjects were recruited and were divided into diarrhea-predominant, constipation predominant, and mixed-symptom groups. Gastrointestinal symptoms and bowel habits were recorded. A total of 86 subjects completed the 6-month study. Each month, the subjects recorded their symptoms that had occurred during a 1-week period. The intensity of abdominal pain, distention, and flatulence was graded on a 0 to 4 scale, and the appearance of stool was recorded. At the conclusion of the trial, the total symptom score (abdominal pain/distension/flatulence/borborygmi) was 7.7 (95% CI: –13.9 to –1.6) points lower in the probiotic group (*P* = .015). This represented a median reduction of 42% in the symptom score of the probiotic group compared with 6% in the placebo group. With respect to individual symptoms, borborygmi were milder in the probiotic group (*P* = .008). Kajander et al[21] carried out a further trial in order to explain the alleviation of symptoms. This study lasted for 6 months and included 55 subjects. Alterations in SCFA concentrations (bacterial metabolic products in feces) did not differ between test and placebo groups, but there was a 67% decrease in fecal β-glucuronidase activity in the group receiving probiotics compared to that receiving placebo. Although all of the ingested probiotic strains were detected in the feces of probiotic-treated subjects, alterations in the composition of the fecal microbiota were not detected.

Prevention of Pouchitis

Chronic pouchitis is the most important long-term complication leading to poor function following ileal pouch-anal anastomosis for UC.[22] Antibiotic administration reduces symptoms of pouchitis, indicating that bacteria have a role in pathogenesis. Elahi et al[23] conducted a meta-analysis of 5 trials on the effect of probiotics on pouchitis (acute, chronic, recurrent, remission). Four of these studies (conducted by the same research group in each case) utilized the multistrain (*L. casei, L. plantarum, L. acidophilus, L. delbrueckii* ssp. *bulgaricus, B. longum, B. breve, B. infantis, S. thermophilus*) probiotic product VSL#3. The outcome of interest in the meta-analysis was for pouchitis, defined as a pouchitis disease activity index of >7.0. Pooling of the results from 5 trials yielded an odds ratio of 0.04 (95% CI 0.01 to 0.14, *P* < .0001) in the probiotic group relative to the placebo group. The need for 8 bacterial strains in the product is not proven because only 2 (*S. thermophilus, B. infantis*) of the strains were detected in the bowel of patients who had been administered VSL#3 during a 6-week period.[24]

SINGLE-STRAIN PROBIOTICS PERMIT EASIER ASSESSMENTS OF MECHANISTIC EFFECTS

Reports of methodical comparisons of the efficacy of specific probiotic strains alone, or in combination, have not been reported in the literature to our knowledge. However, New Zealand researchers have used the same bacterial strains in 2 trials: one in which the strains were administered singly and the other in combination.[25,26] These trials were done to prevent eczema in children. Meta-analysis of 12 eczema trials involving 781 participants conducted by Boyle and colleagues[13] has showed that there was no significant difference in participant- or parent-rated symptom scores in favor of probiotic treatment (5 trials, 313 participants). Symptom severity on a scale from 0 to 20 was 0.90 points lower after probiotic treatment than after placebo treatment (95% CI –1.04, 2.84; P = .36). There was also no significant difference in participant- or parent-rated overall eczema severity in favor of probiotic treatment (3 trials, 150 participants), and there was no significant difference in investigator-rated eczema severity between probiotic and placebo treatments (7 trials, 588 participants). Investigator-rated eczema severity was 2.46 points lower after probiotic treatment than after placebo treatment (95% CI –2.53, 7.45; P = .33). Subgroup analysis by age of participant, severity of eczema, presence of atopy, or presence of food allergy did not identify a population with different treatment outcomes to the population as a whole. These observations led the analysts to conclude that the evidence suggested that probiotics were not an effective treatment for eczema. What the outcomes of eczema trials do point to, however, is that efficacy is related to the bacterial strain administered to the babies and whether the bacteria are consumed during pregnancy by mothers as well as after birth by their infants. In their first study,[25] the New Zealand researchers administered *L. rhamnosus* HN001 and *B. lactis* (*B. animalis* ssp. *lactis*) HN019 to atopic children with eczema. The probiotic group (*n* = 29) received a mixture of the 2 bacteria daily, whereas the placebo group (*n* = 30) did not. Measurement of the extent and severity of atopic eczema (SCORAD) showed that only food-sensitized children benefited marginally from probiotic administration: SCORAD geometric mean ratio 0.73 (95% CI 0.54 to 1.00; P = .047). In the second study,[26] the same 2 bacterial strains were used, but this time singly. Thus, there were 3 groups of subjects: *L. rhamnosus* HN001 as probiotic, *B. lactis* HN019 as probiotic, and placebo. A benefit of probiotic administration was seen only in the *L. rhamnosus* HN001 group; infants receiving this probiotic strain had a significantly reduced risk of eczema by 2 years of age compared with placebo (hazard ratio 0.51, 95% CI 0.30 to 0.85; P = .01). The mothers in this large study (*n* = 474) were administered probiotic or placebo from 35 weeks gestation until 6 months if breastfeeding, and their infants received the same treatment from birth to 2 years of age. The major importance of this study was that it pinpointed that efficacy was specific to a particular strain, in this case *L. rhamnosus* HN001—an achievement that would not have been possible if combinations of bacterial strains had been used. In a supplemental study,[27] the researchers found that more babies (P = .034) born to mothers who had received the *L. rhamnosus* HN001 probiotic had interferon-γ in cord blood and at higher concentration (P = .026) than did those in the placebo or *B. lactis* HN019 groups. Although this observation does not explain the differential effect of the probiotics, it points to the possibility of assigning mechanistic explanations of efficacy if single-strain preparations are used.

CONCLUSION

1. The manufacture of multistrain probiotics is more difficult because of physiological differences and survival attributes between bacterial strains.

2. There does not appear to be any clinical evidence in the literature to favor the use of multistrain probiotics over single-strain preparations. Equally, evidence suggesting that single-strain probiotics are more efficacious than multistrain preparations is lacking.

3. From an experimentalist's point of view, the use of single-strain probiotics should enable easier investigation of the mechanisms by which the probiotic effect is achieved.

REFERENCES

1. Tannock GW. Probiotics: time for a dose of realism. *Curr Issues Intest Microbiol.* 2003;4:33-42.
2. Murch SH. Probiotics as mainstream allergy therapy? *Arch Dis Child.* 2005;90:881-882.
3. Katz JA. Antibiotics, probotics, prebiotics, fish oil and micronutrients (past). *Inflamm Bowel Dis.* 2006;12:S12.
4. Tannock GW. What immunologists should know about bacterial communities of the human bowel. *Seminars Microbiol.* 2007;19:94-105.
5. Tannock GW. The search for disease-associated compositional shifts in bowel bacterial communities. *Trends Microbiol.* 2008;16:488-495.
6. Collado M, Meriluoto J, Salminen S. Development of new probiotics by strain combination: is it possible to improve the adhesion to intestinal mucus? *J Dairy Sci.* 2007;90:2710-2716.
7. Juntunen M, Kirjavainen PV, Ouwehand A, Salminen S, Isolauri E. Adherence of probiotics bacteria to human intestinal mucus in healthy infants and during rotavirus infection. *Clin Diagn Lab Immunol.* 2001;8:293-296.
8. Ouwehand A, Isolauri E, Kirjavainen P, Tolkko S, Salminen S. The mucus binding of *Bifidobacterium lactis* Bb12 is enhanced in presence of *Lactobacillus rhamnosus* GG and *L. delbrueckii* ssp. *bulgaricus. Lett Appl Microbiol.* 2000;30:10-13.
9. Timmerman HM, Niers LE, Ridwan BU, et al. Design of a multispecies probiotic mixture to prevent infectious complications in critically ill patients. *Clin Nutr.* 2006;26:450-459.
10. Temmerman R, Pot B, Huys G, Swings J. Identification and antibiotic susceptibility of bacterial isolates from probiotic products. *Int J Food Microbiol.* 2003;81:1-10.
11. Temmerman R, Scheirlinck I, Huys G, Swings J. Culture independent analysis of probiotic products by denaturing gradient gel electrophoresis. *Appl Environ Micro.* 2003;69:220-226.
12. Kukkonen K, Savilahti E, Haahtela T, et al. Probiotics and prebiotic galacto-oligosaccharides in the prevention of allergic diseases: a randomized, double-blind, placebo-controlled trial. *J Allergy Clin Immunol.* 2007;119:192-198.
13. Boyle RJ, Bath-Hextall FJ, Leonardi-Bee J, Murrell DF, Tang MLK. Probiotics for treating eczema. *Cochrane Database Syst Rev.* 2008;4:CD006135.
14. Kopp MV, Hennemuth I, Heinzmann A, Urbanek R. Randomized, double blind, placebo-controlled trial of probiotics for primary prevention: no clinical effects of *Lactobacillus* GG supplementation. *Pediatrics.* 2008;121:e850-e856.
15. Kalliomaki M, Salminen S, Poussa T, Arvilommi H, Isolauri E. Probiotics in primary prevention of atopic disease: a randomised placebo-controlled trial. *Lancet.* 2001;357:1076-1079.
16. D'Souza AL, Rajkumar C, Cooke J, Bulpitt CJ. Probiotics in prevention of antibiotic associated diarrhea: meta-analysis. *BMJ.* 2002;324:1361-1366.
17. Johnston BC, Supina AL, Vohra S. Probiotcs for pediatric antibiotic-associated diarrhea: a meta-analysis of randomized placebo-controlled trials. *CMAJ.* 2006;175:377-383.
18. Sazawal S, Hiremath G, Dhinga U, Malik P, Deb S, Black RE. Efficacy of probiotics in prevention of acute diarrhea: a meta-analysis of masked, randomized, placebo-controlled trials. *Lancet Infect Dis.* 2006;6:374-382.
19. Rolfe VE, Fortun PJ, Hawkey CJ, Bath-Hextall FJ. Probiotics for maintenance of remission in Crohn's disease. *Cochrane Database Syst Rev.* 2006;4:CD004826.
20. Kajander K, Hatakka K, Poussa T, Farkkila M, Korpela R. A probiotic mixture alleviates symptoms in irritable bowel syndrome patients: a controlled 6-month intervention. *Aliment Pharmacol Ther.* 2005;22:387-394.
21. Kajander K, Krogius-Kurikka L, Rinttila T, Karjalainen H, Palva A, Korpela R. Effect of multispecies probiotic supplementation on intestinal microbiota in irritable bowel syndrome. *Aliment Pharmacol Ther.* 2007;26:463-473.
22. Shen B, Fazio VW, Remzi FH, Lashner BA. Clinical approach to diseases of ileal-anal anastomosis. *Am J Clin Gastrotenterol.* 2005;100:2796-2807.

23. Elahi B, Nikfar S, Derakhshani S, Vafaie M, Abdollahi M. On the benefit of probiotics in the management of pouchitis in patients underwent ileal pouch anal anastomosis: a meta-analysis of controlled clinical trials. *Dig Dis Sci.* 2008;53:1278-1284.

24. Bibiloni R, Fedorak RN, Tannock GW, et al. VSL#3 probiotic-mixture induces remission in patients with active ulcerative colitis. *Am J Gastroenterol.* 2005;100:1539-1546.

25. Sistek D, Kelly R, Wickens K, Stanley T, Fitzharris P, Crane J. Is the effect of probiotics on atopic dermatitis confined to food sensitized children? *Clin Exp Allergy.* 2006;36:629-633.

26. Wickens K, Black PN, Stanley TV, et al. A differential effect of 2 probiotics in the prevention of eczema and atopy: a double-blind, randomized, placebo-controlled trial. *J Allergy Clin Immunol.* 2008;122:788-794.

27. Prescott SL, Wickens K, Westcott L, et al; The Probiotic Study Group. Supplementation with *Lactobacillus rhamnosus* or *Bifidobacterium lactis* probiotics in pregnancy increases cord blood interferon-γ and breast milk transforming growth factor-β and immunoglobulin A detection. *Clin Exp Allergy.* 2008;38:1606-1614.

10

Development of Cultured Dairy Probiotic Food Products

Miguel Freitas, PhD

On the basis of the extensive basic and clinical research that has been conducted on dairy probiotic food products, evidence has accumulated over the recent years to support these products as an important part of the daily diet in many countries. The development of a cultured dairy probiotic food product is a complex process involving years of research. Initial steps include the collection and identification of candidate probiotic strains for a particular beneficial effect. Subsequently, several preclinical approaches, such as in vitro and in vivo models, can be used to select potential candidates. Incorporation of these candidate probiotic strains in dairy foods, including the fermentation process, is also a critical step that requires extensive trials and technical skills. Finally, the beneficial effects of a probiotic food product should be supported by reliable scientific evidence that has been validated in human trials, according to methods recognized by the scientific community. When clinical trials are performed, special attention must be placed on the intended use of the product, the design of the study, and the markers and endpoints selected.

The Joint Food and Agriculture Organization/World Health Organization Working Group (FAO/WHO) defines probiotics as "live microorganisms which, when administered in adequate amounts, confer a health benefit on the host."[1] A dairy probiotic food product can therefore be defined as a dairy food containing specific live microorganisms in a sufficient quantity that have demonstrated beneficial effects on the host.

The specific properties of a cultured dairy probiotic product depend on the type and amount of ingredients, the composition of the milk, the fermentation process, and the cultures, including the probiotic bacteria used. Probiotic benefits are strain specific, and not all live cultures or dairy products containing live cultures are considered probiotics or probiotic-containing foods, because the beneficial effect to the consumer should be clinically proven. This chapter describes the very sophisticated chain leading to the development of a cultured dairy probiotic food, from the collection, identification, and selection process of candidate probiotic strains, to the development of the probiotic-containing food, and performing the human clinical testing of the food.

Floch MH, Kim AS, eds.
Probiotics: A Clinical Guide (pp 131-138)
© 2010 Taylor & Francis Group

COLLECTION AND IDENTIFICATION OF POTENTIAL CANDIDATE PROBIOTIC STRAINS TO USE IN CULTURED DAIRY FOOD PRODUCTS

The candidate probiotic strains must not only provide a beneficial effect to the host when consumed in the dairy product, but also be able to ferment milk and multiply during fermentation. Candidate cultures usually belong to the group of microorganisms known as LAB because they use lactose, the naturally occurring milk sugar, and transform it into lactic acid. LAB have been used for preservation of food by fermentation for thousands of years: however, the term "probiotic" should be reserved for live microorganisms that ultimately have been shown in human studies to provide a benefit.

LAB include, but are not limited to, species of *Lactobacillus* (eg, *L. casei* and *L. acidophilus*), *Lactococcus*, and *Streptococcus thermophilus*. The genus *Bifidobacterium* is taxonomically distinct from the other LAB, but many *Bifidobacterium* species are able to ferment milk; therefore, these are usually included as part of the LAB group. Each species of *Lactobacillus* or *Bifidobacterium* can have many different strains, which increases considerably the number of potential candidates.

Those seeking to develop a probiotic dairy product may collect potential probiotic candidates by isolating microbial strains mainly from traditional fermented dairy products in regions of the world that have been shown to possess particular human health assets and a high consumption of fermented milks (eg, high life expectancy in Japan or Eastern Europe). These assets could be related to the presence of specific LAB with potential beneficial effects. Today, strains of *Lactobacillus* and *Bifidobacterium* are the most commonly used types of probiotics in dairy foods. These bacteria are not considered "probiotics" until the strains are isolated, purified, and proved to benefit when consumed.[2]

The initial characterization of the potential probiotic strain consists of identifying the microorganism's genus and species, which is greatly helped by recent advancements in molecular and genetic sequencing. Identification of the candidate to the strain level is an important step for controlled research and eventually in production quality control. This identification and molecular characterization can be done using techniques that survey the total genomic DNA, such as DNA-DNA hybridization or pulsed field gel electrophoresis, or by using more targeted genomic techniques such as sequencing of DNA encoding 16S rRNA or randomly amplified polymorphic DNA.[3]

It is generally accepted that probiotic benefits are strain specific and that beneficial effects can only be attributed to the strain or strains tested, and not to the species, genus, the whole group of LAB, or other probiotics.[2] Ultimately, if the objective is to make a claim associated to the entire product, human clinical trials and other reliable scientific investigation of benefits must be conducted on the specific probiotic strain, preferably incorporated in the food matrix, or a functional equivalent, that is being sold.

Because each probiotic strain is considered unique, proper identification of a strain includes identification of the genus, species, and strain name (eg, *L. casei* DN-114 001). Some food manufacturers choose to label a product using trademark names for the strains; however, the full scientific designation as identified initially should be made available to any consumer upon request.

Several probiotic industrial suppliers also engage in this collection and characterization process, making their strains commercially available to the food industry. However, in contrast to the food industry approach, probiotic strains made available by supplier companies are rarely tested in the food matrix (eg, milk vs rice cereal) as ingested by consumers, which may limit the ability of a food manufacturer to make claims for its product. Specifically, it creates a challenge with regard to making claims associated directly with the food product consumption as opposed to the benefits associated with the strain. Therefore, the role of the matrix delivering the probiotic strain, the specific manufacturing process for the product (eg, fermentation or absence thereof), and the resulting benefits must be taken into account (eg, yogurt compared to lyophilized strains). Some effects may not be reproduced using a completely different vehicle, for instance, due to a reduced viability of the strain.[4]

In Vitro and In Vivo Screening: Preclinical Selection of Candidate Probiotic Strains

Following the initial identification step, the next stage should involve several screening tests including in vitro functional mapping approaches designed to select promising probiotic strains for specific benefits.

In general, the first step in this selection process consists of identifying the benefit of interest on the basis of consumer expectations and public demands (eg, maintaining a specific body function). Then, several screening tests can be carried out simultaneously to investigate the desired benefit. Historically, researchers used tests such as adherence to intestinal epithelial cells, inhibition of growth, and attachment of pathogens to the bacteria. However, new biomarkers are constantly being identified, and new models are being developed in order to help better select and validate effective candidate probiotics for new benefits. A clear example is the progress made in understanding the human gut microbiota and its implications for obesity and weight management.[5] The choice of biomarkers constitutes an essential step, involving considerable literature research and scientific skills. With this in hand, it is possible to carry out molecular or cellular screening of a large number of LAB using criteria that have been validated and recognized as being representative of the targeted benefit.

Several in vitro and in vivo animal models are relied on to simulate different human body functions. Cell cultures are one in vitro model commonly used in nutrition-related studies. They simplify cellular and molecular physiology by isolating a cell or molecule from a complex organ. These models can be very useful for assessing the candidate probiotic strain's impact on cell functions and biochemical markers such as immune response. However, they cannot replace clinical or animal studies because the interactions between cells, tissues, and organs are multiple and complex. Therefore, these techniques are mainly used as preliminary screening models or complements of in vivo tests and clinical studies. Nevertheless, in vitro models can provide important information about the cellular and molecular mechanisms at play, which can subsequently be useful for developing in vivo and clinical studies. In contrast to in vitro testing, in vivo studies carried out using an animal model can help assess the effects of diet or a complex food product on different body functions. In vivo models can therefore further help in the selection of candidate probiotic strains that exhibit a potential benefit in vitro. The choice of the in vivo model is done in order to get as close as possible to human physiology. The animals most commonly used are rodents. Examples of currently used in vitro and in vivo models include the following:

- Cell lines originated from the intestinal epithelium (eg, HT29, Caco-2, and T84);[6-8]
- Human tissue samples (eg, mucosal explants from healthy or sick patients);[9,10]

- Germ-free mice or mice implanted with human intestinal flora;[11]
- Laboratory models that mimic the digestive system to study survival of the strains when exposed to the aggressive conditions of stomach acids and pancreatic secretions (eg, stomach-small intestine and colon models).

In appropriate circumstances, preclinical data can also serve as the foundation of scientific support along with human clinical trials and other sound scientific methods of investigation.

Food companies are also developing new methods and technologies to obtain probiotics that will result in flavorful products with demonstrated and accepted organoleptic benefits appealing to consumers. Candidate strains with potential probiotic benefits are of no interest unless they can be used for industrial production. Therefore, the candidate strains need to be characterized on the basis of technological criteria, such as (1) the ability of the strain to be propagated, produced on a large scale, and packaged for subsequent use; (2) adaptation to the medium in which it will be used (eg, milk); (3) survival in the finished product for several weeks at the required refrigeration temperature; and (4) the ability to produce the organoleptic characteristics compatible with the intended product. Reproducibility and stability are also important criteria to consider. The survival of the probiotic strains in dairy foods depends on various factors, including the production of lactic acid and sensitivity to pH, the production of bactericidal compounds, the oxygenation of the milk, and the industrial process.

Once characterized and selected, the potential probiotic strains can be further "trained" to better express their potential to the maximum. This can be done by adapting the culture medium and the strains' growth environment during propagation and fermentation of milk (eg, available nutrients, association with other bacterial strains, and temperature).

MILK FERMENTATION PROCESS AND TRADITIONAL YOGURT CULTURES

Milks fermented using LAB can be divided into 2 categories, depending on the microorganisms used and temperature of fermentation. Yogurt and similar products are obtained by the fermentation of milk by a combination of 2 or more, as applicable, thermophilic LAB. Such is the case with traditional yogurt that is fermented by *L. delbrueckii* spp. *bulgaricus* (*L. bulgaricus*) and *S. thermophilus*. Fermentation of milk by these 2 cultures originates the base matrix of a yogurt, to which additional LAB strains, including specific probiotics, can be incorporated at different phases during fermentation. Three different technological ways of incorporating a probiotic strain to a fermented dairy product can be considered: (1) the strain can be used alone to ferment the milk (no traditional yogurt cultures are used); (2) the strain can be used with other strains (probiotic or nonprobiotic) in a mix to ferment the milk; (3) one part of the milk is fermented using the traditional yogurt cultures (*L. bulgaricus* and *S. thermophilus*) and separately another part of the milk is fermented using the probiotic strain, and these 2 parts are combined afterward.

The selection criteria of the specific strains of traditional yogurt cultures (*L. bulgaricus* and *S. thermophilus*) are mainly related to technological suitability, including acidification effect, production of exopolysaccharides for viscosity buildup, proteolysis, and the production of flavoring agents. The choice of these 2 traditional yogurt cultures requires experienced skills. Several combinations of specific strains of both *L. bulgaricus* and *S. thermophilus* have to be tested on a skilled basis to produce the traditional yogurt matrix that will be used in the industrial process. The technological performance of a mix of strains, including the probiotic strains, is first estimated in the laboratory and then tested in the pilot plant before industrialization.

Historically, the purpose of the fermentation was mainly to protect milk from spoilage. The conversion of lactose into lactic acid by LAB, thus considerably lowering the pH of the milk, ensured protection against the growth of many pathogenic and spoilage organisms. Nowadays, the fermentation process is in some cases important for the specific probiotic to deliver the expected benefit. This means that the full benefit for such a probiotic is not solely associated with the strain but with the entire finished food product, including the combination of strains used and the specific fermentation process.

Probiotic food products are unique in that keeping the microbes alive must be a consideration through the stages of product concept, formulation, and the sales/distribution process. The typical issues surrounding product development also apply: products should be tasty, convenient, and priced competitively. But additional considerations must also be addressed: (1) optimizing growth conditions for the probiotic strain or strains, (2) defining a product that can deliver in the right amount the probiotic strain or strains successfully in a viable and functional form to the active site in the human body, and (3) determining the role of the total food in providing the expected benefit. These considerations are not trivial, and unfortunately not all food products marketed as "probiotic" suitably address them.[2]

The final step of this selection involves inserting the strains into a food as it will be produced at industrial level in order to ensure industrial viability and validate their effects through appropriate testing. This step is essential to ensure that changing the scale of production (from the pilot laboratory to the industrial production plant) does not alter the properties studied during the previous stages.

CLINICAL STUDIES THAT SUPPORT THE BENEFITS

It is generally accepted that probiotic benefits have to be supported by well-conducted clinical trials. The quality and results of clinical studies are essential to support the benefits of, and claims made about, a probiotic food product. These studies are viewed as the final proof, and the strength of the claim made on the food as consumed depends on the strength of this body of evidence. Depending on the intended use of the product, there are various degrees of clinical support and strength. If a statistically significant improvement occurs in a subject body function marker, condition, symptom, well-being or quality of life, risk of disease, or reduction of severity or duration of disease, then the evidence should be supportive and convincing for the recommended consumption of that particular probiotic food. The primary and secondary outcomes must be clear and measurable, and the study protocol should preferably involve a randomized, double-blind, placebo-controlled design. The selected placebo must be very similar to the probiotic food in terms of nutritional profile, taste, texture, color, and flavor, but must be devoid of the probiotic strains or LAB strains. In food-related studies, it is sometimes difficult to design a placebo of this type. This is why it is occasionally acceptable to use a control group that receives no product at all during the study. The probiotic food product tested should be administered in its commercial form, or as close as possible to its commercial form, in order to demonstrate the physiological effect under normal conditions of use. Minimal changes in the product formula (eg, fat content, sugar, and flavors) that, based on appropriate investigation, do not have an impact on the product benefit do not need to be specifically tested in additional clinical trials.

The choice of assessment criteria, markers, and endpoints is complex. Options include using exposure markers, markers of target functions (eg, natural killer cells activity for the immune system, intestinal transit time for digestive health), or markers of improvement in the state of health and well-being and/or a reduction of the risk of disease.[12] Regarding the subjects used in the clinical study, certain groups can be targeted because the structure, function, or end point investigated is more accessible in this group than in the general population. For instance, competition athletes are useful for the investigation of immune function benefits because they belong to a population subgroup where the body's defenses are more constantly challenged by physical stress.[13] Results of studies documenting benefits of the probiotic food product or strain should be made available to the consumer or health-care professional via company and product Web sites or other means.

SAFETY ASSESSMENT

It is generally recognized that commercial probiotic strains are safe for the healthy individual. Usually, candidate probiotic strains for a dairy probiotic food product belong to the LAB group, mainly from *Lactobacillus*, *Bifidobacterium*, and *S. thermophilus* species. Their safety for use in foods is accepted because these LAB have a long history of safe use in fermented dairy products such as yogurt, cheese, and milk and these properties are stable during the refrigeration process. Nevertheless, the safety of a cultured probiotic food product should be documented from the early selection of the candidate probiotic strains through their application in human trials and in the final food product in-market consumption. Companies should follow existing international and local guidelines, regulations, and laws for the safety evaluation of the probiotic strain or strains, using widely recognized safety criteria. This evaluation can be done during the different product development steps (eg, identification of candidate strains, pre-clinical selection, and clinical trials).

The FAO/WHO guidelines recommend that LAB probiotic strains be characterized using a series of specific tests, including (1) determination of antibiotic resistance patterns; (2) assessment of certain metabolic activities (eg, D-lactate production and bile salt deconjugation); (3) assessment of side effects during human studies; (4) epidemiological surveillance of adverse incidents in consumers; (5) if not existing, establishing a history of safe use on the basis of intended use of the genus and species in question; (6) conducting toxicity or pathogenicity assessments in validated laboratory or animal models that are relevant to the species being considered, as needed.[1,2]

CHARACTERIZATION OF THE FINISHED FOOD PRODUCT: QUALITY CONTROL

The dairy industry must control the quality of its products, have this quality recognized, and thus gain the confidence of the consumer. Quality assurance involves the manufacturer, the transporter, and the distributor of the product. Various criteria have been defined that can be used to ensure the quality and safety of the finished food products—eg, organoleptic, microbiological, and sensory. In addition, dairy products must comply with the applicable local regulations in force in the country where they are to be sold.

Tests of the organoleptic criteria can be carried out on the production lines using a defined testing schema. Regarding the microbiology criteria, bacterial counts in the finished product and monitoring of process controls relating to these criteria should be ongoing. Today, several independent laboratories can perform appropriate and generally recognized microbiological analysis and enumeration of lactic acid cultures. However, current methods have certain limitations that need to be taken into account such as the reproducibility and repeatability standard deviations associated with any microbiological enumeration. The sensory analysis is intended to describe the sensory characteristics of the products in a measurable way on the basis of clearly defined criteria for texture, appearance, taste, and aroma.

Finally, the logistics chain is now also viewed as a major step to ensure that high-quality products are delivered to the consumer. The limit temperature for the storage of fermented milks is 45°F, a temperature likely to prevent any deterioration and that must be maintained until it is sold to the consumer. Indeed, the temperature can affect the LAB (eg, overdevelopment or overacidification, imbalance between the species present in the product, or mortality of the cultures) and the texture or taste (eg, excessive postacidification).

CONCLUSION

The development of a cultured dairy probiotic food product is a complex process involving years of research. The following is a list of the relevant steps that briefly summarize the suggested requirements for developing a cultured dairy probiotic food product, intended to assist the medical and scientific community in understanding the complexity surrounding this process:

1. Collection and identification of candidate probiotic strains;
2. In vitro and in vivo screening—the preclinical selection;
3. The milk fermentation process;
4. Clinical trial data on finished products to establish and substantiate benefits;
5. Safety assessment;
6. Characterization of the finished product: quality controls.

Acknowledgment
The author would like to thank Raquel Puig, Soline Kintz, Philippe Caradec, Gerard Denariaz, Nancy Dowling, Jean-Michel Antoine, David Obis, and Michael Neuwirth for the fruitful discussions and for helping to review this manuscript.

The views expressed in this article are those of the author only and do not necessarily represent those of The Dannon Company Inc.

REFERENCES

1. United Nations—Food and Agriculture Organization of the United Nations/World Health Organization. Guidelines for the Evaluation of Probiotics in Food. ftp://ftp.fao.org/es/esn/food/wgreport2.pdf. Published 2002. Accessed December 11, 2009.
2. Sanders ME, Gibson G, Gill HS. *Probiotics: Their Potential to Impact Human Health.* Council for Agricultural Science and Technology (CAST). 2007; Issue Paper 36. CAST, Ames, Iowa.
3. Reid G. The importance of guidelines in the development and application of probiotics. *Curr Pharm Des.* 2005;11(1):11-16.
4. American Gastroenterological Association (AGA). Probiotics: what they are and what they can do for you. http://www.gastro.org/wmspage.cfm?parm1=5617. Published 2008. Accessed December 11, 2009.
5. Turnbaugh PJ, Hamady M, Yatsunenko T, et al. A core gut microbiome in obese and lean twins. *Nature.* 2008;457(7228):480-484.
6. Freitas M, Tavan E, Cayuela C, Diop L, Sapin C, Trugnan G. Host-pathogens cross-talk. Indigenous bacteria and probiotics also play the game. *Biol Cell.* 2003;95(8):503-506.
7. Ingrassia I, Leplingard A, Darfeuille-Michaud A. *Lactobacillus casei* DN-114 001 inhibits the ability of adherent-invasive *E. coli* isolated from Crohn's disease patients to adhere to and to invade intestinal epithelial cells. *Appl Environ Microbiol.* 2005;71(6):2880-2887.
8. Parassol N, Freitas M, Thoreux K, Dalmasso G, Bourdet-Sicard R, Rampal P. *Lactobacillus casei* DN-114 001 inhibits the increase of paracellular permeability in enteropathogenic *Escherichia coli*-infected T84 cells. *Res Microbiol.* 2005;156(2):256-262.
9. Borruel N, Carol M, Casellas F, et al. Increased mucosal TNFα production in Crohn's disease can be downregulated ex vivo by probiotic bacteria. *Gut.* 2002;5:659-664.
10. Borruel N, Casellas F, Antolín M, et al. Effects of nonpathogenic bacteria on cytokine secretion by human intestinal mucosa. *Am J Gastro.* 2003;98(4):865-870.
11. Djouzi Z, Andrieux C, Degivry MC, Bouley C, Szylit O. The association of yogurt starters with *Lactobacillus casei* DN-114 001 in fermented milk alters the composition and metabolism of intestinal microflora in germ-free rats and in human flora-associated rats. *J Nutr.* 1997;127:2260-2266.
12. Cummings JH, Antoine JM, Azpiroz F, et al. PASSCLAIM: gut health and immunity. *Eur J Nutr.* 2004;43(suppl 2)43:II118-II173.
13. Pujol P, Huguet J, Drobnic F, et al. The effect of fermented milk containing *Lactobacillus casei* on the immune response to exercise. *Training and Rehab.* 2009;(3):209-223.

SECTION II

USE IN CLINICAL MEDICINE

11

Use of Probiotics and Prebiotics in Children

Jose M. Saavedra, MD, FAAP and Anne M. Dattilo, PhD, RD, CDE

The use of probiotics has arguably had a broader and more profound impact on infants and children than in other populations, and the clinical potential of adding dietary microbes to pregnant women, newborns, infants, and young children is just beginning to be realized. This seemingly major health benefit potential is in part related to the fact that early stages of life offer us a unique opportunity to modify the microbial exposure of an infant. This, in turn, has the effect of modulating host-microbe interaction patterns at a critical stage of a human's immune development, with potentially significant short- and long-term health-related outcomes.

The following review describes interactions between the development of infant microbiota, with influences from diet and other environmental factors, and its effects on health in infancy and early childhood. The use of probiotic bacteria for the purposes of maintaining health, as well as altering the course of illness, is the focus. The use of yeasts as probiotics is not reviewed, but specific strains of probiotic bacteria are identified that have been shown to provide health benefits to pediatric populations. Attention is directed toward bacteria of the genus *Lactobacillus* and *Bifidobacterium*, because these are the most frequently studied probiotic strains with documented impact on human health.

GENERAL CONCEPTS AND RATIONALE FOR PROBIOTIC USE IN PEDIATRICS

For purposes of review, we will discuss the concept of probiotics, focusing on clinical applications and most common uses in pediatrics. As with any probiotic, statements regarding "efficacy" and "safety" in pediatric populations should relate to the specific bacteria, as well as the benefit being discussed, identifying strain-specific properties and effects.[1-3] This allows for valid comparisons for safety and efficacy and prevents inappropriate generalizations.

Floch MH, Kim AS, eds.
Probiotics: A Clinical Guide (pp 141-180)
© 2010 Taylor & Francis Group

In this regard, it is also important to note that the taxonomy and names of probiotic bacteria used in pediatric populations has evolved over time. For example, among the better documented bacteria in pediatric populations, *Lactobacillus paracasei* ssp. *rhamnosus* has been commonly referred to as LGG. *B. animalis* subspecies *lactis* (*B. lactis*) has also been called *B. bifidum*, *B. animalis,* or *Bifidobacterium* Bb12. Although some probiotic species share strong DNA relatedness, it is important to note that even at the species level (*L. casei*), 2 apparently related probiotics (such as *L. casei* ssp. *casei* and *L. casei* ssp. *rhamnosus*) may not have the same effects or confer the same health benefits.[4] Careful attention to selection of probiotics at the strain level, in addition to genus or species designation, is critical for purposes of any generalizations or recommendations.

Probiotic bacteria are dietary microbes that, when given orally, provide the gut with relatively different and larger amounts of bacteria than those that are typically present in modern Western diets. Once consumed, these dietary microbes lead to relatively small but desirable changes in the profile of the host's microbiota, composed of resident microbes. In general, ingested probiotics will not actually colonize the host (ie, do not become resident microbes), but may modify the distal gut bacteria profile, beyond simply increasing the number of the species ingested. For the most part, these changes will persist as long as the probiotic is ingested. However, some reports demonstrate the persistence of probiotics in infants whose mothers were provided a specific bacteria during pregnancy,[5,6] suggesting that there is potential for true colonization by a probiotic when we take advantage of an apparent window of opportunity in the newborn period. In this case, the probiotic is ingested as part of the first oral inocula of maternal bacteria, together with those from the birth canal, breast milk, and the environment, to become part of the resident bacteria in the infant.

Aside from this observed phenomenon, no commercial probiotics have demonstrated the ability to permanently establish themselves in the infant intestine, but adhesion to gut mucosa, or even temporary multiplication, results in an enhanced concentration of probiotics at target sites.[2] Oral supplementation with specific *Lactobacillus* and *Bifidobacterium* strains have been shown to increase fecal counts of these organisms in the gastrointestinal (GI) tract of premature infants[7-10] as well as with full-term infants and children[11-18] and have therefore remained viable through passage in the child's GI tract, allowing probiotics to elicit their effect and potential health benefits either locally, systemically, or, in some cases, both. Most studies have focused on fecal counts in infants and children. However, the relatively small increases in the more sparsely colonized proximal gut in modern humans may be of equal or greater significance in modulating responses to bacteria than changes in the profile of colonic or stool bacteria documented with probiotic consumption, particularly with respect to gut immune responses. In the newborn and young infant, these effects may be of particular relevance, as these immune-related changes in early life may have effects beyond pediatric age.

DETERMINANTS OF INTESTINAL MICROBIOTA IN INFANCY AND CHILDHOOD AND IMPLICATIONS FOR PROBIOTIC USE IN PEDIATRICS

The development and characteristics of intestinal microbiota following birth, and its determining factors, as well as particular association of specific genera—in particular the genus *Bifidobacterium*—have guided some of the interest, choice, and study of specific probiotic bacteria in infants and children. Within hours of the birthing process, bacteria colonize the gut. Early composition of the microbiota of neonates holds a critical role for priming GI immunity and is responsible for postnatal development of the immune system.[19] Moreover, timing and stepwise microbial succession seems to be crucial for immune-related function such as protection against allergic, inflammatory, or autoimmune diseases of childhood, as well as later in life.[20] Such susceptibility to immunomodulation may begin prenatally,[3] occur during the first week of life or within the neonatal period,[21] and continue to adolescence, even to adulthood.[22-24] The potential benefits of early and continued microbial stimulation, as with regular probiotic ingestion, have merit in developing, modulating, and protecting immune function. Therefore, the use of probiotics in pediatrics, starting early in life and through childhood, potentially offers different, unique, and particularly impactful benefits compared to other populations.

The differences in microbiota between infants and adults, as well as the differences between infants who are breastfed versus those who receive breast milk substitutes, have also influenced the rationale for use, as well as the type of probiotics to be used in infants and children, compared to adults. *Bifidobacterium*, isolated over a century ago from infant feces, were teleologically associated with a healthy infant gut because of their predominance in breastfed infants, in comparison to formula-fed babies.[25] Since then, it has been widely accepted that *Bifidobacterium* represent one of the most important bacterial groups of infant microbiota. Several 16S rRNA gene-based libraries have been recently applied to mucosal and fecal samples to assess intestinal bifidobacterial diversity of human microbiota, and quantification of such by real-time PCR has been reported.[26] Type of feeding, mode of delivery (vaginal vs cesarean section [CS]), early medication, environmental surroundings including hospitalization, and other hygiene factors are strong predictors of infant microbiota. Other factors affecting microbial presence and succession in infancy are preterm birth, parenteral nutrition, delayed oral feeding, and neonatal intensive care unit hospitalization. In such cases, the gut is colonized by a small number of typically undesirable bacterial species. *Lactobacillus* and *Bifidobacterium* are less frequently identified in these intensive care hospitalized babies.[27-29] As reviewed below, factors that favor a beneficial microbiota (highest numbers of *Bifidobacterium* and lowest *C. difficile* and *E. coli*) include vaginal delivery, breastfeeding, and less antibiotic use.[30]

Mode of Delivery

Natural birth is not a sterile procedure. Passage through the birth canal provides the infant the first oral inocula of bacteria, some of which will go on to colonize their intestine. Bacteria colonizing the GI tract of neonates delivered by CS are primarily influenced by the hygienic quality of hospitalization.[31] Microbiota of CS babies may be totally devoid of *Bifidobacterium* species,[19] more often colonized with *C. difficile*,[30] or established with *Bifidobacterium* and *Lactobacillus* later than vaginally delivered children.[32-36] Some bacterial colonization patterns may be delayed up to 1 year, compared to vaginally delivered babies.[32]

Respiratory allergies are identified more often in children of CS birth than vaginally delivered infants,[37] and a positive association with the development of asthma has been correlated with CS delivery.[38] CS children supplemented with a mix of probiotics prenatally and the same probiotics with a prebiotic GOS from birth until age 6 months had IgE-associated allergic disease after 5 years nearly half as frequently as controls.[36] Considering that up to one-third of infants in the United States are born via cesarean delivery,[39] and the reported microbial and disease risk to apparently healthy infants born via CS, the concept of giving probiotics to mothers and CS infants would have a sound theoretical basis.

CHAPTER 11

Breastfeeding and Other Dietary Factors

Breastfeeding is not a sterile procedure, and breast milk is not a sterile fluid. Human milk is a ready source of bacteria, including live strains of *Lactobacillus*,[40-43] such as *L. reuteri*,[44,45] *L. plantarum*,[43] and *L. salivarium* CECT 5713.[46] Recent studies have confirmed the abundance of the *Bifidobacterium* genus and *Bifidobacterium* DNA in breast milk samples,[40,47-50] with 85% to 100% of samples from healthy lactating women containing bifidobacteria.[47,48] Species identified with potential probiotic properties include *B. adolescentis*, *B. animalis*, *B. breve*, *B. bifidum*, *B. cantenalatum*, and *B. longum*.[47-49] An average *Bifidobacterium* concentration of approximately 1×10^3 CFU/mL,[48] or an estimated 1×10^6 CFU/800 mL breast milk, has been reported.

The origin of the live bacteria found in breast milk has been controversial and thought to be acquired from skin, or by infant oral contamination with maternal flora via transit through the birth canal, after which newborns would transmit such bacteria during feeding (the so-called vertical mother-to-child transmission). However, in the case of *Bifidobacterium*, an anaerobic genus unlikely to survive on skin,[48] and *Lactobacillus*, which is not readily identified in the birth canal,[42] the hypothesis that breast milk bacteria could originate endogenously has been investigated. An entero-mammary pathway, in which bacteria from the maternal gut circulate to the mammary gland through an endogenous route, has been suggested. Specifically, transfer of intestinal bacteria, involving maternal DCs and macrophages,[51] has been proposed to explain maternal commensal gut bacteria in the mammary gland.[50,52]

Bifidobacterium colonization is rather consistently identified as the most significant difference among breastfed and formula-fed infants. Breastfed infants have a stable intestinal flora rich in bifidobacteria starting from approximately day 7 of life.[27-29] This *Bifidobacterium*-dominant microbiota identified in breastfed infants,[53-57] in which 60% to 90% of microbiota is bifidobacteria,[58,59] may explain, in part, the decreased morbidity in these children, compared to formula-fed infants. Nonbreastfed infants, on the other hand, tend to have a complex microbiota[27] that is more prone to changes and typically contains less *Bifidobacterium*[60] than that of breastfed infants and higher counts of *Bacteroides*, *Clostridium*, and *Enterobacteriaceae*.[30,31,54,57,61-65] Overall, a more diverse, post-weaning-like microbiota has been identified in formula-fed infants compared to breastfed infants. *Lactobacillus*, also an important part of the infant's resident microbiota,[66] appears not as dominant as *Bifidobacterium*.[29] *Lactobacillus* counts are variable in fecal samples of infants provided breast milk, as well as those provided complementary foods to breastfeeding.[56] It is important not only to acknowledge the differences in bacteria found in the stools of infants fed differently, but also to recognize that breastfed infants are regularly consuming bacteria with each feeding, while formula-fed infants receive sterile food during this critical stage of gut immune development.

Breast milk continues to affect microflora composition as complementary foods are introduced to the growing infant. Longitudinal changes in fecal microbiota from birth, through the full weaning process, confirm the dominance of *Bifidobacterium* in infants who had the advantage of exclusive breastfeeding for approximately 5 weeks.[55] Preceding studies also identified that when breast milk was supplemented with solid food, *Bifidobacterium* counts remained constant through the weaning period.[53]

After weaning from breastfeeding entirely, composition of the microbiota becomes more homogenous,[55] and early differences between fecal bacterial counts of breastfed and formula-fed infants tend to even out.[65,67] Although colonic microbiota still evolve through age 17,[68] at weaning, children lose the bacterial and immunologic benefits of breast milk, per se, and increasingly consume more varied, but often processed and sterile foods, leading to a distinct change in the quantity and quality of bacteria to which the gut is exposed. Consequently, the presence and unique characteristics of bacteria in breast milk that provide a regular source of live microorganisms to infants, the differences in microbiota of breast vs sterile formula-fed infants, and the clinical consequences associated with formula feeding (less immune protective benefits, increased risk of infectious and allergic conditions) also provide a solid basis for potential clinical use of probiotic bacteria as part of the diet of infants who do not benefit from exclusive breastfeeding.

Antibiotics

Antibiotic use by pregnant women can adversely affect the newborn microbiota,[69] and antibiotic use during infancy is widely known to alter microbiota and is particularly associated with decreased numbers of fecal *Bifidobacterium*.[30] The entire intestinal flora can be affected by antibiotic treatment[63] with resultant diarrhea and/or with changes to the microbial pattern, suggestive of those predisposing to allergy (both eczema and wheezing).[70] Antibiotic exposure in the first year of life is associated with wheezing,[71,72] and meta-analyses report it as a risk factor for the development of childhood asthma.[73] Thus, in infants who receive antibiotics, there is another potential opportunity for the clinical use of probiotics to minimize GI complications such as AAD or associated consequences such as increased risk of atopy.

PROBIOTIC BACTERIA USED IN PEDIATRIC POPULATIONS

Lactobacillus, *Bifidobacterium*, and *Streptococcus* are the most widely used probiotics in the food supply, and a growing number of species and strains have been studied. A truly complete list of bacteria as potential probiotics is precluded by several factors, including the fact that many studies, especially prior to the past 5 to 10 years, do not adequately specify the strains used. In addition, the documentation of dose and viability is often inadequate, and many bacteria have had very few clinical trials in pediatrics. A summary of clinical outcomes (discussed below) identifies the more frequently studied probiotic agents in infants and children that have demonstrated a specific benefit. These include *Lactobacillus* species, LGG, *L. acidophilus*, *L. casei*, *L. johnsonii*, and *L. reuteri*. Among *Bifidobacterium*, the better studied probiotic agents are *B. breve*, *B. infantis*, *B. lactis*, and *B. longum*, with specific strains identified. Regarding dose, there are very few trials, and very few agents have undergone multiple-dose assessment in pediatric populations, resulting in a wide range of specific amounts or concentrations of bacteria provided in clinical trials that have shown some effect or clinical benefit. Doses of probiotics shown to have clinical effects range from 5×10^5 CFU provided to children on school days[74] to 2×10^{11} CFU each day.[75] A daily intake of 1×10^8 CFU appears effective for consistent beneficial changes in immune and anti-inflammatory markers, as well as overt decreases in allergy symptoms, incidence of diarrhea, and other probiotic health benefits.

Of relevance to the use of probiotics in pediatrics is the form or vehicle in which they are consumed. Foods and beverages containing LAB constitute up to 40% of the food supply worldwide,[76] providing a good vehicle for the delivery of probiotics. With an aim of health maintenance and disease-preventing benefits, foods supplemented with these bacteria provide a practical way of delivering probiotics, rather than use as a daily capsule or pill. The gradual inclusion of probiotic bacteria to the food supply may ultimately be the more logical way of overcoming the lack of microbial stimulus young populations face in increasingly sterile, urban environments, with sterile foods,

TABLE 11-1

SELECTED FOODS AND SUPPLEMENTS WITH PROBIOTICS COMMERCIALIZED FOR INFANTS AND CHILDREN IN THE UNITED STATES

PROBIOTIC	QUANTITY/SERVING	PRODUCT	COMPANY
B. lactis Bb-12	1×10^9 CFU/4 oz serving	Yo-Plus Yogurt	General Mills/ Yoplait
B. lactis Bb-12	1×10^6 CFU/g of powder formula*	Good Start Protect Plus Infant Formula	Nestlé
B. lactis	1×10^9 CFU/30 g serving	Live Active Cheese	Kraft Foods
L. casei DN-114001	1×10^{10} CFU/4 oz serving	DanActive yogurt drink	Dannon
L. reuteri ATCC 55730	1×10^8 CFU/8.25 oz serving	Boost Kid Essentials Nutritional Drink	Nestlé
LGG	1×10^6 CFU/g powder formula*	Nutramigen with Enflora LGG Infant Formula	Mead Johnson
LGG	1×10^{10} CFU/4 oz serving	Danimals Yogurt	Dannon
L. casei shirota	6.5×10^9 CFU/65 mL serving	Yakult (probiotic drink)	Yakult
L. acidophilus L. casei	5×10^6 CFU/1 oz serving	Fruit and Yogurt Snack	Welch's
B. lactis L. acidophilus L. casei	1.8×10^9 CFU/6 oz serving	Yo-Yo Baby Yogurt YoGurt Tubes	Horizon Organic
B. bifidus L. acidophilus L. casei LGG	5×10^9 CFU/4 oz serving	YoBaby YoKids Smoothie	Stonyfield Farms
B. breve B. longum B. infantis L. acidophilus L. plantarum L. paracasei L. bulgaricus S. thermophilus	4.5×10^{10} CFU in total/packet	Supplement: VSL#3 powdered packet	VSL Pharmaceuticals

(continued)

TABLE 11-1 *(continued)*

SELECTED FOODS AND SUPPLEMENTS WITH PROBIOTICS COMMERCIALIZED FOR INFANTS AND CHILDREN IN THE UNITED STATES

PROBIOTIC	QUANTITY/SERVING	PRODUCT	COMPANY
B. longum BB536 B. breve M-16 V B. infantis M-63	1 × 10^9 CFU of each/ packet	Supplement: Baby's Only from powdered packet	Nature's One
LGG	1 × 10^9 CFU/capsule	Supplement: Culturelle tablet or gelatin capsule	ACG Foods

For comparison, probiotic quantity provided as 1 million CFU (colony forming units) = 1 × 10^6; 1 billion CFU = 1 × 10^9.

*Resulting in a minimum intake of 10^8 CFU/day in an exclusively formula-fed infant.

and increasing use of antibiotics (ie, a way to counteract the hygiene hypothesis). In newborns and young infants who do not exclusively breastfeed and lack this protective feeding mode, as well as the bacteria associated with it, the use of probiotics in infant formulas has provided a means for regular delivery of these bacteria and has been shown to be beneficial in decreasing the risk of acute pediatric illnesses. For therapeutic uses, such as the management of acute infantile diarrhea, specific supplement doses over a specified period of time may provide a more practical way to intervene. Probiotics have been documented to have specific benefits when used both as supplements and increasingly in infant formulas, beverages, and yogurts. Table 11-1 provides a select list of food products and supplements of commonly used probiotics in pediatrics in the United States and the forms in which they are available.

CLINICAL BENEFITS OF PROBIOTICS IN INFANCY AND CHILDHOOD

Health-related benefits associated with particular strains of probiotics during infancy and childhood include the following:

(a) Functionally desirable changes related to host defense, maintenance on intestinal barrier function, and modulation of immune response;

(b) Risk reduction (preventive) applications toward specific clinical conditions (eg, acute febrile illness, acute diarrheal disease, atopic disease, AAD, necrotizing enterocolitis [NEC]);

(c) Management (therapeutic) applications of certain clinical conditions (eg, management of acute viral diarrhea, atopic disease, infantile colic).

Specific probiotics offer potentially therapeutic (treatment) alternatives for some conditions, discussed below. However, as with most health-related interventions in pediatrics, health maintenance and prophylaxis are paramount. Increasingly, specific probiotic bacteria are being utilized in this manner, in both healthy pediatric populations as well as at-risk groups (such as premature infants) or in at-risk situations (such as infants receiving antibiotics). Table 11-2 provides a comprehensive summary of published clinical trials that have reported probiotic health benefits with regard to immunity, diarrhea, allergy, as well as selected GI and inflammatory conditions in pediatric populations available at the time of this writing. Trials using combinations of probiotics and oligosaccharides, or yeasts such as *Saccharomyces boulardi*, are not included in this summary. A strength of evidence score, based on definitions provided at the Advances in Clinical Use of Probiotics Workshop (Yale University, November 2007), is provided for each topic area. In addition, the reader is referred to meta-analyses on several of the topic areas for integration of results from individual studies.

Immune Effects and Acute Illness

Desirable functional benefits of specific orally ingested bacteria within pediatric populations include colonization with favorable microbiota, competition with pathogenic bacteria for binding sites and nutrients, increase in secretory IgA production and mucin, production of antimicrobial substances, and decreased gut permeability.[77-79] These effects that demonstrate an enhancement of gut barrier function and immune response help explain the various clinical outcomes documented in a number of studies with probiotic ingestion, particularly improved secretory antibody response (IgA), decreased viral shedding (in rotavirus infection), as well as a preventive risk reduction of acute illness such as decreases in acute respiratory, GI, and febrile illness (Table 11-2A). Several of these studies also document proxies for health maintenance, such as decreased daycare absenteeism and decreased use of antibiotics in pediatric populations receiving probiotics regularly. A significant number of these trials have utilized yogurts, milks, or infant formulas to deliver the probiotic. While various bacteria and daily amounts have been provided in these trials, specific bifidobacteria (*B. breve, B. lactis*) and lactobacilli (LGG, *L. casei, L. reuteri*) are better documented than others in terms of beneficial effects in infants and children.

Management of Acute Diarrhea

By far, the best-studied clinical outcome with use of probiotic bacteria in pediatrics (and in general) has been that of acute diarrheal disease.[78] Individual trials with various probiotic bacteria are summarized in Table 11-2B. One recent meta-analysis specifically assessed the efficacy of LGG for treating acute diarrhea in children,[80] and several other meta-analyses have been conducted that included studies of infants and children utilizing various probiotics.[81-84] Taken together, efficacy has been demonstrated. The most consistent effect reported is a reduction in duration of illness (by one-half) to 2 days of diarrhea, particularly with diarrhea of rotavirus etiology. While the effect may be modest on an individual basis, the overall epidemiologic effect is quite significant. However, cost-benefit analysis for the general therapeutic recommendation of specific probiotic use early in the course of an acute episode of diarrhea is lacking. That said, the amelioration of the clinical course of rotavirus diarrhea infection (as well as decreased incidence discussed below) is the strongest evidence of the immune protective effect of specific probiotic strains.

Prevention of Acute Diarrhea

The first randomized controlled study documenting a clinical benefit of probiotic use in a pediatric population was that of a reduction in incidence of acute viral diarrhea in infants receiving a formula supplemented with *B. lactis* (then termed *"B. bifidum"*) over an extended period of time. Since then, a number of additional studies have shown similar prophylactic benefit with various probiotic bacteria, with varying levels of significance (Table 11-2C). Reduced shedding of rotavirus has been shown with *L. rhamnosus* and *L. reuteri* during treatment[85] and with *B. lactis* when fed regularly and prophylactically.[86] A meta-analysis that reviewed 34 randomized clinical trials for the efficacy of probiotics in the prevention of acute diarrhea concluded that probiotic use significantly reduced the risk of developing diarrhea in infants and children by 57% (95% CI: 35% to 71%).[87] The protective effect did not significantly vary among the probiotic strains used, including *B. lactis*, LGG, and *L. acidophilus*, used alone or in combination with 2 or more strains. No study has documented an increase (significant or not) in diarrheal disease with probiotic use. The use of probiotic bacteria for prevention further bolsters the argument of incorporating specific bacteria into the food supply to foster and facilitate regular consumption in pediatric populations, in this case healthy infants (particularly those who are not breastfed) and children. The "medicinal" use of probiotic supplements (a capsule or pill) on a daily basis is likely to be less economical and is a less practical approach than a dietary modification for the purposes of health maintenance.

Prevention of Antibiotic-Associated Diarrhea

The influence of probiotic supplementation on preventing AAD has been the topic of recent meta-analyses (Table 11-2D).[88,89] Fecal recovery of *Bifidobacterium* has been documented with probiotic supplementation in children while on antibiotic therapy[90] and has been shown to decrease the incidence or severity of diarrhea in infants and children receiving antibiotics.[91-93] The number of children needed to treat with probiotics to prevent one case of diarrhea ranges from 7 to 10.[88,89] In some studies the probiotic was used prophylactically; infants or children received the probiotic as part of their diet (in a formula) over an extended period of time during which they incidentally received antibiotics. In other cases, the probiotic was begun concomitantly with the initiation of an antibiotic for a specific condition.

Prevention and Management of Allergic Conditions

Studies over the past decade have demonstrated that microbiota in infants with allergy differ from those remaining nonallergic.[13,94-98] Not only is the presence of an altered intestinal *Bifidobacterium* microbiota during infancy associated with an increased risk of atopic eczema and atopic sensitization in later life,[70,94,98-100] but also prospective studies assessing neonatal microbiota have identified aberrations in bacterial populations preceding the development of allergy. Colonization with *Bacteroides fragilis* at 3 weeks was more often identified in recurrent wheezing children at risk of persistent asthma at 3 years of age,[21] and more *Clostridia* and fewer *Bifidobacteria* were found in infants at 3 weeks of age who would later develop atopy.[99] Infants colonized with *C. difficile* were at greater risk of developing both eczema or recurrent wheeze.[70] Thus, a therapeutic rationale to prevent allergic disease, particularly in high-risk infants, by modifying the early intestinal microbiota has strong theoretical support.

Probiotic supplementation in infancy favorably influences the development of infants' microbiota that is inconsistent with aberrations in microbiota found in allergic infants. Stool *E. coli* and *Bacteroides* in infants with atopic eczema has been reduced with *B. lactis* supplementation, decreasing potential to develop further allergic inflammation.[13] In addition, identification of favorable immune modulatory outcomes in atopic infants provided probiotic-supplemented infant formula,[101-103] or other supplemental delivery methods (eg, dissolved in food or milk),[104-106] has been demonstrated in several clinical trials (Table 11-2E).

Prevention of overt allergy with probiotic supplementation was initially reported by Kalliomaki and colleagues after administration of LGG to mothers during the last month of pregnancy, and then to infants through 6 months of age.[107] A statistically significant and clinically relevant reduction in atopic eczema persisted to age 7 years.[108] Since that initial study, 4 additional published trials have assessed preventive effects of perinatal administration of probiotics, with results indicating a role for *L. reuteri* in reducing incidence of IgE-mediated atopy[11] and for LGG,[109] as well as for a mixture of probiotics,[110] and a mixture of probiotics plus a prebiotic on the prevention of both eczema and IgE-mediated eczema.[111] One very recent trial[106] concluded that *L. paracasei* ssp. *paracasei* strain F19 supplementation, initiated at weaning, reduced the cumulative incidence of eczema, suggesting that clinical benefit may be extended beyond the prenatal administration of probiotics.

In children with diagnostic atopy, decreased extent and severity after supplementation with LGG or *B. lactis*[101] has been documented. Similarly, studies have also demonstrated improvement in atopic eczema severity scores in infants provided *B. lactis*-supplemented formula in combination with *L. rhamnosus* for food-sensitized children,[112] while a combination of *L. reuteri* and *L. rhamnosus* has been noted to decrease severity of eczema in children with atopy.[113] Improvement in allergy symptom scores in children with allergic rhinitis after supplementation with *Lactobacillus* spp. has been reported in several clinical trials.[114-116]

However, not all studies have documented positive outcomes regarding allergy prevention with specific probiotics[117,118] or have found no effect with probiotic supplementation on decreasing atopic severity.[119] Thus, meta-analyses have attempted to assess effects of administration of probiotics from the prenatal period through to the first months of life and its association with a reduced incidence of eczema.[120-122] Stronger evidence for a preventive benefit, and a lesser strength of evidence for a benefit in allergy treatment, was reported.

EMERGING RESEARCH WITH PROBIOTICS IN PEDIATRIC HEALTH

Children with irritable bowel, CD, and chronic inflammatory conditions have altered microbiota.[123,124] Supplementation with probiotic bacteria has provided not only symptomatic relief,[125-128] but also varying clinical benefit (Table 11-2F).[129-131] Children testing positive for *H. pylori* receiving antibiotic eradication therapy,[132,133] as well as asymptomatic children without concomitant antibiotic use,[134,135] have had various symptomatic relief and eradication success with probiotic supplementation.

Infants with colic have been previously shown to be more frequently colonized with *C. difficile* than age-matched controls,[136] yet a clear and consistent microbiota pattern associated with colic has not been confirmed. The use of *L. reuteri* in infants with the diagnosis of colic has been shown to decrease the frequency of episodes and duration of crying in these babies.[137,138] The mechanism for this potential effect on intestinal motility remains to be elucidated.

Necrotizing Enterocolitis

Premature infants are particularly at risk for a delayed development of a "normal" intestinal microbiota. Often born by CS, not breastfed, and placed in an environment rich in hospital bacteria, these infants typically receive antibiotics and, as routine, sterile formulas that do not contribute any microbial stimulus. Thus, in this population, the potential for a benefit from probiotic agents would be predictably higher. Indeed, several clinical trials using particular individual bacteria, or combinations of these, have documented improved gut permeability and lower antibiotic courses[139] as well as reduction in incidence and/or severity of NEC.[140-143]

The use of probiotic bacteria for NEC is discussed elsewhere in this publication. However, it is becoming increasingly apparent that a significant risk reduction of NEC, with a very low risk-benefit ratio is possible, as documented in 2 recent meta-analyses.[144,145]

Safety of Probiotics in Pediatrics

In general, pediatric populations would be considered vulnerable in terms of potential for a negative effect, particularly bacterial infection from an orally provided bacterium. The safety profile as well as the efficacy of a probiotic agent is species specific and, in some cases, strain specific.

Rare instances of lactobacillemia in children receiving LGG have been documented in immunocompromised patients.[146,147] The mechanisms for these infections and route of contamination in these instances are unclear. Documented correlations between systemic infections and probiotic consumption are few, and all occurred in patients with underlying medical conditions.[148] Nevertheless, if general recommendations are to be made for the use of these bacteria in infants and children, their safety profile should be well characterized. It is important to understand that safety is mainly established by a full assessment of the characteristics of a bacterium (no production of toxins, little production of D-lactate, no transferable antibiotic resistance, no mucosal invasiveness, etc). In addition, history of safe use in large numbers provides a second level of assurance, and finally, use in controlled clinical trials helps ascertain a lack of adverse effects. In particular, use in vulnerable populations helps further decrease any safety concern. From this point of view, the genus *Bifidobacterium* presents a distinct safety profile. Despite being abundant in stools of breastfed newborns, no clear pathogenicity of resident *Bifidobacterium* has been reported. No cases of infections from the consumption of commercial products containing *Bifidobacterium* species have been documented, despite use in milks, yogurts, and infant formulas in extremely large quantities, globally, for many years. And various trials have shown safe use and adequate growth with *Bifidobacterium* in infants from birth,[149] in vulnerable populations including preterm infants,[9,139,150] malnourished infants,[151] and infants born to mothers with HIV disease,[191] making this genus particularly suitable for general and regular use in infants. Currently, *B. lactis* is the only probiotic bacterium assessed by the FDA and with GRAS (generally accepted as safe) status for use in healthy newborns in the United

(text continued on page 169)

TABLE 11-2

CLINICAL TRIALS DOCUMENTING PROBIOTIC BENEFITS IN PEDIATRIC POPULATIONS*

A. Immune Effects and Acute Illness (Strength of Evidence: Level A)

REFERENCE	PATIENT POPULATION	N	PROBIOTICS USED IN INTERVENTION/DOSAGE	SOURCE	BENEFIT IN PROBIOTIC GROUP
Cobo Sanz et al[152]	Healthy children, age 3 to 12 years	251	L. casei DN-114001, 1 × 10¹⁰ CFU, twice daily	Supplemented milk	↓ incidence and duration of lower respiratory tract infection ↓ duration of bronchitis or pneumonia ↓ incidence and duration of fatigue
Cukrowska et al[153]	Preterm infants	61	E. coli Nissle 1917, 1 × 10⁸ CFU/day for 5 days, followed by 3 times weekly for 3 weeks	Oral suspension applied to infants	↑ Anti-E. coli Nissle 1917 IgA and total IgM
Fujii et al[154]	Preterm infants	19	B. breve, 1 × 10⁹ CFU, twice daily	Powder supplement in glucose solution	↑ serum TGF-B 1
Fukushima et al[155]	Healthy children provided polio immunization, average age 2 years	7	B. lactis Bb-12, 1 × 10⁹ CFU/g	Supplemented formula	↑ antibody immune response reflected by: • ↑ total fecal IgA • ↑ antipolio fecal IgA
Hatakka et al[156]	Healthy children attending daycare, average age 4½ years	413	LGG ATCC 53103, 5 to 10 × 10⁵ CFU/mL	Supplemented milk	↓ days absent from daycare due to illness ↓ number of children with respiratory infection ↓ antibiotic treatment for respiratory infection

(continued)

TABLE 11-2 (continued)

REFERENCE	PATIENT POPULATION	N	PROBIOTICS USED IN INTERVENTION/DOSAGE	SOURCE	BENEFIT IN PROBIOTIC GROUP
Hatakka et al[157]	Healthy children prone to otitis infection with average age 2½ years	269	LGG, L. rhamnosus LC 705, B. breve 99, Propionibacterium freudenreichii ssp. Shermanii JS, 8 to 9 × 10⁹ CFU of each strain/day	Capsule	↓ occurrence of recurrent respiratory infections
Isolauri et al[158]	Healthy infants	46	L. casei strain GG, 5 × 10⁵ CFU, twice daily	Powder supplement in water	↑ rotavirus IgA seroconversion and rotavirus-specific IgM after oral vaccination
Kaila et al[75]	Children with acute diarrhea, average age nearly 1½ years	39	Lactobacillus GG, 1 × 10¹⁰ to 1 × 10¹¹ CFU, twice daily	Supplemented milk	↑ antibody immune response reflected by: • ↑ IgA, IgG, and IgM secreting cell numbers • ↑ IgA specific antibody to rotavirus • ↓ duration of diarrhea
Majamaa et al[4]	Children with rotavirus diarrhea, average age 1½ years	49	Lactobacillus GG or L. casei rhamnosus, 2.2 × 10⁸ CFU/g	Powder supplement in water	↑ antibody immune response reflected by: • ↑ IgA secreting cells and ↑ specific antibody to rotavirus for LGG group • ↓ duration of diarrhea for LGG group

(continued)

TABLE 11-2 (continued)

CLINICAL TRIALS DOCUMENTING PROBIOTIC BENEFITS IN PEDIATRIC POPULATIONS*

A. Immune Effects and Acute Illness (Strength of Evidence: Level A)

REFERENCE	PATIENT POPULATION	N	PROBIOTICS USED IN INTERVENTION/DOSAGE	SOURCE	BENEFIT IN PROBIOTIC GROUP
Mohan et al[150]	Preterm infants	69	B. lactis Bb-12, 1.6 × 10⁹ CFU/day for 3 days and 4 × 10⁹ CFU for 18 days	Supplemented formula	↑ immune response (fecal IgA) ↓ markers of inflammation (calprotectin)
Nase et al[74]	Healthy children, average age of 4½ years	451	LGG, 5 to 10 × 10⁵ CFU/mL, 5 times/week	Supplemented milk	↓ risk of dental caries
Phuapradit et al[159]	Children residing in an orphanage, average age 1½ years	97	B. lactis, 1 × 10⁸ CFU/g; and S. thermophilus (dose not specified)	Supplemented formula	↓ antibody titers to rotavirus, indicating reduced subclinical infection
Rautava et al[160]	Healthy infants, age less than 2 months	72	B. lactis and Lactobacillus GG, 1 × 10¹⁰ CFU/day	Supplemented formula	↑ Milk-specific IgA secreting cells ↑ Serum TGF-β and sCD14
Saavedra et al[86]	Infants hospitalized for reasons other than diarrhea with average age nearly 1 year	55	B. lactis, 1 × 10⁸ CFU/g powder formula; S. thermophilus, 1 × 10⁷ CFU/g powder formula	Supplemented formula	↓ rotavirus shedding ↓ incidence of diarrhea
Saavedra et al[161]	Healthy infants, average age 7 months	118	B. lactis Bb-12, 1 × 10⁷ CFU/g powder formula; S. thermophilus, 1 × 10⁷ CFU/g powder formula	Supplemented formula	↓ frequency of antibiotic use

(continued)

TABLE 11-2 (continued)

REFERENCE	PATIENT POPULATION	N	PROBIOTICS USED IN INTERVENTION/DOSAGE	SOURCE	BENEFIT IN PROBIOTIC GROUP
Saran et al[162]	Undernourished children from urban area in India, age 2 to 5 years	100	L. acidophilus, 1×10^8 CFU/g	Supplement added to yogurt	↓ incidence of febrile episodes and duration of fever ↑ height and weight
Stratiki et al[139]	Preterm infants	75	B. lactis Bb-12, 2×10^7 CFU/g powder formula	Supplemented formula	↓ intestinal permeability ↓ use of antibiotics
Weizman et al[163]	Healthy infants, attending child care, age 4 to 10 months	201	L. reuteri ATCC 55730, 1×10^7 CFU/ g powder formula; or B. lactis Bb-12, 1×10^7 CFU/g powder formula	Supplemented formula	L. reuteri or B. lactis: • ↓ febrile episodes • ↓ diarrhea episodes and duration L. reuteri: • ↓ antibody prescriptions and clinic visits • ↓ days with fever • ↓ child care absences

B. Management of Acute Diarrhea (Strength of Evidence: Level A)

REFERENCE	PATIENT POPULATION	N	PROBIOTICS USED IN INTERVENTION/DOSAGE	SOURCE	BENEFIT IN PROBIOTIC GROUP
Boudraa et al[164]	Hospitalized infants and children with acute diarrhea, age 3 to 24 months	112	L. bulgaricus, 1×10^8 CFU/day; S. thermophilus, 1×10^8 CFU/day	Supplemented formula	↓ duration of diarrhea ↓ stool frequency

(continued)

TABLE 11-2 (continued)

CLINICAL TRIALS DOCUMENTING PROBIOTIC BENEFITS IN PEDIATRIC POPULATIONS*

REFERENCE	PATIENT POPULATION	N	PROBIOTICS USED IN INTERVENTION/DOSAGE	SOURCE	BENEFIT IN PROBIOTIC GROUP
Canani et al[165]	Children with acute diarrhea, average age 15 to 20 months	571	*L. casei rhamnosus* GG, 6 × 10⁹ CFU, twice daily; or *S. boulardii*, 5 × 10⁹ CFU, twice daily; or *Bacillus clausii*, 1 × 10⁹ CFU, twice daily; or mixture of *L. delbrueckii bulgaricus* (LMG-P17550), 1 × 10⁹ CFU, twice daily, *L. acidophilus* (LMG-P 17549), 1 × 10⁹ CFU, twice daily, *S. thermophilus*, (LMG-P 17503), 1 × 10⁹ CFU, twice daily; *B. bifidum* (LMG-P 17500), 5 × 10⁸ CFU, twice daily; or *Enterococcus faecium* (SF 68), 7.5 × 10⁷ CFU, twice daily	Supplement, added to water	↓ duration of diarrhea for LGG and probiotic mix groups
Gaon et al[166]	Hospitalized infants with acute diarrhea, average age 1 year	89	*L. casei* and *L. acidophilus* (CERELA), 1 × 10¹⁰ to 1 × 10¹² CFU/g, twice daily	Supplemented formula	↓ duration of diarrhea
Guandalini et al[167]	Children with acute diarrhea, age 1 to 36 months	287	LGG, 4 × 10¹⁰ CFU, daily	Supplemented formula	↓ duration of diarrhea ↓ duration of hospital stay
Guarino et al[168]	Children with mild diarrhea, age 1½ years	100	*L. casei* strain GG, 3 × 10⁹ CFU, twice daily	Supplemented milk	↓ duration of diarrhea ↓ rotavirus shedding

(continued)

TABLE 11-2 (continued)

REFERENCE	PATIENT POPULATION	N	PROBIOTICS USED IN INTERVENTION/DOSAGE	SOURCE	BENEFIT IN PROBIOTIC GROUP
Isolauri et al[169]	Hospitalized infants and children with acute diarrhea, age 4 to 45 months	71	*Lactobacillus* GG, 2×10^{10} to 2×10^{11} CFU, twice daily	Supplemented formula	↓ duration of diarrhea
Isolauri et al[170]	Infants and children with acute rotavirus diarrhea, age 5 to 28 months	42	*L. casei* GG, 2×10^{10} CFU, daily	Supplement	↓ duration of diarrhea
Kaila et al[75]	Children with acute diarrhea, average age nearly 1½ years	39	*Lactobacillus* GG, 1×10^{10} to 1×10^{11} CFU, twice daily	Supplemented milk	↓ duration of diarrhea ↑ antibody immune response reflected by: • ↑ IgA, IgG, and IgM secreting cell numbers • ↑ IgA specific antibody to rotavirus
Lee et al[171]	Infants and children with acute diarrhea, age 6 to 60 months	100	*L. acidophilus* and *B. infantis*, 6×10^9 CFU, daily	Capsules	↓ duration of diarrhea in both rotavirus positive and negative diarrhea

(continued)

TABLE 11-2 (continued)

CLINICAL TRIALS DOCUMENTING PROBIOTIC BENEFITS IN PEDIATRIC POPULATIONS*

REFERENCE	PATIENT POPULATION	N	PROBIOTICS USED IN INTERVENTION/DOSAGE	SOURCE	BENEFIT IN PROBIOTIC GROUP
Majamaa et al[4]	Children with rotavirus diarrhea, average age 1½ years	49	*Lactobacillus* GG or *L. casei rhamnosus*, 2.2 × 10⁸ CFU/g	Powder supplement mixed with water	↑ antibody immune response reflected by: • ↑ IgA secreting cells and ↑ specific antibody to rotavirus for LGG group • ↓ duration of diarrhea for LGG group
Mao et al[172]	Children with severe, acute diarrhea, average age 1 year	142	*B. lactis* (Bb-12), 1 × 10⁹ CFU/g; and *S. thermophilus*, 5 × 10⁸ CFU/g	Supplemented formula	↓ rotavirus shedding
Pant et al[173]	Hospitalized infants with acute diarrhea, average age 8 months	39	LGG, 2 × 10¹⁰ to 2 × 10¹¹ CFU/day	Supplement added to oral rehydration solution	↓ duration of diarrhea ↓ stool frequency
Raza et al[174]	Hospitalized infants with acute diarrhea, average age 13 months	40	LGG, 2 × 10¹⁰ to 2 × 10¹¹ CFU/day	Supplement added to oral rehydration solution	↓ duration of diarrhea ↓ stool frequency

(continued)

TABLE 11-2 (continued)

REFERENCE	PATIENT POPULATION	N	PROBIOTICS USED IN INTERVENTION/DOSAGE	SOURCE	BENEFIT IN PROBIOTIC GROUP
Rosenfeldt et al[85]	Hospitalized children with acute diarrhea, average age 1½ years old	69	L. rhamnosus 19070-2, 1.7 × 10¹⁰ CFU, twice daily; and L. reuteri DSM 12246, 0.5 × 10¹⁰ CFU, twice daily	Powder supplement, reconstituted	↓ length of hospital stay In children treated within 60 hours of diarrheal onset: • ↓ duration of diarrhea • ↓ rotavirus excretion
Rosenfeldt et al[175]	Children attending daycare with acute diarrhea, average age nearly 2 years	43	L. rhamnosus 19070-2, 1 × 10¹⁰ CFU, twice daily; and L. reuteri DSM 12246, 1 × 10¹⁰ CFU, twice daily	Powder supplement, reconstituted	↓ duration of diarrhea ↑ number of children with resolution of diarrhea within 5 days of supplementation
Shornikova et al[176]	Children hospitalized for rotavirus diarrhea with an average age of nearly 1½ years	66	L. reuteri ATCC 55730, 5 × 10⁸ to 2 × 10⁹ CFU, twice daily at enrollment, followed by once daily	Capsule, reconstituted	↓ duration of diarrhea ↑ number of children without watery diarrhea within 48 hours of supplementation ↑ fecal L. reuteri
Shornikova et al[177]	Children hospitalized for acute diarrhea (75% rotavirus) with an average age of 1½ years	40	L. reuteri SD 2112, 1 × 10¹⁰ to 1 × 10¹¹ CFU/day	Powder supplement reconstituted	↓ number of children with diarrhea ↓ number of children with vomiting ↓ duration of diarrhea ↑ fecal L. reuteri

(continued)

TABLE 11-2 *(continued)*

CLINICAL TRIALS DOCUMENTING PROBIOTIC BENEFITS IN PEDIATRIC POPULATIONS*

REFERENCE	PATIENT POPULATION	N	PROBIOTICS USED IN INTERVENTION/DOSAGE	SOURCE	BENEFIT IN PROBIOTIC GROUP
Shornikova et al[178]	Children hospitalized for acute diarrhea with an average age of 1½ years	123	LGG, 5 × 10⁹ CFU, twice daily	Reconstituted powder supplement	↓ duration of rotaviral diarrhea
Szymanski et al[179]	Children hospitalized with infectious diarrhea, average age 1½ years	87	L. rhamnosus strains 573L/1, 2, and 3, 1.2 × 10¹⁰ CFU, twice daily	Ampoule mixed with 10% glucose solution	↓ duration of diarrhea in rotavirus infection group; ↓ duration of parenteral rehydration in rotavirus infection group

C. Prevention of Acute Diarrhea (Strength of Evidence: Level A)

REFERENCE	PATIENT POPULATION	N	PROBIOTICS USED IN INTERVENTION/DOSAGE	SOURCE	BENEFIT IN PROBIOTIC GROUP
Chouraqui et al[180]	Healthy infants with average age less than 4 months	90	B. lactis (Bb-12), 1 × 10⁶ CFU/g powder formula resulting in 1.5 × 10⁸ CFU/L and S. thermophilus and L. helveticus used for acidification	Supplemented formula	↓ daily probability and risk of diarrhea; ↓ number of days with diarrhea per child-year
Oberhelman et al[181]	Undernourished infants and children, 6 to 24 months	204	LGG, 3.7 × 10¹⁰ CFU, 6 days/week	Added to liquid gelatin	↓ episodes of diarrhea
Pedone et al[182]	Healthy children, attending daycare, average age 1½ years	287	L. casei DN114 001, 3.2 × 10⁸ CFU, 5 days per week	Supplemented yogurt	↓ duration of diarrhea

(continued)

TABLE 11-2 *(continued)*

REFERENCE	PATIENT POPULATION	N	PROBIOTICS USED IN INTERVENTION/DOSAGE	SOURCE	BENEFIT IN PROBIOTIC GROUP
Pedone et al[183]	Healthy children attending daycare, age 6 to 24 months	779	L. casei DN114 001, 3.2×10^8 CFU, 5 days per week	Supplemented yogurt	↓ incidence of diarrhea
Saavedra et al[86]	Infants hospitalized for reasons other than diarrhea with average age nearly 1 year	55	B. lactis, 1×10^8 CFU/g powder formula; and S. thermophilus, 1×10^7 CFU/g powder formula	Supplemented formula	↓ rotaviral shedding ↓ incidence of diarrhea
Saran et al[162]	Undernourished children from urban area in India, age 2 to 5 years	100	L. acidophilus, 1×10^8 CFU/g	Supplement added to yogurt	↓ incidence of diarrhea
Szajewska et al[184]	Children, age 1 to 36 months, hospitalized for reasons other than diarrhea	81	LGG, 6×10^9 CFU; twice daily	Reconstituted sachet	↓ incidence of diarrhea ↓ incidence of rotavirus gastroenteritis
Weizman et al[163]	Healthy infants, age 4 to 10 months	201	L. reuteri 55730 or B. lactis Bb-12, 1×10^9 CFU/day	Supplemented formula	↓ diarrhea episodes and duration
Ziegler et al[185]	Healthy newborns	88	B. lactis Bb-12, 3.6×10^7 CFU/g powder formula resulting in 4.8×10^9 CFU/L	Supplemented formula	↓ number of days with diarrhea ↓ number of diarrheal episodes

(continued)

TABLE 11-2 *(continued)*

CLINICAL TRIALS DOCUMENTING PROBIOTIC BENEFITS IN PEDIATRIC POPULATIONS*

REFERENCE	PATIENT POPULATION	N	PROBIOTICS USED IN INTERVENTION/DOSAGE	SOURCE	BENEFIT IN PROBIOTIC GROUP
D. Prevention of Antibiotic-Associated Diarrhea					
Strength of Evidence: Level B					
Arvola et al[91]	Children on antibiotic therapy for acute respiratory infection; average age age 4½ years	119	LGG ATCC 53103, 2 × 10^{10} CFU, twice daily	Capsules	↓ incidence of diarrhea
Correa et al[92]	Children on antibiotic therapy, average age 2 years	157	B. lactis (Bb-12) 1 × 10^{7} CFU/g and S. thermophilus 1 × 10^{6} CFU/g	Supplemented formula	↓ incidence of diarrhea; ↓ incidence of dehydration
Vanderhoof et al[93]	Children on antibiotic therapy for common childhood infections, average age 4 years	188	Lactobacillus GG, 1 to 2 × 10^{10} CFU/day	Capsule	↓ incidence of diarrhea
E. Prevention and Management of Allergic Conditions					
Strength of Evidence: Level B					
Giovannini et al[114]	Children with allergic rhinitis, age 2 to 5 years	187	L. casei DN-114 001, 1 × 10^{8} CFU/mL; and yogurt cultures (L. bulgaricus, S. thermophilus)	Supplemental milk	↓ rhinitis episodes; ↓ duration of diarrhea

(continued)

TABLE 11-2 (continued)

REFERENCE	PATIENT POPULATION	N	PROBIOTICS USED IN INTERVENTION/DOSAGE	SOURCE	BENEFIT IN PROBIOTIC GROUP
Isolauri et al[101]	Breastfed atopic infants	27	B. lactis, 1×10^9 CFU/day; or LGG, 3×10^8 CFU/day	Supplemented formula	Improved skin condition ↓ atopic score B. lactis: ↓ serum sCD4, IL-2, TGF-B1 and urinary eosinophil protein X LGG: ↓ serum sCD4 and urinary eosinophil protein
Kirjavainen et al[13]	Atopic infants, average age 5 months	21	B. lactis, 8×10^{10} CFU/kg body weight	Supplemented formula	Positive correlation between Serum IgE and E. coli or Bacteroides in highly sensitized infants ↓ fecal Bacteroides and E. coli in supplemented group
Majamaa and Isolauri[102]	Atopic infants	37	LGG, 5×10^8 CFU/g	Supplemented formula	↓ fecal alpha 1 antitrypsin ↓ fecal TNF alpha
Peng and Hsu[115]	Children with allergic rhinitis, average age 15 years	90	L. paracasei 33 (LP33), 5×10^9 CFU/capsule, twice daily	Capsule	Improved allergy symptom score with regard to frequency of symptoms, level of bother, and overall quality of life

(continued)

TABLE 11-2 *(continued)*

CLINICAL TRIALS DOCUMENTING PROBIOTIC BENEFITS IN PEDIATRIC POPULATIONS*

REFERENCE	PATIENT POPULATION	N	PROBIOTICS USED IN INTERVENTION/DOSAGE	SOURCE	BENEFIT IN PROBIOTIC GROUP
Pessi et al[103]	Children with atopic dermatitis and cow's milk allergy, average age nearly 2 years	9	LGG ATTC 53103, 1 × 10^10 CFU, twice daily	Delivery method not specified	↑ serum Il-10
Pohjavuori et al[104]	Atopic infants with cow's milk allergy	119	LGG, 5 × 10^9 CFU/day; or mixture of LGG, 5 × 10^9 CFU, L. rhamnosus 5 × 10^9 CFU, B. breve, 2 × 10^8 CFU, and P. freudenreichii spp. shermanii, 2 × 10^9 CFU/day	Powder supplement mixed with food	Probiotic Mix: ↑ IFN-gamma; no change in Il-4, Il-5, and Il-12, in infants with IgE-associated dermatitis receiving LGG
Rosenfeldt et al[113]	Children with atopy, average age 5 years	43	L. reuteri DSM 122460 and L. rhamnosus 190702, 1 × 10^10 CFU each, twice daily	Supplement dissolved in liquid	↓ severity of eczema ↓ eosinophil cationic protein
Rosenfeldt et al[186]	Children with moderate to severe atopy, average age 4 years	41	L. reuteri DSM 122460 and L. rhamnosus 190702, 1 × 10^10 CFU each, twice daily	Supplement dissolved in liquid	Improved intestinal barrier function ↓ symptoms of diarrhea, vomiting, abdominal pain
Sistek et al[112]	Children with atopy, age 3 to 4 years	59	B. lactis and L. rhamnosus for total dose of 2 × 10^10 CFU/g	Supplement	↓ atopic score among food-sensitized children

(continued)

TABLE 11-2 (continued)

REFERENCE	PATIENT POPULATION	N	PROBIOTICS USED IN INTERVENTION/DOSAGE	SOURCE	BENEFIT IN PROBIOTIC GROUP
Viljanen et al[105]	Atopic infants	230	LGG, 5×10^9 CFU/day; or mixture of LGG, 5×10^9 CFU, L. rhamnosus 5×10^9 CFU, B. breve 2×10^8 CFU, and P. freudenreichii spp. shermanii, 2×10^9 CFU/day	Powder supplement mixed with food	LGG: ↑ fecal IgA Mixture of probiotics: nonsignificant ↑ fecal IgA
Weston et al[187]	Atopic infants age 6 to 18 months	56	L. fermentum VRI-033, 1×10^9 CFU/g, twice daily	Powder supplement mixed with water	↓ atopic score
Wang et al[116]	Children with perennial allergic rhinitis; average age 15 years	80	L. paracasei, 1×10^7 CFU/mL; and yogurt cultures (L. bulgaricus, S. thermophilus)	Supplemental milk	Improved allergy symptom scores with regard to nose symptoms, activity limitations, and overall quality of life
West et al[106]	Healthy infants at the initiation of weaning, age 4 to 13 months	179	L. paracasei ssp. paracasei, strain F19, 1×10^8 CFU/day	Supplement added to cereal	↓ incidence of eczema ↑ IFN-c/IL4 mRNA ratio Ratio reflective of enhanced T cell-mediated immune response

(continued)

TABLE 11-2 (continued)

CLINICAL TRIALS DOCUMENTING PROBIOTIC BENEFITS IN PEDIATRIC POPULATIONS*

F. Emerging Areas of Research with Probiotics in Pediatric Health (Strength of Evidence: Level C)

REFERENCE	PATIENT POPULATION	N	PROBIOTICS USED IN INTERVENTION/DOSAGE	SOURCE	BENEFIT IN PROBIOTIC GROUP
Bausserman and Michail[125]	Children with irritable bowel syndrome, average age 12 years	50	*Lactobacillus* GG, 1×10^{10} CFU/day	Capsule	↓ perceived abdominal distention
Bekkali et al[126]	Children with constipation, age 4 to 16 years	20	Probiotic mixture of *B. bifidum*, *B. longum*, *B. infantis*, *L. casei*, *L. plantarum*, *L. rhamnosus* totaling 4×10^9 CFU/day	Delivery method not specified	↑ stool frequency and improved stool consistency ↓ incontinence episodes ↓ abdominal pain
Bruzzese et al[129]	Children with cystic fibrosis, average age 13 years	38	LGG, 6×10^9 CFU/day	Dissolved in oral rehydration solution	↓ number pulmonary exacerbations and improved pulmonary function ↓ number of hospitalizations ↑ body weight
Bu et al[127]	Children with chronic constipation, age ≤10 years	45	*L. casei rhamnosus* Lcr35, 8×10^8 CFU/day	Supplement	↑ stool frequency ↓ abdominal pain ↓ enema usage
Cruchet et al[134]	Asymptomatic children testing positive for *H. pylori*, age nearly 10 years	326	*L. johnsonii* (La 1), >1×10^7 CFU/mL, 5 times weekly	Supplemented beverage	↓ *H. pylori* colonization

(continued)

TABLE 11-2 (continued)

REFERENCE	PATIENT POPULATION	N	PROBIOTICS USED IN INTERVENTION/DOSAGE	SOURCE	BENEFIT IN PROBIOTIC GROUP
Gawronska et al[128]	Children with diagnosed irritable bowel syndrome, average age 11½ years	37	LGG, 3×10^9 CFU, twice daily	Capsule	↓ frequency of abdominal pain
Gotteland et al[135]	Asymptomatic children, testing positive for H. pylori, age 6 to 16 years	271	L. johnsonii (La 1), $>1 \times 10^7$ CFU/mL	Supplemented beverage	↑ H. pylori eradication rate
Gupta et al[130]	Children with mild to moderate Crohn's disease	4	Lactobacillus GG, 1×10^{10} CFU, twice daily	Tablet	↓ intestinal permeability; Improvement in clinical status reflected by ↓ Crohn's disease index score
Indrio et al[137]	Preterm infants	30	L. reuteri ATCC 55730, 1×10^8 CFU/day	Supplemental drops	↓ inconsolable crying; ↓ regurgitation
Kanamori et al[131]	Malnourished children with short bowel syndrome, average age 9 years	7	B. breve Yakult, and L. casei Shirota, totaling 1×10^9 CFU, 3 times daily	Supplement	↑ short fecal chain fatty acids; ↑ stool Bifidobacterium and Lactobacillus; ↑ serum prealbumin; ↑ body weight
Malin et al[188]	Children with chronic inflammatory conditions, average age 10 years	23	L. casei strain LGG ATTC 53103, 1×10^{10} CFU, twice daily	Powder supplement mixed with liquid	↑ antibody immune response as reflected by ↑ antigen-specific IgA

(continued)

TABLE 11-2 *(continued)*

CLINICAL TRIALS DOCUMENTING PROBIOTIC BENEFITS IN PEDIATRIC POPULATIONS*

REFERENCE	PATIENT POPULATION	N	PROBIOTICS USED IN INTERVENTION/DOSAGE	SOURCE	BENEFIT IN PROBIOTIC GROUP
Malin et al[189]	Children with juvenile chronic arthritis, average age age 8 years	16	*Lactobacillus* GG ATCC 53103, 1×10^{10} CFU, twice daily	Powder, mixed with liquid	↓ stool urease activity, used as an indicator for reduction in altered fecal bacteria
Lionetti et al[132]	*H. pylori*-positive children receiving antibiotic eradication therapy, average age 12 years	40	*L. reuteri* ATCC 55730, 1×10^8 CFU/ day	Pills	Improved Gastrointestinal Symptom Rating Scale score during *H. pylori* eradication therapy and after treatment
Savino et al[138]	Breastfed infants with diagnosed colic	46	*L. reuteri* ATCC 55730, 1×10^8 CFU/ day	Supplemental drops	↓ inconsolable crying within 1 week of treatment
Sykora et al[133]	*H. pylori* positive children receiving antibiotic eradication therapy, average age 12½ years	86	*L. casei* DN-114001, 1×10^{10} CFU/day	Fermented milk supplement	↑ *H. pylori* eradication rate
Tabbers et al[190]	Children with functional constipation, age 3 to 16 years	160	*B. lactis* DN-173 010, 6×10^9 CFU, twice daily	Supplemented yogurt	↑ stool frequency

*Results shown are those reported as significant in the individual studies.
Studies in which probiotic dose was not provided, or those utilizing yeasts (*S. boulardii*) as a sole intervention, heat killed probiotics, synbiotics, or probiotics provided during gestation are excluded.

(continued from page 151)

States. *Lactobacillus*, particularly LGG, despite very rare instances of bacteremia, may be a probiotic appropriate for the older infant or child. Having been approved by the FDA for use in therapeutic infant formulas and in foods or beverages for older children, LGG appears generally safe. The use of probiotics, in general, cannot be recommended in immunocompromised populations, unless specific bacteria show particular benefits that outweigh concerns. However, as safety is better documented for individual probiotic bacteria or combinations, some of these populations (such as premature infants) may actually be those who benefit most from their use.

PREBIOTIC USE IN PEDIATRICS

The definitions and criteria for prebiotics have continued to evolve. However, the basic concept behind a prebiotic dietary substance is that it can provide health benefits to the host by stimulating the growth or activity of colonic bacteria such as *Lactobacillus* or *Bifidobacterium*, which in turn contribute to health and well-being.[192] Dietary probiotics, by definition, improve host health. The basic effect of a prebiotic substance is that it can be shown to increase fecal counts of these desirable species. As opposed to probiotics, the potential specific effect or benefit on the host has not commonly been part of the definition of a prebiotic. Several prebiotic substances, mostly oligosaccharides, have well-documented benefits relating to their effect in the gut lumen as a nonabsorbable carbohydrate, thereby conveying digestive benefits such as those of soluble fiber, increased substrate for fermentation, leading to production of SCFAs that favor epithelial trophism, and lowering distal gut pH, which is inhibitory to pathogens, all of which contribute to gut and, particularly, colonic health. The comments below are limited to the prebiotic effects mediated by compositional microbiota changes and their potential for a clinical benefit via this mechanism in infants and young children.

The best-documented substances with bifidogenic effects include inulin and fructans (oligofructoses) and GOS. Most studies assessing prebiotic effects of these substances have been done in adults and the elderly, and the majority have documented fecal flora changes with dietary fructans.[192,193] Compared to research with probiotics in pediatric populations, only a limited number of studies have assessed health benefits with prebiotic supplementation. On the basis of the fact that human milk contains GOS, the vast majority of these studies utilize a mixture of short-chain GOS, often combined with FOS of varying polymeric lengths, for supplementation to infant formula and other foods. The effective amount or dose of prebiotic varies among studies. The goal of bifidogenicity with these prebiotic blends has been documented after assessing increased *Bifidobacterium* number in stool of preterm infants,[194,195] full-term infants,[196-199] and those of weaning age.[200] However, the initial numbers of *Bifidobacterium* in the gut may be the limiting factor influencing the prebiotic effect, rather than the quantity of prebiotic provided. The increase in new bifidobacteria, expressed as an absolute number, has been described as a "prebiotic index" associated with dietary prebiotics[193] and may be a useful indicator for comparing prebiotic effects of various ingredients.

Via anaerobic fermentation, probiotic bacteria use nondigestible colonic contents (eg, specific prebiotics) to multiply and typically create an acidic, potentially less pathogenic environment in the distal gut. However, in addition to increasing *Bifidobacterium*, FOS can also be fermented by most species of *Enterobacteriacia* present in the human intestine,[201] and increased concentrations of *Enterobacteriacia* and *Salmonella* have been demonstrated with both dietary FOS and inulin supplementation in strictly controlled animal studies.[202-204] Other bacterial groups, including *Clostridium*-related species, may also be stimulated by dietary fructans,[205] possibly through a mechanism described as cross-feeding[206] in which metabolic products produced from the dietary addition of some fermentable carbohydrates by one bacterial species yield substrates enabling the growth of other microbial communities[207] or modifying colonic barrier function.[208] However, no negative outcomes in this regard have been documented in clinical trials, which supports the safe and already broad use of these oligosaccharides in foods and beverages.

Some data suggest that combinations of GOS and FOS may yield immune-related benefits in infants. A reduced incidence of atopic dermatitis with high-risk infants supplemented with a GOS-FOS mixture during the first 6 months of life has been documented,[209] and a follow-up study of some of the children through age 2 years showed a continued protective effect on atopy as well as recurrent wheezing.[210] This cohort of children also had decreased incidence of upper respiratory tract infections, antibiotic prescriptions, and episodes of fever. A trend toward increased fecal sIgA with a prebiotic mixture has been reported in another group of supplemented infants.[211]

The stools of infants consuming GOS- or GOS-FOS-supplemented formulas may be softer and more frequent than those consuming unsupplemented formula.[198,212-214] While no general recommendations on supplementation or prebiotic addition to infant foods and beverages have been made to date,[215] the clinical benefits of prebiotics, particularly from the immunomodulatory point of view, are emerging.

CONCLUSION

Early and continued exposure to bacterial species is essential for proper immune system development. Our contemporary lifestyle is leading to decreases in vaginal births (the first source of bacteria for an infant), substitution of breast milk (another common source of bacteria) for sterile formulas, increased antibiotic use, and a general environmental decrease in microbial experience in infants and children. Environmental sanitation and the advent of pasteurization (sterilization of the most common source of dietary bacteria in humans until a century ago) perpetuate this decreased level of host-microbe interaction later in life. This appears to have health consequences, many of which can be explained by an altered or inappropriate development and maintenance of immune response. The use of probiotics (specific dietary bacteria that show a specific benefit) on a regular basis for health maintenance, and in instances for managing illness, has a sound foundation. The oral consumption of certain microbes in early life with an adequate safety profile, and the positive effect of these microbes on gut barrier function and immune response are increasingly being documented in pediatric populations, and the potential for long-term health benefits is increasingly tangible.

REFERENCES

1. Collado MC, Isolauri E, Salminen S, Sanz Y. The impact of probiotic on gut health. *Curr Drug Metab.* 2009;10(1):68-78.
2. Salminen S, Benno Y, de Vos W. Intestinal colonisation, microbiota and future probiotics? *Asia Pac J Clin Nutr.* 2006;15(4):558-562.
3. Salminen S, Isolauri E. Opportunities for improving the health and nutrition of the human infant by probiotics. *Nestle Nutr Workshop Ser Pediatr Program.* 2008;62:223-233.
4. Majamaa H, Isolauri E, Saxelin M, Vesikari T. Lactic acid bacteria in the treatment of acute rotavirus gastroenteritis. *J Pediatr Gastroenterol Nutr.* 1995;20(3):333-338.

5. Gueimonde M, Sakata S, Kalliomaki M, Isolauri E, Benno Y, Salminen S. Effect of maternal consumption of *Lactobacillus* GG on transfer and establishment of fecal bifidobacterial microbiota in neonates. *J Pediatr Gastroenterol Nutr.* 2006;42(2):166-170.

6. Schultz M, Gottl C, Young RJ, Iwen P, Vanderhoof JA. Administration of oral probiotic bacteria to pregnant women causes temporary infantile colonization. *J Pediatr Gastroenterol Nutr.* 2004;38(3):293-297.

7. Kitajima H, Sumida Y, Tanaka R, Yuki N, Takayama H, Fujimura M. Early administration of *Bifidobacterium breve* to preterm infants: randomised controlled trial. *Arch Dis Child Fetal Neonatal Ed.* 1997;76(2):F101-F107.

8. Li Y, Shimizu T, Hosaka A, Kaneko N, Ohtsuka Y, Yamashiro Y. Effects of *Bifidobacterium breve* supplementation on intestinal flora of low birth weight infants. *Pediatr Int.* 2004;46(5):509-515.

9. Mohan R, Koebnick C, Schildt J, et al. Effects of *Bifidobacterium lactis* Bb12 supplementation on intestinal microbiota of preterm infants: a double-blind, placebo-controlled, randomized study. *J Clin Microbiol.* 2006;44(11):4025-4031.

10. Uhlemann M, Heine W, Mohr C, Plath C, Pap S. Effects of oral administration of *bifidobacteria* on intestinal microflora in premature and newborn infants (translation from German). *Z Geburtshilfe Neonatol.* 1999;203(5):213-217.

11. Abrahamsson TR, Jakobsson T, Bottcher MF, et al. Probiotics in prevention of IgE-associated eczema: a double-blind, randomized, placebo-controlled trial. *J Allergy Clin Immunol.* 2007;119:1174-1180.

12. Fukushima Y, Li S-T, Hara H, Terada A, Mitsuoka T. Effect of follow-up formula containing Bifidobacteria (NAN BF) on fecal flora and fecal metabolites in healthy children. *Bioscience Microflora.* 1997;16(2):65-72.

13. Kirjavainen PV, Arvola T, Salminen SJ, Isolauri E. Aberrant composition of gut microbiota of allergic infants: a target of bifidobacterial therapy at weaning? *Gut.* 2002;51(1):51-55.

14. Langhendries JP, Detry J, Van Hees J, et al. Effect of a fermented infant formula containing viable bifidobacteria on the fecal flora composition and pH of healthy full-term infants. *J Pediatr Gastroenterol Nutr.* 1995;21(2):177-181.

15. Mah KW, Chin VI, Wong WS, et al. Effect of a milk formula containing probiotics on the fecal microbiota of Asian infants at risk of atopic diseases. *Pediatr Res.* 2007;62(6):674-679.

16. Martino DJ, Currie H, Taylor A, Conway P, Prescott SL. Relationship between early intestinal colonization, mucosal immunoglobulin A production and systemic immune development. *Clin Exp Allergy.* 2008;38(1):69-78.

17. Petschow BW, Figueroa R, Harris CL, Beck LB, Ziegler E, Goldin B. Effects of feeding an infant formula containing *Lactobacillus* GG on the colonization of the intestine: a dose-response study in healthy infants. *J Clin Gastroenterol.* 2005;39(9):786-790.

18. Sepp E, Mikelsaar M, Salminen S. Effect of administration of *Lactobacillus casei* strain GG on the gastrointestinal microbiota of newborns. *Microbial Ecology Health Dis.* 1993;6:309-314.

19. Biasucci G, Benenati B, Morelli L, Bessi E, Boehm G. Cesarean delivery may affect the early biodiversity of intestinal bacteria. *J Nutr.* 2008;138(9):1796S-1800S.

20. Cebra JJ. Influences of microbiota on intestinal immune system development. *Am J Clin Nutr.* 1999;69(5):1046S-1051S.

21. Vael C, Nelen V, Verhulst SL, Goossens H, Desager KN. Early intestinal *Bacteroides fragilis* colonisation and development of asthma. *BMC Pulm Med.* 2008;8:19.

22. Kemp A, Bjorksten B. Immune deviation and the hygiene hypothesis: a review of the epidemiological evidence. *Pediatr Allergy Immunol.* 2003;14(2):74-80.

23. Linneberg A. Hypothesis: urbanization and the allergy epidemic—a reverse case of immunotherapy? *Allergy.* 2005;60(4):538-539.

24. Matricardi PM, Yazdanbakhsh M. Mycobacteria and atopy, 6 years later: a fascinating, still unfinished, business. *Clin Exp Allergy.* 2003;33(6):717-720.

25. Tissier H. Traitement des infections intestinales par la methode de la flore bacterienne de l'intestin. *C R Soc Biol.* 1906;60:359-361.

26. Turroni F, van Sinderen D, Ventura M. Bifidobacteria: from ecology to genomics. *Front Biosci.* 2009;14:4673-4684.

27. Edwards CA, Parrett AM. Intestinal flora during the first months of life: new perspectives. *Br J Nutr.* 2002;88(suppl 1):S11-S18.

28. Fanaro S, Chierici R, Guerrini P, Vigi V. Intestinal microflora in early infancy: composition and development. *Acta Paediatr Suppl.* 2003;91(441):48-55.

29. Mitsuoka T. The human gastrointestinal tract. In: Wood BJB, ed. *The Lactic Acid Bacteria in Health and Disease.* Vol. 1. London: Elsevier Applied Science; 1992:69-114.

30. Penders J, Thijs C, Vink C, et al. Factors influencing the composition of the intestinal microbiota in early infancy. *Pediatrics.* 2006;118(2):511-521.

31. Bezirtzoglou E. The intestinal microflora during the first weeks of life. *Anaerobe.* 1997;3(2-3):173-177.
32. Adlerberth I, Lindberg E, Aberg N, et al. Reduced enterobacterial and increased staphylococcal colonization of the infantile bowel: an effect of hygienic lifestyle? *Pediatr Res.* 2006;59(1):96-101.
33. Adlerberth I, Strachan DP, Matricardi PM, et al. Gut microbiota and development of atopic eczema in 3 European birth cohorts. *J Allergy Clin Immunol.* 2007;120(2):343-350.
34. Gronlund MM, Lehtonen OP, Eerola E, Kero P. Fecal microflora in healthy infants born by different methods of delivery: permanent changes in intestinal flora after cesarean delivery. *J Pediatr Gastroenterol Nutr.* 1999;28(1):19-25.
35. Huurre A, Kalliomaki M, Rautava S, Rinne M, Salminen S, Isolauri E. Mode of delivery—effects on gut microbiota and humoral immunity. *Neonatology.* 2008;93(4):236-240.
36. Kuitunen M, Kukkonen K, Juntunen-Backman K, et al. Probiotics prevent IgE-associated allergy until age 5 years in cesarean-delivered children but not in the total cohort. *J Allergy Clin Immunol.* 2009;123(2):335-341.
37. Renz-Polster H, David MR, Buist AS, et al. Caesarean section delivery and the risk of allergic disorders in childhood. *Clin Exp Allergy.* 2005;35(11):1466-1472.
38. Bager P, Melbye M, Rostgaard K, Benn CS, Westergaard T. Mode of delivery and risk of allergic rhinitis and asthma. *J Allergy Clin Immunol.* 2003;111(1):51-56.
39. Hamilton BE, Martin JA, Ventura SJ, Sutton PD, Menacker F. Births: preliminary data for 2004. *Natl Vital Stat Rep.* 2005;54(8):1-17.
40. Collado MC, Delgado S, Maldonado A, Rodriguez JM. Assessment of the bacterial diversity of breast milk of healthy women by quantitative real-time PCR. *Lett Appl Microbiol.* 2009;48:523-528.
41. Heikkila MP, Saris PE. Inhibition of *Staphylococcus aureus* by the commensal bacteria of human milk. *J Appl Microbiol.* 2003;95(3):471-478.
42. Martin R, Langa S, Reviriego C, et al. Human milk is a source of lactic acid bacteria for the infant gut. *J Pediatr.* 2003;143(6):754-758.
43. Martin R, Heilig HG, Zoetendal EG, et al. Cultivation-independent assessment of the bacterial diversity of breast milk among healthy women. *Res Microbiol.* 2007;158(1):31-37.
44. Casas IA, Dobrogosz WJ. Validation of the probiotic concept: *Lactobacillus reuteri* confers broad-spectrum protection against disease in humans and animals. *Microbiol Ecology Health Dis.* 2000;12:247-285.
45. Sinkiewicz G, Nordstrom E. Occurrence of *Lactobacillus reuteri*, lactobacilli and bifidobacteria in human breast milk. *Ped Research.* 2005;58(2):415.
46. Martin R, Jimenez E, Olivares M, et al. *Lactobacillus salivarius* CECT 5713, a potential probiotic strain isolated from infant feces and breast milk of a mother-child pair. *Int J Food Microbiol.* 2006;112(1):35-43.
47. Gronlund MM, Gueimonde M, Laitinen K, et al. Maternal breast-milk and intestinal bifidobacteria guide the compositional development of the *Bifidobacterium* microbiota in infants at risk of allergic disease. *Clin Exp Allergy.* 2007;37(12):1764-1772.
48. Gueimonde M, Laitinen K, Salminen S, Isolauri E. Breast milk: a source of bifidobacteria for infant gut development and maturation? *Neonatology.* 2007;92(1):64-66.
49. Martin R, Jimenez E, Heilig H, et al. Isolation of bifidobacteria from breast milk and assessment of the bifidobacterial population by PCR-denaturing gradient gel electrophoresis and quantitative real-time PCR. *Appl Environ Microbiol.* 2009;75(4):965-969.
50. Perez PF, Dore J, Leclerc M, et al. Bacterial imprinting of the neonatal immune system: lessons from maternal cells? *Pediatrics.* 2007;119(3):e724-e732.
51. Martin R, Langa S, Reviriego C, et al. The commensal microflora of human milk: new perspectives for food bacterio-therapy and probiotics. *Trends Food Sci Technol.* 2004;15:121-127.
52. Qutaishat SS, Stemper ME, Spencer SK, et al. Transmission of salmonella enterica serotype typhimurium DT104 to infants through mother's breast milk. *Pediatrics.* 2003;111(6, pt 1):1442-1446.
53. George M, Nord KE, Ronquist G, Hedenstierna G, Wiklund L. Faecal microflora and urease activity during the first six months of infancy. *J Med Sci.* 1996;101(3):233-250.
54. Harmsen HJ, Wildeboer-Veloo AC, Raangs GC, et al. Analysis of intestinal flora development in breast-fed and formula-fed infants by using molecular identification and detection methods. *J Pediatr Gastroenterol Nutr.* 2000;30(1):61-67.
55. Magne F, Hachelaf W, Suau A, et al. A longitudinal study of infant faecal microbiota during weaning. *FEMS Microbiol Ecol.* 2006;58(3):563-571.
56. Vlkova E, Nevoral J, Jencikova B, et al. Detection of infant faecal bifidobacteria by enzymatic methods. *J Microbiol Methods.* 2005;60(3):365-373.
57. Yoshioka H, Iseki K, Fujita K. Development and differences of intestinal flora in the neonatal period in breast-fed and bottle-fed infants. *Pediatrics.* 1983;72(3):317-321.
58. Favier CF, Vaughan EE, De Vos WM, Akkermans AD. Molecular monitoring of succession of bacterial communities in human neonates. *Appl Environ Microbiol.* 2002;68(1):219-226.

59. Vaughan EE, de Vries MC, Zoetendal EG, Ben Amor K, Akkermans AD, De Vos WM. The intestinal LABs. *Antonie Van Leeuwenhoek.* 2002;82(1-4):341-352.
60. Mullie C, Romond MB, Izard D. Establishment and follow-up of bifidobacterial species in the gut of healthy bottle-fed infants of 1-4 months age. *Folia Microbiol (Praha).* 2006;51(5):473-477.
61. Haarman M, Knol J. Quantitative real-time PCR assays to identify and quantify fecal *Bifidobacterium* species in infants receiving a prebiotic infant formula. *Appl Environ Microbiol.* 2005;71(5):2318-2324.
62. Mackie RI, Sghir A, Gaskins HR. Developmental microbial ecology of the neonatal gastrointestinal tract. *Am J Clin Nutr.* 1999;69(5):1035S-1045S.
63. Penders J, Vink C, Driessen C, London N, Thijs C, Stobberingh EE. Quantification of *Bifidobacterium* spp., *Escherichia coli* and *Clostridium difficile* in faecal samples of breast-fed and formula-fed infants by real-time PCR. *FEMS Microbiol Lett.* 2005;243(1):141-147.
64. Rubaltelli FF, Biadaioli R, Pecile P, Nicoletti P. Intestinal flora in breast- and bottle-fed infants. *J Perinat Med.* 1998;26(3):186-191.
65. Stark PL, Lee A. The microbial ecology of the large bowel of breast-fed and formula-fed infants during the first year of life. *J Med Microbiol.* 1982;15(2):189-203.
66. Guerin-Danan C, Andrieux C, Popot F, et al. Pattern of metabolism and composition of the fecal microflora in infants 10 to 18 months old from day care centers. *J Pediatr Gastroenterol Nutr.* 1997;25(3):281-289.
67. Wang M, Ahrne S, Antonsson M, Molin G. T-RFLP combined with principal component analysis and 16S rRNA gene sequencing: an effective strategy for comparison of fecal microbiota in infants of different ages. *J Microbiol Methods.* 2004;59(1):53-69.
68. Balamurugan R, Janardhan HP, George S, Chittaranjan SP, Ramakrishna BS. Bacterial succession in the colon during childhood and adolescence: molecular studies in a southern Indian village. *Am J Clin Nutr.* 2008;88(6):1643-1647.
69. Neu J. Perinatal and neonatal manipulation of the intestinal microbiome: a note of caution. *Nutr Rev.* 2007;65(6 Pt 1):282-285.
70. Penders J, Thijs C, van den Brandt PA, et al. Gut microbiota composition and development of atopic manifestations in infancy: the KOALA Birth Cohort Study. *Gut.* 2007;56(5):661-667.
71. Alm B, Erdes L, Mollborg P, et al. Neonatal antibiotic treatment is a risk factor for early wheezing. *Pediatrics.* 2008;121(4):697-702.
72. Verhulst SL, Vael C, Beunckens C, Nelen V, Goossens H, Desager K. A longitudinal analysis on the association between antibiotic use, intestinal microflora, and wheezing during the first year of life. *J Asthma.* 2008;45(9):828-832.
73. Marra F, Lynd L, Coombes M, et al. Does antibiotic exposure during infancy lead to development of asthma?: a systematic review and metaanalysis. *Chest.* 2006;129(3):610-618.
74. Nase L, Hatakka K, Savilahti E, et al. Effect of long-term consumption of a probiotic bacterium, *Lactobacillus rhamnosus* GG, in milk on dental caries and caries risk in children. *Caries Res.* 2001;35(6):412-420.
75. Kaila M, Isolauri E, Soppi E, Virtanen E, Laine S, Arvilommi H. Enhancement of the circulating antibody secreting cell response in human diarrhea by a human *Lactobacillus* strain. *Pediatr Res.* 1992;32(2):141-144.
76. Campbell-Platt G. Fermented foods: a world perspective. *Food Research International.* 1994;27:253-257.
77. Bailey M, Haverson K, Inman C, et al. The development of the mucosal immune system pre- and post-weaning: balancing regulatory and effector function. *Proc Nutr Soc.* 2005;64(4):451-457.
78. Saavedra JM. Use of probiotics in pediatrics: rationale, mechanisms of action, and practical aspects. *Nutr Clin Pract.* 2007;22(3):351-365.
79. Salminen SJ, Gueimonde M, Isolauri E. Probiotics that modify disease risk. *J Nutr.* 2005;135(5):1294-1298.
80. Szajewska H, Skorka A, Ruszczynski M, Gieruszczak-Bialek D. Meta-analysis: *Lactobacillus* GG for treating acute diarrhoea in children. *Aliment Pharmacol Ther.* 2007;25(8):871-881.
81. Huang JS, Bousvaros A, Lee JW, Diaz A, Davidson EJ. Efficacy of probiotic use in acute diarrhea in children: a meta-analysis. *Dig Di Sci.* 2002;47(11):2625-2634.
82. McFarland LV, Elmer GW, McFarland M. Meta-analysis of probiotics for the prevention and treatment of acute pediatric diarrhea. *Int J Probiotics Prebiotics.* 2006;1(1):63-76.
83. Szajewska H, Mrukowicz JZ. Probiotics in the treatment and prevention of acute infectious diarrhea in infants and children: a systematic review of published randomized, double-blind, placebo-controlled trials. *J Pediatr Gastroenterol Nutr.* 2001;33(suppl 2):S17-S25.
84. Van Niel CW, Feudtner C, Garrison MM, Christakis DA. *Lactobacillus* therapy for acute infectious diarrhea in children: a meta-analysis. *Pediatrics.* 2002;109(4):678-684.
85. Rosenfeldt V, Michaelsen KF, Jakobsen M, et al. Effect of probiotic *Lactobacillus* strains in young children hospitalized with acute diarrhea. *Pediatr Infect Dis J.* 2002;21(5):411-416.

86. Saavedra JM, Bauman NA, Oung I, Perman JA, Yolken RH. Feeding of *Bifidobacterium bifidum* and *Streptococcus thermophilus* to infants in hospital for prevention of diarrhoea and shedding of rotavirus. *Lancet.* 1994;344(8929):1046-1049.

87. Sazawal S, Hiremath G, Dhingra U, Malik P, Deb S, Black RE. Efficacy of probiotics in prevention of acute diarrhoea: a meta-analysis of masked, randomised, placebo-controlled trials. *Lancet Infect Dis.* 2006;6(6):374-382.

88. Szajewska H, Ruszczynski M, Radzikowski A. Probiotics in the prevention of antibiotic-associated diarrhea in children: a meta-analysis of randomized controlled trials. *J Pediatr.* 2006:367-373.

89. Johnston BC, Supina AL, Ospina M, Vohra S. Probiotics for the prevention of pediatric antibiotic-associated diarrhea. *Cochrane Database Syst Rev.* 2007;(2):CD004827.

90. Hotta M, Sato Y, Iwata S, et al. Clinical effects of *Bifidobacterium* preparations on pediatric intractable diarrhea. *Keio J Med.* 1987;36(3):298-314.

91. Arvola T, Laiho K, Torkkeli S, et al. Prophylactic *Lactobacillus* GG reduces antibiotic-associated diarrhea in children with respiratory infections: a randomized study. *Pediatrics.* 1999;104(5):64-67.

92. Correa NB, Peret Filho LA, Penna FJ, Lima FM, Nicoli JR. A randomized formula controlled trial of *Bifidobacterium lactis* and *Streptococcus thermophilus* for prevention of antibiotic-associated diarrhea in infants. *J Clin Gastroenterol.* 2005;39(5):385-389.

93. Vanderhoof JA, Whitney DB, Antonson DL, Hanner TL, Lupo JV, Young RJ. *Lactobacillus* GG in the prevention of antibiotic-associated diarrhea in children. *J Pediatr.* 1999;135(5):564-568.

94. Bjorksten B, Sepp E, Julge K, Voor T, Mikelsaar M. Allergy development and the intestinal microflora during the first year of life. *J Allergy Clin Immunol.* 2001;108(4):516-520.

95. Gore C, Munro K, Lay C, et al. *Bifidobacterium pseudocatenulatum* is associated with atopic eczema: a nested case-control study investigating the fecal microbiota of infants. *J Allergy Clin Immunol.* 2008;121:135-140.

96. Kirjavainen PV, Apostolou E, Arvola T, Salminen SJ, Gibson GR, Isolauri E. Characterizing the composition of intestinal microflora as a prospective treatment target in infant allergic disease. *FEMS Immunol Med Microbiol.* 2001;32(1):1-7.

97. Mah KW, Bjorksten B, Lee BW, et al. Distinct pattern of commensal gut microbiota in toddlers with eczema. *Int Arch Allergy Immunol.* 2006;140(2):157-163.

98. Suzuki S, Shimojo N, Tajiri Y, Kumemura M, Kohno Y. Differences in the composition of intestinal *Bifidobacterium* species and the development of allergic diseases in infants in rural Japan. *Clin Exp Allergy.* 2007;37(4):506-511.

99. Kalliomaki M, Kirjavainen P, Eerola E, Kero P, Salminen S, Isolauri E. Distinct patterns of neonatal gut microflora in infants in whom atopy was and was not developing. *J Allergy Clin Immunol.* 2001;107(1):129-134.

100. Stsepetova J, Sepp E, Julge K, Vaughan E, Mikelsaar M, De Vos WM. Molecularly assessed shifts of *Bifidobacterium* ssp. and less diverse microbial communities are characteristic of 5-year-old allergic children. *FEMS Immunol Med Microbiol.* 2007;51(2):260-269.

101. Isolauri E, Arvola T, Sutas Y, Moilanen E, Salminen S. Probiotics in the management of atopic eczema. *Clin Exp Allergy.* 2000;30(11):1604-1610.

102. Majamaa H, Isolauri E. Probiotics: a novel approach in the management of food allergy. *J Allergy Clin Immunol.* 1997;99(2):179-185.

103. Pessi T, Sutas Y, Hurme M, Isolauri E. Interleukin-10 generation in atopic children following oral *Lactobacillus rhamnosus* GG. *Clin Exp Allergy.* 2000;30(12):1804-1808.

104. Pohjavuori E, Viljanen M, Korpela R, et al. *Lactobacillus* GG effect in increasing IFN-gamma production in infants with cow's milk allergy. *J Allergy Clin Immunol.* 2004;114(1):131-136.

105. Viljanen M, Kuitunen M, Haahtela T, Juntunen-Backman K, Korpela R, Savilahti E. Probiotic effects on faecal inflammatory markers and on faecal IgA in food allergic atopic eczema/dermatitis syndrome infants. *Pediatr Allergy Immunol.* 2005;16(1):65-71.

106. West CE, Hammarstrom ML, Hernell O. Probiotics during weaning reduce the incidence of eczema. *Pediatr Allergy Immunol.* 2009;20(5):430-437.

107. Kalliomaki M, Salminen S, Arvilommi H, Kero P, Koskinen P, Isolauri E. Probiotics in primary prevention of atopic disease: a randomised placebo-controlled trial. *Lancet.* 2001;357(9262):1076-1079.

108. Kalliomaki M, Salminen S, Poussa T, Isolauri E. Probiotics during the first 7 years of life: a cumulative risk reduction of eczema in a randomized, placebo-controlled trial. *J Allergy Clin Immunol.* 2007;119:1019-1021.

109. Wickens K, Black PN, Stanley TV, et al. A differential effect of 2 probiotics in the prevention of eczema and atopy: a double-blind, randomized, placebo-controlled trial. *J Allergy Clin Immunol.* 2008;122(4):788-794.

110. Marschan E, Kuitunen M, Kukkonen K, et al. Probiotics in infancy induce protective immune profiles that are characteristic for chronic low-grade inflammation. *Clin Exp Allergy.* 2008;38(4):611-618.

111. Kukkonen K, Savilahti E, Haahtela T, et al. Probiotics and prebiotic galacto-oligosaccharides in the prevention of allergic diseases: a randomized, double-blind, placebo-controlled trial. *J Allergy Clin Immunol.* 2007;119(1):192-198.
112. Sistek D, Kelly R, Wickens K, Stanley T, Fitzharris P, Crane J. Is the effect of probiotics on atopic dermatitis confined to food sensitized children? *Clin Exp Allergy.* 2006;36(5):629-633.
113. Rosenfeldt V, Benfeldt E, Nielsen SD, et al. Effect of probiotic *Lactobacillus* strains in children with atopic dermatitis. *J Allergy Clin Immunol.* 2003;111(2):389-395.
114. Giovannini M, Agostoni C, Riva E, et al. A randomized prospective double blind controlled trial on effects of long-term consumption of fermented milk containing *Lactobacillus casei* in pre-school children with allergic asthma and/or rhinitis. *Pediatr Res.* 2007;62(2):215-220.
115. Peng GC, Hsu CH. The efficacy and safety of heat-killed *Lactobacillus paracasei* for treatment of perennial allergic rhinitis induced by house-dust mite. *Pediatr Allergy Immunol.* 2005;16(5):433-438.
116. Wang MF, Lin HC, Wang YY, Hsu CH. Treatment of perennial allergic rhinitis with lactic acid bacteria. *Pediatr Allergy Immunol.* 2004;15(2):152-158.
117. Kopp MV, Hennemuth I, Heinzmann A, Urbanek R. Randomized, double-blind, placebo-controlled trial of probiotics for primary prevention: no clinical effects of *Lactobacillus* GG supplementation. *Pediatrics.* 2008;121(4):e850-e856.
118. Taylor AL, Dunstan JA, Prescott SL. Probiotic supplementation for the first 6 months of life fails to reduce the risk of atopic dermatitis and increases the risk of allergen sensitization in high-risk children: a randomized controlled trial. *J Allergy Clin Immunol.* 2007;119(1):184-191.
119. Brouwer ML, Wolt-Plompen SA, Dubois AE, et al. No effects of probiotics on atopic dermatitis in infancy: a randomized placebo-controlled trial. *Clin Exp Allergy.* 2006;36(7):899-906.
120. Boyle RJ, Bath-Hextall FJ, Leonardi-Bee J, Murrell DF, Tang ML. Probiotics for treating eczema. *Cochrane Database Syst Rev.* 2008;(4):CD006135.
121. Lee J, Seto D, Bielory L. Meta-analysis of clinical trials of probiotics for prevention and treatment of pediatric atopic dermatitis. *J Allergy Clin Immunol.* 2008;121:116-121.
122. Osborn DA, Sinn JK. Probiotics in infants for prevention of allergic disease and food hypersensitivity (review). *Cochrane Database Syst Rev.* 2007;(4):CD006475.
123. Collado MC, Donat E, Ribes-Koninckx C, Calabuig M, Sanz Y. Specific duodenal and faecal bacterial groups associated with paediatric coeliac disease. *J Clin Pathol.* 2009;62(3):264-269.
124. Guarner F. The intestinal flora in inflammatory bowel disease: normal or abnormal? *Curr Opin Gastroenterol.* 2005;21(4):414-418.
125. Bausserman M, Michail S. The use of *Lactobacillus* GG in irritable bowel syndrome in children: a double-blind randomized control trial. *J Pediatr.* 2005;147(2):197-201.
126. Bekkali N, Bongers ME, Van den Berg MM, Liem O, Benninga MA. The role of a probiotics mixture in the treatment of childhood constipation: a pilot study. *Nutr J.* 2007;6(1):17.
127. Bu LN, Chang MH, Ni YH, Chen HL, Cheng CC. *Lactobacillus casei rhamnosus* Lcr35 in children with chronic constipation. *Pediatr Int.* 2007;49(4):485-490.
128. Gawronska A, Dziechciarz P, Horvath A, Szajewska H. A randomized double-blind placebo-controlled trial of *Lactobacillus* GG for abdominal pain disorders in children. *Aliment Pharmacol Ther.* 2007;25(2):177-184.
129. Bruzzese E, Raia V, Spagnuolo MI, et al. Effect of *Lactobacillus* GG supplementation on pulmonary exacerbations in patients with cystic fibrosis: a pilot study. *Clin Nutr.* 2007;26(3):322-328.
130. Gupta P, Andrew H, Kirschner BS, Guandalini S. Is *Lactobacillus* GG helpful in children with Crohn's disease? Results of a preliminary, open-label study. *J Pediatr Gastroenterol Nutr.* 2000;31(4):453-457.
131. Kanamori Y, Sugiyama M, Hashizume K, Yuki N, Morotomi M, Tanaka R. Experience of long-term synbiotic therapy in seven short bowel patients with refractory enterocolitis. *J Pediatr Surg.* 2004;39(11):1686-1692.
132. Lionetti E, Miniello VL, Castellaneta SP, et al. *Lactobacillus reuteri* therapy to reduce side-effects during anti-*Helicobacter pylori* treatment in children: a randomized placebo controlled trial. *Aliment Pharmacol Ther.* 2006;24(10):1461-1468.
133. Sykora J, Valeckova K, Amlerova J, et al. Effects of a specially designed fermented milk product containing probiotic *Lactobacillus casei* DN-114 001 and the eradication of *H. pylori* in children: a prospective randomized double-blind study. *J Clin Gastroenterol.* 2005;39(8):692-698.
134. Cruchet S, Obregon MC, Salazar G, Diaz E, Gotteland M. Effect of the ingestion of a dietary product containing *Lactobacillus johnsonii* La1 on *Helicobacter pylori* colonization in children. *Nutrition.* 2003;19(9):716-721.
135. Gotteland M, Andrews M, Toledo M, et al. Modulation of *Helicobacter pylori* colonization with cranberry juice and *Lactobacillus johnsonii* La1 in children. *Nutrition.* 2008;24(5):421-426.

136. Lehtonen L, Korvenranta H, Eerola E. Intestinal microflora in colicky and noncolicky infants: bacterial cultures and gas-liquid chromatography. *J Pediatr Gastroenterol Nutr.* 1994;19(3):310-314.

137. Indrio F, Riezzo G, Raimondi F, Bisceglia M, Cavallo L, Francavilla R. The effects of probiotics on feeding tolerance, bowel habits, and gastrointestinal motility in preterm newborns. *J Pediatr.* 2008;152(6): 801-806.

138. Savino F, Pelle E, Palumeri E, Oggero R, Miniero R. *Lactobacillus reuteri* (American Type Culture Collection Strain 55730) versus simethicone in the treatment of infantile colic: a prospective randomized study. *Pediatrics.* 2007;119(1):e124-e130.

139. Stratiki Z, Costalos C, Sevastiadou S, et al. The effect of a bifidobacter supplemented bovine milk on intestinal permeability of preterm infants. *Early Hum Dev.* 2007;83(9):575-579.

140. Bin-Nun A, Bromiker R, Wilschanski M, et al. Oral probiotics prevent necrotizing enterocolitis in very low birth weight neonates. *J Pediatr.* 2005;147(2):192-196.

141. Hoyos AB. Reduced incidence of necrotizing enterocolitis associated with enteral administration of *Lactobacillus acidophilus* and *Bifidobacterium infantis* to neonates in an intensive care unit. *Int J Infect Dis.* 1999;3(4):197-202.

142. Lin HC, Su BH, Chen AC, et al. Oral probiotics reduce the incidence and severity of necrotizing enterocolitis in very low birth weight infants. *Pediatrics.* 2005;115(1):1-4.

143. Lin HC, Hsu CH, Chen HL, et al. Oral probiotics prevent necrotizing enterocolitis in very low birth weight preterm infants: a multicenter, randomized, controlled trial. *Pediatrics.* 2008;122(4):693-700.

144. Alfaleh K, Bassler D. Probiotics for prevention of necrotizing enterocolitis in preterm infants. *Cochrane Database Syst Rev.* 2008;(1):CD005496.

145. Barclay AR, Stenson B, Simpson JH, Weaver LT, Wilson DC. Probiotics for necrotizing enterocolitis: a systematic review. *J Pediatr Gastroenterol Nutr.* 2007;45(5):569-576.

146. Kunz AN, Noel JM, Fairchok MP. Two cases of *Lactobacillus bacteremia* during probiotic treatment of short gut syndrome. *J Pediatr Gastroenterol Nutr.* 2004;38(4):457-458.

147. Land MH, Rouster-Stevens K, Woods CR, Cannon ML, Cnota J, Shetty AK. *Lactobacillus* sepsis associated with probiotic therapy. *Pediatrics.* 2005;115(1):178-181.

148. Food and Agriculture Organization, World Health Organization. The Food and Agriculture Organization of the United Nations and the World Health Organization Joint FAO/WHO working group report on drafting guidelines for the evaluation of probiotics in food. FAO/WHO Report No 4-30- 2002.

149. Weizman Z, Alsheikh A. Safety and tolerance of a probiotic formula in early infancy comparing two probiotic agents: a pilot study. *J Am Coll Nutr.* 2006;25(5):415-419.

150. Mohan R, Koebnick C, Schildt J, Mueller M, Radke M, Blaut M. Effects of *Bifidobacterium lactis* supplementation on body weight, fecal pH, acetate, lactate, calprotectin and IgA in preterm infants. *Pediatr Res.* 2008;64(4):418-422.

151. Nopchinda S, Varavithya W, Phuapradit P, et al. Effect of *Bifidobacterium* Bb12 with or without *Streptococcus thermophilus* supplemented formula on nutritional status. *J Med Assoc Thai.* 2002;85(suppl 4): S1225-S1231.

152. Cobo Sanz JM, Mateos JA, Munoz CA. Effect of *Lactobacillus casei* on the incidence of infectious conditions in children. *Nutr Hosp.* 2006;21(4):547-551.

153. Cukrowska B, Lodlnova-Zadnlkova R, Enders C, Sonnenborn U, Schulze J, Tlaskalova-Hogenova H. Specific proliferative and antibody responses of premature infants to intestinal colonization with nonpathogenic probiotic *E. coli* strain Nissle 1917. *Scand J Immunol.* 2002;55(2):204-209.

154. Fujii T, Ohtsuka Y, Lee T, et al. *Bifidobacterium breve* enhances transforming growth factor beta1 signaling by regulating Smad7 expression in preterm infants. *J Pediatr Gastroenterol Nutr.* 2006;43(1):83-88.

155. Fukushima Y, Kawata Y, Hara H, Terada A, Mitsuoka T. Effect of a probiotic formula on intestinal immunoglobulin A production in healthy children. *Int J Food Microbiol.* 1998;42(1-2):39-44.

156. Hatakka K, Savilahti E, Ponka A, et al. Effect of long term consumption of probiotic milk on infections in children attending day care centres: double blind, randomised trial. *BMJ.* 2001;322:1-5.

157. Hatakka K, Blomgren K, Pohjavuori S, et al. Treatment of acute otitis media with probiotics in otitis-prone children—a double-blind, placebo-controlled randomised study. *Clin Nutr.* 2007;26(3):314-321.

158. Isolauri E, Joensuu J, Suomalainen H, Luomala M, Vesikari T. Improved immunogenicity of oral D × RRV reassortant rotavirus vaccine by *Lactobacillus casei* GG. *Vaccine.* 1995;13(3):310-312.

159. Phuapradit P, Varavithya W, Vathanophas K, et al. Reduction of rotavirus infection in children receiving bifidobacteria-supplemented formula. *J Med Assoc Thai.* 1999;82(suppl 1):S43-S48.

160. Rautava S, Arvilommi H, Isolauri E. Specific probiotics in enhancing maturation of IgA responses in formula-fed infants. *Pediatr Res.* 2006;60(2):222-225.

161. Saavedra JM, Abi-Hanna A, Moore N, Yolken RH. Long-term consumption of infant formulas containing live probiotic bacteria: tolerance and safety. *Am J Clin Nutr.* 2004;79(2):261-267.

162. Saran S, Gopalan S, Krishna TP. Use of fermented foods to combat stunting and failure to thrive. *Nutrition.* 2002;18(5):393-396.

163. Weizman Z, Asli G, Alsheikh A. Effect of a probiotic infant formula on infections in child care centers: comparison of two probiotic agents. *Pediatrics*. 2005;115(1):5-9.
164. Boudraa G, Benbouabdellah M, Hachelaf W, Boisset M, Desjeux JF, Touhami M. Effect of feeding yogurt versus milk in children with acute diarrhea and carbohydrate malabsorption. *J Pediatr Gastroenterol Nutr*. 2001;33(3):307-313.
165. Canani RB, Cirillo P, Terrin G, et al. Probiotics for treatment of acute diarrhoea in children: randomised clinical trial of five different preparations. *BMJ*. 2007;335(7615):340.
166. Gaon D, Garcia H, Winter L, et al. Effect of *Lactobacillus* strains and *Saccharomyces boulardii* on persistent diarrhea in children. *Medicina (B Aires)*. 2003;63(4):293-298.
167. Guandalini S, Pensabene L, Zikri MA, et al. *Lactobacillus* GG administered in oral rehydration solution to children with acute diarrhea: a multicenter European trial. *J Pediatr Gastroenterol Nutr*. 2000;30(1):54-60.
168. Guarino A, Canani RB, Spagnuolo MI, Albano F, Di BL. Oral bacterial therapy reduces the duration of symptoms and of viral excretion in children with mild diarrhea. *J Pediatr Gastroenterol Nutr*. 1997;25(5):516-519.
169. Isolauri E, Juntunen M, Rautanen T, Sillanaukee P, Koivula T. A human *Lactobacillus* strain (*Lactobacillus casei* sp strain GG) promotes recovery from acute diarrhea in children. *Pediatrics*. 1991;88(1):90-97.
170. Isolauri E, Kaila M, Mykkanen H, Ling WH, Salminen S. Oral bacteriotherapy for viral gastroenteritis. *Dig Dis Sci*. 1994;39(12):2595-2600.
171. Lee MC, Lin LH, Hung KL, Wu HY. Oral bacterial therapy promotes recovery from acute diarrhea in children. *Acta Paediatr Taiwan*. 2001;42(5):301-305.
172. Mao M, Yu T, Xiong Y, et al. Effect of a lactose-free milk formula supplemented with bifidobacteria and streptococci on the recovery from acute diarrhoea. *Asia Pac J Clin Nutr*. 2008;17(1):30-34.
173. Pant AR, Graham SM, Allen SJ, et al. *Lactobacillus* GG and acute diarrhoea in young children in the tropics. *J Trop Pediatr*. 1996;42(3):162-165.
174. Raza S, Graham SM, Allen SJ, Sultana S, Cuevas L, Hart CA. *Lactobacillus* GG promotes recovery from acute nonbloody diarrhea in Pakistan. *Pediatr Infect Dis J*. 1995;14(2):107-111.
175. Rosenfeldt V, Michaelsen KF, Jakobsen M, et al. Effect of probiotic *Lactobacillus* strains on acute diarrhea in a cohort of nonhospitalized children attending day-care centers. *Pediatr Infect Dis J*. 2002;21(5):417-419.
176. Shornikova AV, Casas IA, Mykkanen H, Salo E, Vesikari T. Bacteriotherapy with *Lactobacillus reuteri* in rotavirus gastroenteritis. *Pediatr Infect Dis J*. 1997;16(12):1103-1107.
177. Shornikova AV, Casas IA, Isolauri E, Mykkanen H, Vesikari T. *Lactobacillus reuteri* as a therapeutic agent in acute diarrhea in young children. *J Pediatr Gastroenterol Nutr*. 1997;24(4):399-404.
178. Shornikova AV, Isolauri E, Burkanova L, Lukovnikova S, Vesikari T. A trial in the Karelian Republic of oral rehydration and *Lactobacillus* GG for treatment of acute diarrhoea. *Acta Paediatr*. 1997;86(5):460-465.
179. Szymanski H, Pejcz J, Jawien M, Chmielarczyk A, Strus M, Heczko PB. Treatment of acute infectious diarrhoea in infants and children with a mixture of three *Lactobacillus rhamnosus* strains—a randomized, double-blind, placebo-controlled trial. *Aliment Pharmacol Ther*. 2006;23(2):247-253.
180. Chouraqui JP, Van Egroo LD, Fichot MC. Acidified milk formula supplemented with *Bifidobacterium lactis*: impact on infant diarrhea in residential care settings. *J Pediatr Gastroenterol Nutr*. 2004;38(3):288-292.
181. Oberhelman RA, Gilman RH, Sheen P, et al. A placebo-controlled trial of *Lactobacillus* GG to prevent diarrhea in undernourished Peruvian children. *J Pediatr*. 1999;134(1):15-20.
182. Pedone CA, Bernabeu AO, Postaire ER, Bouley CF, Reinert P. The effect of supplementation with milk fermented by *Lactobacillus casei* (strain DN-114 001) on acute diarrhoea in children attending day care centres. *Int J Clin Pract*. 1999;53(3):179-184.
183. Pedone CA, Arnaud CC, Postaire ER, Bouley CF, Reinert P. Multicentric study of the effect of milk fermented by *Lactobacillus casei* on the incidence of diarrhoea. *Int J Clin Pract*. 2000;54(9):568-571.
184. Szajewska H, Kotowska M, Mrukowicz JZ, Armanska M, Mikolajczyk W. Efficacy of *Lactobacillus* GG in prevention of nosocomial diarrhea in infants. *J Pediatr*. 2001;138(3):361-365.
185. Ziegler EE, Jeter JM, Drulis JM, et al. Formula with reduced content of improved, partially hydrolyzed protein and probiotics: infant growth and health. *Monatsschr Kinderheilkd*. 2003;1(151):S65-S71.
186. Rosenfeldt V, Benfeldt E, Valerius NH, Paerregaard A, Michaelsen KF. Effect of probiotics on gastrointestinal symptoms and small intestinal permeability in children with atopic dermatitis. *J Pediatr*. 2004;145(5):612-616.
187. Weston S, Halbert A, Richmond P, Prescott SL. Effects of probiotics on atopic dermatitis: a randomised controlled trial. *Arch Dis Child*. 2005;90(9):892-897.
188. Malin M, Suomalainen H, Saxelin M, Isolauri E. Promotion of IgA immune response in patients with Crohn's disease by oral bacteriotherapy with *Lactobacillus* GG. *Ann Nutr Metab*. 1996;40(3):137-145.

189. Malin M, Verronen P, Mykkanen H, Salminen S, Isolauri E. Increased bacterial urease activity in faeces in juvenile chronic arthritis: evidence of altered intestinal microflora? *Br J Rheumatol.* 1996;35(7):689-694.

190. Tabbers MM, Chmielewska A, Roseboom MG, et al. Effect of the consumption of a fermented dairy product containing *Bifidobacterium lactis* DN-173 010 on constipation in childhood: a multicentre randomised controlled trial (NTRTC: 1571). *BMC Pediatr.* 2009;9:22.

191. Velaphi SC, Cooper PA, Bolton KD, et al. Growth and metabolism of infants born to women infected with human immunodeficiency virus and fed acidified whey-adapted starter formulas. *Nutrition.* 2008;24:203-211.

192. Roberfroid M. Inulin-type fructans: functional food ingredients. *J Nutr.* 2007;137:2493S-2502S.

193. Roberfroid M. Prebiotics: the concept revisited. *J Nutr.* 2007;137(3 suppl 2):830S-837S.

194. Boehm G, Lidestri M, Casetta P, et al. Supplementation of a bovine milk formula with an oligosaccharide mixture increases counts of faecal bifidobacteria in preterm infants. *Arch Dis Child Fetal Neonatal Ed.* 2002;86(3):F178-F181.

195. Kapiki A, Costalos C, Oikonomidou C, Triantafyllidou A, Loukatou E, Pertrohilou V. The effect of a fructo-oligosaccharide supplemented formula on gut flora of preterm infants. *Early Hum Dev.* 2007;83(5):335-339.

196. Knol J, Scholtens P, Kafka C, et al. Colon microflora in infants fed formula with galacto- and fructo-oligosaccharides: more like breast-fed infants. *J Pediatr Gastroenterol Nutr.* 2005;40(1):36-42.

197. Magne F, Hachelaf W, Suau A, et al. Effects on faecal microbiota of dietary and acidic oligosaccharides in children during partial formula feeding. *J Pediatr Gastroenterol Nutr.* 2008;46(5):580-588.

198. Moro G, Minoli I, Mosca M, et al. Dosage-related bifidogenic effects of galacto- and fructooligosaccharides in formula-fed term infants. *J Pediatr Gastroenterol Nutr.* 2002;34(3):291-295.

199. Schmelzle H, Wirth S, Skopnik H, et al. Randomized double-blind study of the nutritional efficacy and bifidogenicity of a new infant formula containing partially hydrolyzed protein, a high beta-palmitic acid level, and nondigestible oligosaccharides. *J Pediatr Gastroenterol Nutr.* 2003;36(3):343-351.

200. Fanaro S, Marten B, Bagna R, et al. Galacto-oligosaccharides are bifidogenic and safe at weaning: a double-blind randomized multicenter study. *J Pediatr Gastroenterol Nutr.* 2009;48(1):82-88.

201. Hartemink R, Van Laere KM, Rombouts FM. Growth of enterobacteria on fructo-oligosaccharides. *J Appl Microbiol.* 1997;83(3):367-374.

202. Ten Bruggencate SJ, Bovee-Oudenhoven IM, Lettink-Wissink ML, Van der Meer R. Dietary fructo-oligosaccharides dose-dependently increase translocation of salmonella in rats. *J Nutr.* 2003;133(7):2313-2318.

203. Ten Bruggencate SJ, Bovee-Oudenhoven IM, Lettink-Wissink ML, Katan MB, Van der Meer R. Dietary fructo-oligosaccharides and inulin decrease resistance of rats to salmonella: protective role of calcium. *Gut.* 2004;53(4):530-535.

204. Ten Bruggencate SJ, Bovee-Oudenhoven IM, Lettink-Wissink ML, Van der Meer R. Dietary fructooligosaccharides increase intestinal permeability in rats. *J Nutr.* 2005;135(4):837-842.

205. Kleessen B, Hartmann L, Blaut M. Oligofructose and long-chain inulin: influence on the gut microbial ecology of rats associated with a human faecal flora. *Br J Nutr.* 2001;86(2):291-300.

206. Duncan SH, Scott KP, Ramsay AG, et al. Effects of alternative dietary substrates on competition between human colonic bacteria in an anaerobic fermentor system. *Appl Environ Microbiol.* 2003;69(2):1136-1142.

207. Salazar N, Gueimonde M, Hernandez-Barranco AM, Ruas-Madiedo P, de los Reyes-Gavilan CG. Exopolysaccharides produced by intestinal *Bifidobacterium* strains act as fermentable substrates for human intestinal bacteria. *Appl Environ Microbiol.* 2008;74(15):4737-4745.

208. Rodenburg W, Keijer J, Kramer E, Vink C, Van der Meer R, Bovee-Oudenhoven IM. Impaired barrier function by dietary fructo-oligosaccharides (FOS) in rats is accompanied by increased colonic mitochondrial gene expression. *BMC Genomics.* 2008;9:144.

209. Moro G, Arslanoglu S, Stahl B, Jelinek J, Wahn U, Boehm G. A mixture of prebiotic oligosaccharides reduces the incidence of atopic dermatitis during the first six months of age. *Arch Dis Child.* 2006;91(10):814-819.

210. Arslanoglu S, Moro GE, Schmitt J, Tandoi L, Rizzardi S, Boehm G. Early dietary intervention with a mixture of prebiotic oligosaccharides reduces the incidence of allergic manifestations and infections during the first two years of life. *J Nutr.* 2008;138(6):1091-1095.

211. Bakker-Zierikzee AM, Tol EA, Kroes H, Alles MS, Kok FJ, Bindels JG. Faecal SIgA secretion in infants fed on pre- or probiotic infant formula. *Pediatr Allergy Immunol.* 2006;17(2):134-140.

212. Ben XM, Zhou XY, Zhao WH, et al. Supplementation of milk formula with galacto-oligosaccharides improves intestinal micro-flora and fermentation in term infants. *Chin Med J (Engl).* 2004;117(6):927-931.

213. Ben XM, Li J, Feng ZT, et al. Low level of galacto-oligosaccharide in infant formula stimulates growth of intestinal bifidobacteria and lactobacilli. *World J Gastroenterol.* 2008;14(42):6564-6568.
214. Costalos C, Kapiki A, Apostolou M, Papathoma E. The effect of a prebiotic supplemented formula on growth and stool microbiology of term infants. *Early Hum Dev.* 2008;84(1):45-49.
215. Agostoni C, Axelsson I, Goulet O, et al. Prebiotic oligosaccharides in dietetic products for infants: a commentary by the ESPGHAN Committee on Nutrition. *J Pediatr Gastroenterol Nutr.* 2004;39(5):465-473.

12

Neonatal Necrotizing Enterocolitis

Erika C. Claud, MD and W. Allan Walker, MD

Neonatal necrotizing enterocolitis (NEC) is an inflammatory bowel necrosis that primarily afflicts premature infants after the initiation of enteral feeding. It is the most common gastrointestinal emergency in the neonatal intensive care unit, affecting approximately 10% of premature infants <1500 g.[1-4] The risk factors for this disease are prematurity, bacterial colonization, enteral feeding, and altered intestinal blood flow. However, the link between these risk factors and the pathogenesis of the disease has been elusive, and the pathophysiology is poorly understood. This chapter will focus on the role of bacteria in neonatal NEC, both pathogenic and potentially preventative. Factors that affect colonization of the preterm gut, means by which beneficial bacteria may play a role in optimizing the gastrointestinal health of preterm infants, and specific evidence supporting the use of probiotics to decrease the incidence of NEC will be reviewed.

NEONATAL NECROTIZING ENTEROCOLITIS

NEC affects patients characteristically between 7 and 14 days of life,[1,3,4] although increasingly NEC has been documented several weeks after birth, particularly in very low-birth weight infants.[2] In addition, susceptibility to NEC appears inversely related to gestational age.[5] Thus, more immature infants have an increased incidence of this disease and a longer window of risk for the disease. There does not appear to be a gender or race predilection.

The inflammation in NEC can be focal, segmental, or diffuse, and it primarily affects the terminal ileum and proximal colon. Pathologic and histologic specimens have shown a combination of ischemic necrosis, acute and chronic inflammation, bacterial overgrowth, and tissue repair, suggesting that NEC is an evolving process rather than an acute event. Inflammation can be limited to the mucosa and submucosa of the intestine, or progress to transmural involvement in the most severe cases.

Floch MH, Kim AS, eds.
Probiotics: A Clinical Guide (pp 181-194)
© 2010 Taylor & Francis Group

NEC presents with variable symptoms that may include nonspecific signs of gastrointestinal dysfunction such as abdominal distension, feeding intolerance, gastric aspirates, bilious vomiting, and hematochezia, with progression to pneumoperitoneum and/or systemic signs of shock and rapid death in severe cases.[6,7] The pathognomonic feature is pneumatosis intestinalis on abdominal radiograph, which indicates air tracking within the bowel wall and may represent bacterial fermentation of intraluminal substrates. NEC has been classically described by the Bell's staging criteria in which Stage 1 or suspect NEC presents with mild systemic and gastrointestinal signs, such as hemoccult positive stools, abdominal distension, and gastric residuals after feedings. Stage 2 or definite NEC is the presence of pneumatosis intestinalis or portal venous air in addition to Stage 1 findings. Stage 3 or advanced NEC is Stage 2 plus progression to shock, disseminated intravascular coagulation, acidosis, thrombocytopenia, neutropenia, peritonitis, or pneumoperitoneum.[8]

BACTERIAL COLONIZATION AND NEONATAL NECROTIZING ENTEROCOLITIS

Bacteria are known to be important in the pathophysiology of NEC. However, although clusters of cases of NEC have been reported suggesting an infectious etiology, no specific organism has been linked to this disease. Isolated studies have demonstrated associations with organisms including enterobacteriaceae,[9,10] delta-toxin-producing methicillin-resistant *Staphylococcus aureus*,[11] *Clostridium*,[12,13] *E. coli*, and *Klebsiella pneumoniae*,[14] but none has been proven causative. Other studies have found no specific organism linked to this disease, but rather that each infant—with or without NEC—has his or her own distinct flora.[15] Thus, it is unknown if a specific pathogen causes this disease or if certain bacterial patterns predispose to NEC. Furthermore, it is unclear whether bacteria are a primary effector of NEC or are passive participants, entering the bowel wall through a breach in the intestinal mucosal barrier induced by other factors. Presence of bacteria is a prerequisite for NEC, and indeed studies have shown that prophylactic antibiotics may decrease the incidence of NEC.[16] However, NEC is not believed to be an infection in the classical sense, but rather an exaggerated inflammatory response to the presence of bacteria, with or without concomitant true sepsis, because only about 30% of infants with this disease have positive blood cultures.[17-19]

Bacterial Colonization of the Preterm Gut

The newborn gut is initially sterile. Thereafter, a rapid colonization by a wide variety of organisms ensues. This is a normal part of development and is important for gut maturation, containment of pathogenic organisms, as well as normal metabolism.[20,21] This begins a complex cross talk between the gut and its microflora. It is not merely the existence of bacteria but the balance of bacteria that affects a variety of signaling pathways and immune responses.

The intestine is generally initially colonized with a complex flora that reflects maternal flora.[22,23] However, further colonization of the bacteria in the intestine of a newborn is affected by a variety of factors including mode of delivery, type of feeding, hospitalization, and antibiotic use.[24] A variety of organisms, both beneficial and potentially harmful, can colonize the gut. Anaerobes such as *Bifidobacterium* and *Lactobacillus* are generally considered beneficial. Organisms such as *Escherichia coli* and *Bacteroides* are sometimes beneficial and sometimes harmful. In contrast, *Pseudomonas aerugi-*

nosa, clostridia, and *Staphylococcus* species are generally opportunistic pathogens. The KOALA Birth Cohort study in the Netherlands found that the most "beneficial" gut microbiota, defined as the highest numbers of bifidobacteria and the lowest number of *C. difficile* and *E. coli*, was found in term infants born vaginally at home and exclusively breastfed.[24]

Studies have shown that delivery method can have an influence. Infants delivered vaginally have earlier colonization with both *Bifidobacterium* and *Lactobacillus*, while infants delivered by cesarean section can have colonization with these beneficial organisms delayed by up to 30 days.[22,25] Feeding can also affect patterns. In breastfed infants, *Bifidobacterium* is a primary organism with *Lactobacillus* and *Streptococcus* as minor components. In formula-fed infants, similar amounts of *Bacteroides* and *Bifidobacterium* are found with minor components of the more pathogenic species *Staphylococcus*, *E. coli*, and clostridia.[23,26-29] In addition, while numbers of *Bifidobacterium* slowly increase in formula-fed infants, their levels remain significantly lower than those of breastfed infants even at 1 month of age.[30]

Colonization is also affected by gestational age. Although a wide range of aerobic and anaerobic flora colonizes normal full-term infants by 10 days of age, premature infants in the neonatal intensive care unit undergo a delayed colonization with a limited number of bacterial species that tend to be virulent, including *E. coli*, *Enterococcus* species, and *K. pneumoniae*.[1,31-34] Specifically, Gewolb et al noted that extremely low-birth weight infants were rarely colonized with *Lactobacillus* and bifidobacteria species.[26] There are several potential explanations for this phenomenon.[35] The common use of broad-spectrum antibiotics in premature infants leads to a loss of resistance to colonization by opportunistic pathogens that are more prevalent in the hospital environment to which these infants are exposed.[36] Instrumentation with nasogastric tubes for feeding and suction catheters introduces organisms. Use of medications such as opioids delays intestinal transit time, affecting bacterial adherence and colonization, while use of acid-neutralizing drugs removes a known intestinal host defense mechanism. Thus, colonization of the blank slate of the preterm intestine is influenced by iatrogenic manipulations of neonatal intensive care. Resulting altered microbial flora may contribute to a unique vulnerability to NEC and have significant implications for the development of the immature preterm gut.

Immature Intestinal Host Defense in the Preterm Infant

Microbial flora is determined not only by the organisms to which the intestine is exposed, but also by intrinsic intestinal host defense mechanisms. The premature infant population, expecting the conditions of the intrauterine environment, has the complicating challenge of being ill prepared for coexisting with an extensive microflora. The mature intestine has many physical barriers to bacteria including peristalsis, gastric acid, proteolytic enzymes, intestinal mucus, cell surface glycoconjugates, and tight junctions between intestinal epithelial cells. These are designed to limit bacteria to the gut lumen and prevent attachment and translocation across the intestinal epithelium. However, animal studies have shown that pathogenic organisms adhere to and translocate across the intestine to a greater extent in immature animals than in mature animals, and the adherence of bacterial strains may affect the ability to induce diseases such as NEC.[37] Abnormal peristaltic activity in immature infants may increase bacterial adherence, allowing for increased bacterial attachment and bacterial overgrowth.[38-40] Cell surface glycoconjugates serve as adhesion sites for a variety of microbes, and the immature intestine has a different pattern of carbohydrate residues, which may result in increased pathogenic colonization in preterm infants.[41,42] Furthermore, it is known that intestinal mucus, which protects against bacterial and toxin invasion, is different in developing animals and perhaps in premature infants in terms of carbohydrate composition, density, and possibly in inclusion of secretory immunoglobulin.[43]

Next, there is immaturity of the functional barrier that limits the growth of bacteria that breach the physical barrier. This functional barrier is comprised of the immunologic host defense and various biochemical factors. It is known that numbers of intestinal B and T lymphocytes are decreased in neonates and do not approach adult levels until 3 to 4 weeks of life. Newborns also have reduced levels of secretory IgA in salivary samples, presumably reflecting decreased activity in the intestine.[44-46] Additionally, premature infants have lower gastric acid production than do older children, and immature proteolytic enzyme activity may lead to incomplete breakdown of toxins.[44]

Finally, key proteins secreted from the intestinal epithelium, such as intestinal trefoil factor, are developmentally regulated and deficient in premature infants.[47-49] Human defensins (or cryptidins) synthesized and secreted from Paneth cells protect against bacterial translocation and are also altered in premature infants and those with NEC.[50,51]

Response of Immature Gut to Bacteria

An exacerbating condition for the preterm infant is the immaturity of the response to bacteria. It is potentially an important developmental step for enterocytes to decrease inflammatory responsiveness in order to prevent immune defense mechanisms against normal flora. Preterm infants may not have completed this maturation when initially fed and colonized by bacteria.

Evidence suggests that the premature neonate may be predisposed to intestinal inflammation. Studies have demonstrated that compared to adult intestinal epithelial cells (IEC), human fetal IEC have an exaggerated production of inflammatory cytokines in response to both pathogenic and commensal bacteria, as well as to endogenous inflammatory mediators such as TNF-α and IL-1β.[52,53]

TLR are a highly conserved family of pathogen-associated molecular pattern receptors that recognize bacterial components. TLR4 specifically recognizes the bacterial cell wall component lipopolysaccharide. Interestingly, TLR4 expression decreases after birth in the intestines of healthy mother-fed rat pups, but expression increases in the intestinal epithelium when pups are exposed to stresses common to preterm infants such as formula feeding and asphyxia.[54]

TLR activation, as well as TNFα and IL-1β, can activate nuclear factor kappaB (NF-κB) proteins, which leads to transcription of a wide variety of genes important in inflammatory and immune responses. In its resting state, NF-κB dimers are bound in the cytoplasm to inhibitory κB (IκB) proteins.[55] Cell stimulation can trigger signaling pathways, leading to degradation of IκB by the 26S proteasome.[56,57] NF-κB, thus liberated, moves to the nucleus where it activates gene transcription. Interestingly, NF-κB binding sites are located on the inhibitory IκBα promoter. Thus, an elegant autoregulatory feedback loop exists in which NF-κB activation leads to IκBα synthesis, which terminates the NF-κB response.[58,59] However, it has been shown that immature enterocytes have increased NF-κB activity associated with decreased baseline expression of IκB isoforms and compounded by more rapid IκBα degradation in stimulated immature enterocytes.[60,61] This suggests a developmental difference in a key inflammatory pathway common to many stimuli. Taken together, these results indicate that the preterm gut may be weighted toward proinflammatory responses, predisposing it to NEC.

CURRENT TREATMENTS

Because the pathogenesis for NEC is poorly understood, current treatment options are nonspecific and merely supportive—bowel rest with immediate cessation of enteral feeds and institution of nasogastric suction, fluid resuscitation, close monitoring of acid/base and electrolyte balance, broad-spectrum parenteral antibiotics, and parenteral nutrition. Frequent abdominal radiographs are required to document progression to pneumoperitoneum, and surgery is indicated for pneumoperitoneum, peritonitis, or intestinal obstruction. However, recent studies have demonstrated that patients who require surgery for NEC have a 50% mortality rate, require prolonged parenteral nutrition, and are at significant increased risk for neurodevelopmental impairment, including cerebral palsy as well as low mental development and psychomotor development indices.[62-64] Thus, it appears that by the time an infant progresses to surgery, significant irreversible damage has already been done. Current treatment modalities are often inadequate because of the rapid progression of NEC from its initial diagnosis. Thus, prevention of NEC may be a more important goal than NEC treatment. Intervention is required at a proximal step in the pathophysiologic cascade leading to NEC, which once started is very difficult to stop — the most proximal component being prematurity or the immature intestine itself.

PROBIOTICS AND NECROTIZING ENTEROCOLITIS: RATIONALE

The preterm infant appears predisposed to NEC due to (1) pathogenic bacterial colonization, (2) immature intestinal host defense mechanisms, and (3) a heightened proinflammatory response to colonizing organisms. Evidence from studies in cell culture and animal models suggests that while pathogenic bacterial colonization patterns may predispose preterm infants to NEC, specific beneficial bacteria have the potential to ameliorate the risk factors for NEC (Figure 12-1).

It is known that certain bacteria can provide interference resulting in competitive colonization against pathogenic organisms. A study using adherent *E. coli* strains from infants to induce NEC in a rabbit model found that coinfection with Gram-positive isolates from healthy children was able to block induction of disease.[37] The situation of the preterm infant could be considered comparable to that of the germ-free mouse. Studies have demonstrated that coliform organisms multiply rapidly and persistently colonize all organs of the GI tract in germ-free animals, in contrast to mice raised under ordinary conditions in which extensive invasion of the GI tract is transient.[65] Interestingly, when germ-free mice were fed the intestinal contents of healthy, pathogen-free mice, the coliform content dramatically decreased, suggesting that microbial balance is key in containment of pathogenic organisms. Commensal flora can interfere with infection by pathogenic organisms by competition for host-binding sites, stimulation of host defense mechanisms, production of bacteriocins, competition for nutrients, and triggering of cell-signaling events that limit the production of virulence factors; thus, the growth of competitive nonpathogenic strains of bacteria may be protective.[66]

It has been hypothesized that the injury in NEC begins with a breach in the intestinal mucosal barrier, leading to bacterial translocation across the epithelium and exacerbation of the inflammatory cascade, resulting in the clinical signs of NEC. A breach could be caused by disruption of connections between cells such as a loss of tight junctions or by loss of cells themselves by cell death such as apoptosis. In intestinal epithelial cell monolayers, probiotic mixtures containing *S. thermophilus* and *Lactobacillus* and

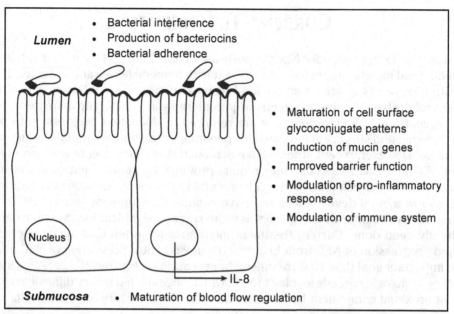

Figure 12-1. Means by which probiotic agents may decrease susceptibility of the preterm gut to neonatal NEC. Printed with permission from Claud EC, Walker WA. Bacterial colonization, probiotics, and necrotizing enterocolitis. *J Clin Gastroenterol.* 2008;42(suppl 2):S46-S52.

Bifidobacterium species have been shown to increase transepithelial resistance, which is one means of evaluating the intactness of the intestinal barrier.[67] This effect was accompanied by protection against cell death induced by a pathogenic *Salmonella* strain.[67,68]

The specific probiotic organism LGG has been shown to counteract cow milk-induced increases in intestinal permeability in suckling rats, as well as to decrease apoptosis and promote cytoprotective responses in developing murine gut.[69,70] Furthermore, studies have shown that using only factors secreted by LGG without live organisms led to protection against cytokine-induced apoptosis and from hydrogen peroxide-induced alterations in permeability and tight junction protein distribution, as well as promotion of IEC growth, thus preserving the key host defense mechanism—the intestinal barrier.[71,72]

Intestinal mucus is another physical barrier to infection that has been shown in animal studies to be developmentally mediated. Probiotic mixtures have been shown to induce the specific mucus genes MUC2, MUC3, and MUC5AC, reducing pathogenic bacterial attachment.[67,73] Furthermore, maturation patterns of cell surface glycoconjugates, which are the adhesion sites for a variety of microbes, are influenced by bacterial colonization. In a study that compared the cell surface glycoconjugate patterns in maturing germ-free and conventional mice, it was shown that fucosyltransferase increases with maturity while sialyltransferase decreases over time in conventional mice. In contrast, in germ-free mice the immature pattern of low fucosyltransferase and high sialyltransferase is maintained. However, colonization of the germ-free animals with conventional bacteria was sufficient to shift these patterns to normal "mature patterns" within 2 weeks, suggesting that commensal bacteria are important regulators of the maturational development of glycosyltransferase activity in the intestinal brush border.[74]

Lastly, while preterm infants have an exaggerated inflammatory response associated with increased NF-κB activity, it has been shown that combinations of probiotic organisms can decrease NF-κB activation. This appears to occur via inhibition of the proteasome, preventing degradation of the inhibitor IκB, thus keeping NF-κB in the cytoplasm and blocking nuclear translocation.[75] Preserving IκB may be specifically important as this is a key point of developmental differentiation between immature and mature enterocytes, with immature enterocytes having less baseline expression of IκB.[60]

PROBIOTICS AND NECROTIZING ENTEROCOLITIS: CLINICAL TRIALS

Because bacteria are necessary for maturation of the intestine and appropriate containment of inflammatory responses, it may be important to influence bacterial colonization. Health may not hinge on the presence of bad vs good bacteria, but on the creation of optimal bacterial communities vs pathogenic bacterial communities. Thus, for a premature infant, it has been suggested that optimizing the bacterial flora can enhance intestinal maturation and decrease the incidence of NEC.[76]

The promise of a potential benefit from probiotic organisms and/or their products has led to multiple studies. Initial animal studies of NEC in rodent, quail, and pig models have shown protection against NEC using *Bifidobacterium* and *Lactobacillus* species as well as *Saccharomyces boulardii*.[77-79] Initial studies in preterm infants used various organisms and evaluated varied responses. Cukrowska et al administered the nonpathogenic *E. coli* Nissle 1917 strain and found that it enhanced natural immune responses by inducing systemic humoral and cellular immunity.[80] Two studies evaluated *Lactobacillus* species—LGG and *L. acidophilus*—and found that *Lactobacillus* administration was well tolerated and successfully colonized the preterm gut; however, this colonization did not reduce the numbers of potential pathogens or appear to have clinical benefit.[81,82] Other studies of LGG in preterm infants documented that administered LGG had no adverse effects on SCFA production.[83] A larger double-blind multicenter study in Italy on the effects of LGG did not document successful colonization and also did not find a significant decrease in the primary outcomes of urinary tract infection, NEC, or sepsis.[84] Two studies have evaluated *B. breve* and found that early administration—beginning less than 24 hours after birth—resulted in earlier establishment of a *Bifidobacterium*-predominant flora compared to supplementation beginning 24 hours after birth or no supplementation, and further documented improved weight gain, decreased abnormal abdominal signs, and no adverse side effects.[85,86]

Despite variable results, these preliminary studies have led to 4 recent clinical studies that have specifically suggested a beneficial effect of probiotics on the incidence of NEC (Table 12-1).

Hoyos et al administered Infloran Berna7 (Swiss Serum and Vaccine Institute, Berne, Switzerland) containing a mixture of *L. acidophilus* and *B. infantis* to all newborns admitted to the neonatal intensive care unit at Hospital Simon Bolivar in Bogota, Colombia between October 15, 1994, and October 15, 1995.[87] All infants received one quarter capsule of Infloran (1000 million live *L. acidophilus* and 1000 million live *B. infantis* per capsule) in sterile water or dextrose solution daily for the entire hospital stay. A total of 1237 newborns received the probiotic treatment, and incidence of NEC in this cohort was compared to the incidence of NEC in historical controls from the previous year. This study did not document colonization of the infant gut with the probiotic organisms administered, but did find a significantly lower incidence of NEC—2.9% in the probiotic-treated infants vs 6.6 % in historical controls—and no adverse events. However, there were many concerns raised about this study, including the controls used and the larger babies that were included.

TABLE 12-1

Summary of Clinical Trials Utilizing Probiotic Preparations to Specifically Decrease the Incidence of Neonatal NEC

STUDY	SITE/PATIENT POPULATION	PROBIOTIC ADMINISTRATION	DECREASE IN NEC
Hoyos et al[87]	Bogota, Columbia All admitted newborns Historical controls	Daily Infloran until D/C (*L. acidophilus, B. infantis*)	2.9% vs 6.6%
Lin et al[88]	Taiwan VLBW <1500 g Prospective, masked, randomized controlled trial	2x/day Infloran until D/C (*L. acidophilus, B. infantis*)	1.1% vs 5.3%
Bin-Nun et al[89]	Israel Preterm infants <1500 g Prospective, blinded, randomized controlled trial	Daily ABC Dophilus until 36 weeks postconceptual age (*B. infantis, S. thermophilus, B. bifidus*)	1% vs 14%
Lin et al[90]	Taiwan VLBW <1500 g Multicenter, prospective, masked, randomized controlled trial	2x/day Infloran until D/C (*L. acidophilus, B. bifidum*)	1.8% vs 6.5%

Level of recommendation: Level C: Positive studies but clearly inadequate amount of work to establish level A or B.

Based on definitions agreed upon during the "Advances in Clinical Use of Probiotics Workshop," held at Yale University in November 2007.
Level A: Strong, positive, well-conducted, controlled studies in the primary literature, not abstract form.
Level B: Positive, controlled studies but some negative studies are present.
Level C: Positive studies but clearly inadequate amount of work to establish level A or B.

Lin et al also evaluated the efficacy of the probiotic product Infloran (Swiss Serum and Vaccine Institute, Berne, Switzerland) in a prospective, masked, randomized controlled trial of 367 infants <1500 g at China Medical University Hospital in Taiwan from July 1, 1999, to Dec 31, 2003.[88] All infants received breast milk with or without Infloran 125 mg/kg twice daily from study entry when enterally feeding, clinically stable and ≥7 days of life, until discharge. Daily treatment with *L. acidophilus* and *B. infantis* again decreased the incidence of NEC (≥ Bell Stage 2) from 5.3% to 1.1% (*P* = .04) with no reported adverse effect. This study also did not report evidence of colonization with the administered organisms. This trial was recently repeated as a prospective, blinded, randomized, multicenter controlled trial at 7 neonatal intensive care units in Taiwan from April 1, 2005 to May 30, 2007, and enrolled 434 infants <1500 g.[90] Patients received regular feeds of breast milk, or a combination of breast milk and formula with or without Infloran with a new formulation containing a combination of *L. acidophilus* 10^9 CFU and *B. bifidum* 10^9 CFU (National Collection of Dairy Organisms, Reading, United Kingdom and Laboratorio, Farmaceutico, Mede, Italy) at a dose of 125 mg/kg per dose twice daily. A pilot study was reported to have been performed using this probiotic product, which confirmed colonization with the administered organisms. The incidence of NEC (≥ Bell Stage 2) was again decreased from 6.5% to 1.8% in the probiotic treatment group with no reported adverse events.

Last, Bin-nun et al conducted a trial at the Shaare Zedek Medical Center in Israel between September 2001 and September 2004. One hundred forty-five infants <1500 g were enrolled in a prospective, randomized, double-blind study. In addition to their regular feedings, patients received an additional 3 mL feeding daily that did or did not contain the probiotic product ABC Dophilus (Solgar, division of Wyeth Consumer Healthcare, Bergen County, NJ). This probiotic mixture contained *B. infantis*, *S. thermophilus*, and *B. bifidus*.[89] Infants received 0.35×10^9 CFU of each organism for a total of 1.05×10^9 total CFU daily from the first day of feeds until the infants reached 36 weeks postconceptual age. This study did not report evidence of colonization with the administered organisms but did demonstrate a significant decrease in incidence of NEC (≥ Bell Stage 2) from 14% to 1% (*P* = .013) with no adverse effects.

CONCERNS

The previously cited clinical studies of probiotics and NEC were not sufficiently powered to fully assess the safety of administration of live bacteria to preterm infants. Thus, despite persuasive suggestion of efficacy and potential biologic plausibility for the use of probiotics in the treatment of NEC, safety is a primary concern. First, is it really safe to give live organisms to relatively "immunocompromised" preterm patients? Cases of *Lactobacillus* sepsis have been documented and prompt caution.[91] Studies reporting increased infant mortality in probiotic-treated animal models have also raised questions as to the prudence of using live bacteria in premature infants.[92]

Another concern is efficacy and means of administration. In the clinical studies of the effect of probiotics on preterm infants, varied probiotic preparations were used, and populations used may or may not be generalizable. Further, no mechanism of action, dosage, or timing specifics in the immature intestine are known. The optimal probiotic organism or combination of organisms to use is also unclear. Multiple studies have shown that different organisms have different effects, and even different strains of the same organism may behave differently.[93] Thus, our understanding is complicated by the use of different organisms in various clinical studies of probiotics.

Live probiotic bacteria have the potential to become pathogenic when host defenses are compromised, be it from immune deficiencies or illness.[94-97] Although some protective effects of probiotics require direct bacterial-epithelial cell-to-cell contact with live bacteria, other studies have shown that beneficial effects can be conferred by synthesized bioactive factors. Use of these secreted factors is currently under study.[75,98] Use of prebiotics or factors to promote growth of beneficial organisms is another option for conferring protection against the development of NEC without the risk of administration of live organisms.

CONCLUSION

NEC is a devastating condition without a precise etiology; however, it is known that prematurity is the primary risk factor for NEC. The premature infant differs from term infants and older patients in multiple ways, including an immature host defense system, an exaggerated intestinal inflammatory response by the immature enterocyte, and altered intestinal flora. Bacteria have been shown to play a key role in intestinal maturation. It is not merely the presence of bacteria but the balance of "beneficial" and "pathogenic" bacterial communities that makes a difference. Appropriate colonization can lead to appropriate maturation of glycoconjugate pathways, improved barrier function, improved intestinal epithelial cell survival, competitive exclusion of pathogenic organisms, and appropriate maturation of the immune system. This may be of particular importance to the fundamentally immature preterm gut. Administration of probiotics is an intriguing therapeutic option with evidence for clinical benefit, which warrants further study into the mechanism of action of specific organisms in models of immature intestine, in order to identify a potential means of optimizing intestinal colonization and influencing outcome of these vulnerable infants. However, until a single protocol using a specific probiotic preparation at the same dose, administered at the same time to a large number of premature infants across multiple nurseries, shows an effect, specific recommendations to practicing neonatologists for the routine use of probiotics to prevent NEC cannot be made.

In the neonatal population, microbial patterns are not yet established. Thus, in this patient group, one has the unique opportunity to initiate and influence colonization. Probiotic treatment in this patient population may not only temporarily affect bacterial colonization, but influence long-term bacterial pattern imprinting in a naïve host.

REFERENCES

1. Kosloske AM. Epidemiology of necrotizing enterocolitis. *Acta Paediatr Suppl.* 1994;396:2-7.
2. Lemons JA, Bauer CR, Oh W, et al. Very low birth weight outcomes of the National Institute of Child health and human development neonatal research network, January 1995 through December 1996. NICHD Neonatal Research Network. *Pediatrics.* 2001;107(1):E1.
3. MacKendrick W, Caplan M. Necrotizing enterocolitis. New thoughts about pathogenesis and potential treatments. *Pediatr Clin North Am.* 1993;40(5):1047-1059.
4. Rayyis SF, Ambalavanan N, Wright L, Carlo WA. Randomized trial of "slow" vs "fast" feed advancements on the incidence of necrotizing enterocolitis in very low birth weight infants. *J Pediatr.* 1999;134(3):293-297.
5. Stoll BJ, Kanto WP Jr, Glass RI, Nahmias AJ, Brann AW Jr. Epidemiology of necrotizing enterocolitis: a case control study. *J Pediatr.* 1980;96(3 Pt 1):447-451.
6. Walsh MC, Kliegman RM. Necrotizing enterocolitis: treatment based on staging criteria. *Pediatr Clin North Am.* 1986;33(1):179-201.

7. Faix RG, Adams JT. Neonatal necrotizing enterocolitis: current concepts and controversies. *Adv Pediatr Infect Dis.* 1994;9:1-36.
8. Bell MJ, Ternberg JL, Feigin RD, et al. Neonatal necrotizing enterocolitis. Therapeutic decisions based upon clinical staging. *Ann Surg.* 1978;187(1):1-7.
9. Bell MJ, Shackelford PG, Feigin RD, Ternberg JL, Brotherton T. Alterations in gastrointestinal microflora during antimicrobial therapy for necrotizing enterocolitis. *Pediatrics.* 1979;63(3):425-428.
10. Millar MR, MacKay P, Levene M, Langdale V, Martin C. Enterobacteriaceae and neonatal necrotising enterocolitis. *Arch Dis Child.* 1992;67(1 Spec No):53-56.
11. Overturf GD, Sherman MP, Scheifele DW, Wong LC. Neonatal necrotizing enterocolitis associated with delta toxin-producing methicillin-resistant *Staphylococcus aureus. Pediatr Infect Dis J.* 1990;9(2):88-91.
12. Sturm R, Staneck JL, Stauffer LR, Neblett WW III. Neonatal necrotizing enterocolitis associated with penicillin-resistant, toxigenic *Clostridium butyricum. Pediatrics.* 1980;66(6):928-931.
13. Blakey JL, Lubitz L, Campbell NT, Gillam GL, Bishop RF, Barnes GL. Enteric colonization in sporadic neonatal necrotizing enterocolitis. *J Pediatr Gastroenterol Nutr.* 1985;4(4):591-595.
14. Bell MJ, Feigin RD, Ternberg JL. Changes in the incidence of necrotizing enterocolitis associated with variation of the gastrointestinal microflora in neonates. *Am J Surg.* 1979;138(5):629-631.
15. Gupta S, Morris JG Jr, Panigrahi P, Nataro JP, Glass RI, Gewolb IH. Endemic necrotizing enterocolitis: lack of association with a specific infectious agent. *Pediatr Infect Dis J.* 1994;13(8):728-734.
16. Krediet TG, van Lelyveld N, Vijlbrief DC, et al. Microbiological factors associated with neonatal necrotizing enterocolitis: protective effect of early antibiotic treatment. *Acta Paediatr.* 2003;92(10):1180-1182.
17. Duffy LC, Zielezny MA, Carrion V, et al. Bacterial toxins and enteral feeding of premature infants at risk for necrotizing enterocolitis. *Adv Exp Med Biol.* 2001;501:519-527.
18. Duffy LC, Zielezny MA, Carrion V, et al. Concordance of bacterial cultures with endotoxin and interleukin-6 in necrotizing enterocolitis. *Dig Dis Sci.* 1997;42(2):359-365.
19. Hoy C, Millar MR, MacKay P, Godwin PG, Langdale V, Levene MI. Quantitative changes in faecal microflora preceding necrotising enterocolitis in premature neonates. *Arch Dis Child.* 1990;65(10 Spec No):1057-1059.
20. Stappenbeck TS, Hooper LV, Gordon JI. Developmental regulation of intestinal angiogenesis by indigenous microbes via Paneth cells. *Proc Natl Acad Sci U S A.* 2002;99(24):15451-15455.
21. Hooper LV, Wong MH, Thelin A, Hansson L, Falk PG, Gordon JI. Molecular analysis of commensal host-microbial relationships in the intestine. *Science.* 2001;291(5505):881-884.
22. Gronlund MM, Lehtonen OP, Eerola E, Kero P. Fecal microflora in healthy infants born by different methods of delivery: permanent changes in intestinal flora after cesarean delivery. *J Pediatr Gastroenterol Nutr.* 1999;28(1):19-25.
23. Harmsen HJ, Wildeboer-Veloo AC, Raangs GC, et al. Analysis of intestinal flora development in breast-fed and formula-fed infants by using molecular identification and detection methods. *J Pediatr Gastroenterol Nutr.* 2000;30(1):61-67.
24. Penders J, Thijs C, Vink C, et al. Factors influencing the composition of the intestinal microbiota in early infancy. *Pediatrics.* 2006;118(2):511-521.
25. Chen J, Cai W, Feng Y. Development of intestinal bifidobacteria and lactobacilli in breast-fed neonates. *Clin Nutr.* 2007;26(5):559-566.
26. Gewolb IH, Schwalbe RS, Taciak VL, Harrison TS, Panigrahi P. Stool microflora in extremely low birth-weight infants. *Arch Dis Child Fetal Neonatal Ed.* 1999;80(3):F167-F173.
27. Rubaltelli FF, Biadaioli R, Pecile P, Nicoletti P. Intestinal flora in breast- and bottle-fed infants. *J Perinat Med.* 1998;26(3):186-191.
28. Tomkins AM, Bradley AK, Oswald S, Drasar BS. Diet and the faecal microflora of infants, children and adults in rural Nigeria and urban U.K. *J Hyg (Lond).* 1981;86(3):285-293.
29. Wold AE, Adlerberth I. Breast feeding and the intestinal microflora of the infant: implications for protection against infectious diseases. *Adv Exp Med Biol.* 2000;478:77-93.
30. Yoshioka H, Iseki K, Fujita K. Development and differences of intestinal flora in the neonatal period in breast-fed and bottle-fed infants. *Pediatrics.* 1983;72(3):317-321.
31. Orrhage K, Nord CE. Factors controlling the bacterial colonization of the intestine in breast-fed infants. *Acta Paediatr Suppl.* 1999;88(430):47-57.
32. Goldmann DA, Leclair J, Macone A. Bacterial colonization of neonates admitted to an intensive care environment. *J Pediatr.* 1978;93(2):288-293.
33. Long SS, Swenson RM. Development of anaerobic fecal flora in healthy newborn infants. *J Pediatr.* 1977;91(2):298-301.
34. Schwiertz A, Gruhl B, Lobnitz M, Michel P, Radke M, Blaut M. Development of the intestinal bacterial composition in hospitalized preterm infants in comparison with breast-fed, full-term infants. *Pediatr Res.* 2003;54(3):393-399.

35. Hall MA, Cole CB, Smith SL, Fuller R, Rolles CJ. Factors influencing the presence of faecal lactobacilli in early infancy. *Arch Dis Child*. 1990;65(2):185-188.
36. Bennet R, Eriksson M, Nord CE. The fecal microflora of 1-3-month-old infants during treatment with eight oral antibiotics. *Infection*. 2002;30(3):158-160.
37. Panigrahi P, Gupta S, Gewolb IH, Morris JG Jr. Occurrence of necrotizing enterocolitis may be dependent on patterns of bacterial adherence and intestinal colonization: studies in Caco-2 tissue culture and weanling rabbit models. *Pediatr Res*. 1994;36(1, pt 1):115-121.
38. Berseth CL. Gestational evolution of small intestine motility in preterm and term infants. *J Pediatr*. 1989;115(4):646-651.
39. Berseth CL. Neonatal small intestinal motility: motor responses to feeding in term and preterm infants. *J Pediatr*. 1990;117(5):777-782.
40. Berseth CL. Gut motility and the pathogenesis of necrotizing enterocolitis. *Clin Perinatol*. 1994;21(2):263-270.
41. Dai D, Nanthkumar NN, Newburg DS, Walker WA. Role of oligosaccharides and glycoconjugates in intestinal host defense. *J Pediatr Gastroenterol Nutr*. 2000;30(suppl 2):S23-S33.
42. Chu SH, Walker WA. Developmental changes in the activities of sialyl- and fucosyltransferases in rat small intestine. *Biochim Biophys Acta*. 1986;883(3):496-500.
43. Snyder JD, Walker WA. Structure and function of intestinal mucin: developmental aspects. *Int Arch Allergy Appl Immunol*. 1987;82(3-4):351-356.
44. Udall JN, Jr. Gastrointestinal host defense and necrotizing enterocolitis. *J Pediatr*. 1990;117(1, pt 2):S33-S43.
45. Eibl MM, Wolf HM, Furnkranz H, Rosenkranz A. Prevention of necrotizing enterocolitis in low-birth-weight infants by IgA-IgG feeding. *N Engl J Med*. 1988;319(1):1-7.
46. Roberts SA, Freed DL. Neonatal IgA secretion enhanced by breast feeding. *Lancet*. 1977;2(8048):1131.
47. Tan XD, Hsueh W, Chang H, Wei KR, Gonzalez-Crussi F. Characterization of a putative receptor for intestinal trefoil factor in rat small intestine: identification by in situ binding and ligand blotting. *Biochem Biophys Res Commun*. 1997;237(3):673-677.
48. Sands BE, Podolsky DK. The trefoil peptide family. *Annu Rev Physiol*. 1996;58:253-273.
49. Lin J, Holzman IR, Jiang P, Babyatsky MW. Expression of intestinal trefoil factor in developing rat intestine. *Biol Neonate*. 1999;76(2):92-97.
50. Ouellette AJ. Paneth cells and innate immunity in the crypt microenvironment. *Gastroenterology*. 1997;113(5):1779-1784.
51. Salzman NH, Polin RA, Harris MC, et al. Enteric defensin expression in necrotizing enterocolitis. *Pediatr Res*. 1998;44(1):20-26.
52. Claud EC, Savidge T, Walker WA. Modulation of human intestinal epithelial cell IL-8 secretion by human milk factors. *Pediatr Res*. 2003;53(3):419-425.
53. Nanthakumar NN, Fusunyan RD, Sanderson I, Walker WA. Inflammation in the developing human intestine: A possible pathophysiologic contribution to necrotizing enterocolitis. *Proc Natl Acad Sci U S A*. 2000;97(11):6043-6048.
54. Jilling T, Simon D, Lu J, et al. The roles of bacteria and TLR4 in rat and murine models of necrotizing enterocolitis. *J Immunol*. 2006;177(5):3273-3282.
55. Ghosh S, Karin M. Missing pieces in the NF-kappaB puzzle. *Cell*. 2002;109(suppl):S81-S96.
56. DiDonato JA, Hayakawa M, Rothwarf DM, Zandi E, Karin M. A cytokine-responsive IkappaB kinase that activates the transcription factor NF-kappaB. *Nature*. 1997;388(6642):548-554.
57. Roff M, Thompson J, Rodriguez MS, et al. Role of IkappaBalpha ubiquitination in signal-induced activation of NFkappaB in vivo. *J Biol Chem*. 1996;271(13):7844-7850.
58. Chiao PJ, Miyamoto S, Verma IM. Autoregulation of I kappa B alpha activity. *Proc Natl Acad Sci U S A*. 1994;91(1):28-32.
59. Sun SC, Ganchi PA, Ballard DW, Greene WC. NF-kappa B controls expression of inhibitor I kappa B alpha: evidence for an inducible autoregulatory pathway. *Science*. 1993;259(5103):1912-1915.
60. Claud EC, Lu L, Anton PM, Savidge T, Walker WA, Cherayil BJ. Developmentally regulated IkappaB expression in intestinal epithelium and susceptibility to flagellin-induced inflammation. *Proc Natl Acad Sci U S A*. 2004;101(19):7404-7408.
61. Claud EC, Zhang X, Petrof EO, Sun J. Developmentally regulated tumor necrosis factor-alpha induced nuclear factor-kappaB activation in intestinal epithelium. *Am J Physiol Gastrointest Liver Physiol*. 2007;292(5):G1411-G1419.
62. Blakely ML, Tyson JE, Lally KP, et al. Laparotomy vs peritoneal drainage for necrotizing enterocolitis or isolated intestinal perforation in extremely low birth weight infants: outcomes through 18 months adjusted age. *Pediatrics*. 2006;117(4):e680-e687.
63. Hintz SR, Kendrick DE, Stoll BJ, et al. Neurodevelopmental and growth outcomes of extremely low birth weight infants after necrotizing enterocolitis. *Pediatrics*. 2005;115(3):696-703.

64. Moss RL, Dimmitt RA, Barnhart DC, et al. Laparotomy vs peritoneal drainage for necrotizing enterocolitis and perforation. *N Engl J Med.* 2006;354(21):2225-2234.
65. Schaedler RW, Dubos R, Costello R. The development of the bacterial flora in the gastrointestinal tract of mice. *J Exp Med.* 1965;122:59-66.
66. Bernet MF, Brassart D, Neeser JR, Servin AL. *Lactobacillus acidophilus* LA 1 binds to cultured human intestinal cell lines and inhibits cell attachment and cell invasion by enterovirulent bacteria. *Gut.* 1994;35(4):483-489.
67. Otte JM, Podolsky DK. Functional modulation of enterocytes by gram-positive and gram-negative microorganisms. *Am J Physiol Gastrointest Liver Physiol.* 2004;286(4):G613-G626.
68. Resta-Lenert S, Barrett KE. Probiotics and commensals reverse TNF-alpha- and IFN-gamma-induced dysfunction in human intestinal epithelial cells. *Gastroenterology.* 2006;130(3):731-746.
69. Isolauri E, Majamaa H, Arvola T, Rantala I, Virtanen E, Arvilommi H. *Lactobacillus casei* strain GG reverses increased intestinal permeability induced by cow milk in suckling rats. *Gastroenterology.* 1993;105(6):1643-1650.
70. Lin PW, Nasr TR, Berardinelli AJ, Kumar A, Neish AS. The probiotic *Lactobacillus* GG may augment intestinal host defense by regulating apoptosis and promoting cytoprotective responses in the developing murine gut. *Pediatr Res.* 2008;64(5):511-516.
71. Seth A, Yan F, Polk DB, Rao RK. Probiotics ameliorate the hydrogen peroxide-induced epithelial barrier disruption by a PKC- and MAP kinase-dependent mechanism. *Am J Physiol Gastrointest Liver Physiol.* 2008;294(4):G1060-G1069.
72. Yan F, Polk DB. Probiotic bacterium prevents cytokine-induced apoptosis in intestinal epithelial cells. *J Biol Chem.* 2002;277(52):50959-50965.
73. Mack DR, Michail S, Wei S, McDougall L, Hollingsworth MA. Probiotics inhibit enteropathogenic *E. coli* adherence in vitro by inducing intestinal mucin gene expression. *Am J Physiol.* 1999;276(4, pt 1): G941-G950.
74. Nanthakumar NN, Dai D, Newburg DS, Walker WA. The role of indigenous microflora in the development of murine intestinal fucosyl- and sialyltransferases. *Faseb J.* 2003;17(1):44-46.
75. Petrof EO, Kojima K, Ropeleski MJ, et al. Probiotics inhibit nuclear factor-kappaB and induce heat shock proteins in colonic epithelial cells through proteasome inhibition. *Gastroenterology.* 2004;127(5):1474-1487.
76. Lawrence G, Bates J, Gaul A. Pathogenesis of neonatal necrotising enterocolitis. *Lancet.* 1982;1(8264): 137-139.
77. Akisu M, Baka M, Yalaz M, Huseyinov A, Kultursay N. Supplementation with *Saccharomyces boulardii* ameliorates hypoxia/reoxygenation-induced necrotizing enterocolitis in young mice. *Eur J Pediatr Surg.* 2003;13(5):319-323.
78. Butel MJ, Waligora-Dupriet AJ, Szylit O. Oligofructose and experimental model of neonatal necrotising enterocolitis. *Br J Nutr.* 2002;87(suppl 2):S213-S219.
79. Caplan MS, Miller-Catchpole R, Kaup S, et al. Bifidobacterial supplementation reduces the incidence of necrotizing enterocolitis in a neonatal rat model. *Gastroenterology.* 1999;117(3):577-583.
80. Cukrowska B, LodInova-Zadnlkova R, Enders C, Sonnenborn U, Schulze J, Tlaskalova-Hogenova H. Specific proliferative and antibody responses of premature infants to intestinal colonization with non-pathogenic probiotic *E. coli* strain Nissle 1917. *Scand J Immunol.* 2002;55(2):204-209.
81. Millar MR, Bacon C, Smith SL, Walker V, Hall MA. Enteral feeding of premature infants with *Lactobacillus* GG. *Arch Dis Child.* 1993;69(5 Spec No):483-487.
82. Reuman PD, Duckworth DH, Smith KL, Kagan R, Bucciarelli RL, Ayoub EM. Lack of effect of *Lactobacillus* on gastrointestinal bacterial colonization in premature infants. *Pediatr Infect Dis.* 1986;5(6):663-668.
83. Stansbridge EM, Walker V, Hall MA, et al. Effects of feeding premature infants with *Lactobacillus* GG on gut fermentation. *Arch Dis Child.* 1993;69(5 Spec No):488-492.
84. Dani C, Biadaioli R, Bertini G, Martelli E, Rubaltelli FF. Probiotics feeding in prevention of urinary tract infection, bacterial sepsis and necrotizing enterocolitis in preterm infants. A prospective double-blind study. *Biol Neonate.* 2002;82(2):103-108.
85. Li Y, Shimizu T, Hosaka A, Kaneko N, Ohtsuka Y, Yamashiro Y. Effects of *Bifidobacterium breve* supplementation on intestinal flora of low birth weight infants. *Pediatr Int.* 2004;46(5):509-515.
86. Kitajima H, Sumida Y, Tanaka R, Yuki N, Takayama H, Fujimura M. Early administration of *Bifidobacterium breve* to preterm infants: randomised controlled trial. *Arch Dis Child Fetal Neonatal Ed.* 1997;76(2):F101-F107.
87. Hoyos AB. Reduced incidence of necrotizing enterocolitis associated with enteral administration of *Lactobacillus acidophilus* and *Bifidobacterium infantis* to neonates in an intensive care unit. *Int J Infect Dis.* 1999;3(4):197-202.
88. Lin HC, Su BH, Chen AC, et al. Oral probiotics reduce the incidence and severity of necrotizing enterocolitis in very low birth weight infants. *Pediatrics.* 2005;115(1):1-4.

89. Bin-Nun A, Bromiker R, Wilschanski M, et al. Oral probiotics prevent necrotizing enterocolitis in very low birth weight neonates. *J Pediatr.* 2005;147(2):192-196.

90. Lin HC, Hsu CH, Chen HL, et al. Oral probiotics prevent necrotizing enterocolitis in very low birth weight preterm infants: a multicenter, randomized, controlled trial. *Pediatrics.* 2008;122(4):693-700.

91. Land MH, Rouster-Stevens K, Woods CR, Cannon ML, Cnota J, Shetty AK. *Lactobacillus* sepsis associated with probiotic therapy. *Pediatrics.* 2005;115(1):178-181.

92. Wagner RD, Warner T, Roberts L, Farmer J, Balish E. Colonization of congenitally immunodeficient mice with probiotic bacteria. *Infect Immun.* 1997;65(8):3345-3351.

93. Christensen HR, Frokiaer H, Pestka JJ. Lactobacilli differentially modulate expression of cytokines and maturation surface markers in murine dendritic cells. *J Immunol.* 2002;168(1):171-178.

94. Antony SJ. Lactobacillemia: an emerging cause of infection in both the immunocompromised and the immunocompetent host. *J Natl Med Assoc.* 2000;92(2):83-86.

95. Horwitch CA, Furseth HA, Larson AM, Jones TL, Olliffe JF, Spach DH. Lactobacillemia in three patients with AIDS. *Clin Infect Dis.* 1995;21(6):1460-1462.

96. Schlegel L, Lemerle S, Geslin P. *Lactobacillus* species as opportunistic pathogens in immunocompromised patients. *Eur J Clin Microbiol Infect Dis.* 1998;17(12):887-888.

97. De Groote MA, Frank DN, Dowell E, Glode MP, Pace NR. *Lactobacillus rhamnosus* GG bacteremia associated with probiotic use in a child with short gut syndrome. *Pediatr Infect Dis J.* 2005;24(3):278-280.

98. Zhang L, Li N, des Robert C, et al. *Lactobacillus rhamnosus* GG decreases lipopolysaccharide-induced systemic inflammation in a gastrostomy-fed infant rat model. *J Pediatr Gastroenterol Nutr.* 2006;42(5):545-552.

13

The Role of Probiotics in Diarrheal Diseases

Stefano Guandalini, MD

Diarrheal diseases continue to represent a major threat to global health. In spite of more widespread use of oral rehydration solutions and slowly improving hygienic standards in developing countries, mortality from acute diarrhea, especially in young children, continues to be unacceptably high in these areas. In developed countries, on the other hand, while the burden of mortality from diarrheal diseases has largely regressed to be now considered marginal, these disorders still retain a high impact in terms of morbidity and associated financial and social costs that range from hospitalizations to absenteeism from work and/or school, and so on. While there is hope that the relatively recent introduction of the vaccination against rotavirus (the single most common cause of acute-onset diarrhea in children worldwide) would help in reducing such a burden, it is clear that even in developed countries, there is currently an unmet need for preventative and therapeutic strategies aimed at reducing the incidence, severity, and duration of acute diarrheal episodes. In this regard, in the past several years, a considerable amount of research work has been done to verify whether appropriate utilization of some probiotic strains may represent the answer to this need.

This chapter focuses largely on the status of the evidence for the efficacy of probiotics in acute-onset diarrhea. Most of the evidence currently available stems from studies on infants and young children; in fact, it is in this age group that diarrhea is more problematic, due to the higher risk of dehydration and electrolyte imbalances, as compared to the adult. As a consequence, much fewer studies have been performed in adults. Other gastrointestinal conditions also associated with diarrhea such as IBDs, NEC, AAD, and irritable bowel diseases are dealt with in separate chapters of this book.

Floch MH, Kim AS, eds.
Probiotics: A Clinical Guide (pp 195-206)
© 2010 Taylor & Francis Group

TABLE 13-1

Probiotics Investigated in Humans for Prevention and/or Treatment of Diarrhea

STRAIN	TYPE
Lactobacilli	L. acidophilus*
	L. bulgaricus*
	L. casei*
	L. rhamnosus GG
	L. johnsonii
	L. paracasei
	L. plantarum*
	L. reuteri
	L. salivarius
Bifidobacteria	B. animalis
	B. bifidum
	B. breve*
	B. infantis*
	B. lactis
	B. longum*
E. coli	Nissle 1917
Streptococci	Salivarius subsp.thermophilus*
Enterococci	E. faecium
Yeasts	S. boulardii

*Present in combination in the preparation VSL#3.

Probiotics Utilized in Clinical Trials in the Prevention and/or Treatment of Diarrhea

As in many other inflammatory disorders, not only gastrointestinal but also extra-intestinal, the most studied probiotics for children and adults with acute diarrhea are bacteria of the genus *Lactobacillus* or *Bifidobacterium*, used either as single species or in mixed cultures with other bacteria (Table 13-1). Other nonpathogenic genera, including *Escherichia*, *Enterococcus*, and *Bacillus*, and nonbacterial organisms, such as the nonpathogenic yeast *Saccharomyces boulardii*, have also been quite extensively investigated. The yogurt-producing bacteria, *L. bulgaricus* and *Streptococcus thermophilus*, also have received some attention, especially in preventing diarrhea.

PREVENTION OF COMMUNITY-, DAYCARE-, HOSPITAL-ACQUIRED, OR TRAVELER'S DIARRHEA

Community-Acquired Diarrhea

Very few studies are available addressing the efficacy of probiotics, administered to healthy children or adults, to prevent the onset or mitigate the severity of sporadic diarrhea acquired in the community. Oberhelman et al[1] conducted such a prospective study in a rural community in Peru. The study followed more than 200, mostly malnourished, infants and young children receiving LGG or placebo for 15 months, and Oberhelman et al found that there were significantly fewer diarrheal episodes in children treated with LGG compared with those treated with placebo (5.2 vs 6.0 episodes per child per year; $P = .028$). The benefit was particularly evident in nonbreastfed children aged 18 to 29 months, as they experienced one fewer episode per child per year ($P = .005$).

In adults, Pereg et al[2] followed for 8 weeks 500 individuals receiving in a yogurt either *L. casei* 10^{10} CFU per day or placebo. The incidence of diarrhea in the probiotic group and the control group was 12.2% and 16.1%, respectively, but the difference was not significant.

Daycare-Acquired Diarrhea

Infants and young children attending daycare centers are notoriously exposed to a higher risk of common infectious diseases, including upper respiratory infections and diarrhea. Several randomized, placebo-controlled trials (RCTs) have been published on the capacity of probiotics to prevent incidence, duration, or severity of diarrheal episodes in these settings.

In a study published in the year 2000,[3] the probiotic *L. casei* was administered in a yogurt to healthy children attending daycare centers between the ages of 6 and 24 months for 12 weeks, followed by 6 weeks with no supplementation. A total of 779 children completed the study. The incidence of diarrhea between the 2 treated and placebo groups was significantly different, with 22% of the control children having at least one attack of diarrhea compared to 15.8% of the children consuming probiotic-containing yogurt.

In the subsequent year, the efficacy of LGG was evaluated in preschool children in a multicenter trial conducted in Finland.[4] The probiotic was provided in milk containing 5×10^{10} CFU/mL, and the intake reported was at least 200 mL/day for 30 weeks. No significant difference was observed between the study and the control groups in terms of frequency or severity of the episodes of diarrhea.

In an RCT, French investigators assessed the prevalence of acute diarrhea in more than 900 infants (4 to 6 months of age) who were fed for a prolonged period a formula rich in *B. breve* and *S. thermophilus*.[5] Again, no significant difference was found in the incidence or duration of the episodes of diarrhea, as well as in the number of hospital admissions. It must be noted, however, that the children in the probiotic-supplemented group suffered less severe episodes. They, in fact, had fewer instances of dehydration (2.5% vs 6.1%, $P = .01$), and required fewer medical consultations (46% vs 57%, $P = .003$), fewer oral rehydration solution prescriptions (42% vs 52%, $P = .003$), and fewer formula changes (59% vs 75%, $P = .0001$).

The same year, another group of investigators also based in France[6] reported the results of a multicenter RCT to evaluate the efficacy of a formula supplemented with *B. lactis* strain Bb 12 in the prevention of acute diarrhea in infants younger than 8 months living in residential nurseries or foster-care centers. Ninety healthy children received either the Bb12 or a standard formula daily throughout their stay in the residential center for a total of almost 5 months. Also in this trial, the probiotic did not reduce the prevalence of diarrhea when compared with placebo (28.3% vs 38.7%). The only significant difference noticed was in the number of days with diarrhea: the Bb12 group had in fact 1.15 ± 2.5 days of diarrhea, with a daily probability of diarrhea of 0.84, vs 2.3 ± 4.5 days and 1.55 days, respectively, in the control group ($P = .0002$ and .001).

Saavedra et al[7] working in the United States compared 2 different concentrations of *B. lactis* Bb12 + *S. thermophilus* in formulas either 1×10^7 or 1×10^6 CFU/g in 118 children, 8 to 24 months of age. Also, in this study, no significant differences were found between groups in growth, health-care attention seeking, daycare absenteeism, or other health variables, including prevalence of diarrheal episodes.

An interesting RCT was reported in 2005.[8] The study was conducted in Israel by Weizman et al, which compared 2 different probiotics: *B. lactis* Bb12 vs *L. reuteri* provided in formula as 1×10^7 CFU/g. The study was carried out for 3 months on almost 200 infants of 4 to 10 months of age. In this case, both probiotics performed better than placebo with regard to number of diarrheal episodes (0.3 ± 0.1 vs 0.1 ± 0.08 for Bb12 and 0.02 ± 0.01 for *L. reuteri*, $P < .001$) and days with diarrhea (0.6 ± 0.2 vs 0.4 ± 0.1 for Bb12 and 0.15 ± 0.10 for *L. reuteri*, $P < .001$).

Finally, in 2007, Binns et al[9] evaluated the efficacy of a milk product containing probiotics and prebiotics on the incidence of diarrhea in almost 500 children attending 29 daycare centers in Perth, Australia. The probiotic employed was *B. lactis* (1.2×10^{10} CFU/day administered with a prebiotic blend) for 5 months. Even though the prevalence of diarrhea was not significantly different between the study and the control group, the children in the study group had significantly fewer days of diarrhea with 4 or more stools, representing a reduction of about 20% in diarrheal rate.

In summary, while all probiotics tested were found to be completely safe, the evidence of their efficacy in preventing diarrheal episodes in infants and children attending daycare centers, or similar institutions where they are more exposed to the risk of acquiring infectious diarrhea, is overall quite modest. Although it is statistically significant for some strains and for some parameters, so far it appears to be of somewhat doubtful clinical relevance.

Hospital-Acquired Diarrhea

Diarrhea can spread among patients admitted to hospital wards. In children, this event is actually not infrequent and well known. In most instances, these episodes are due to a rapidly spreading rotavirus infection and, in fewer instances, are due to the spreading of *Clostridium difficile*. Both agents can cause serious consequences, especially in ill infants and children who are already weak because of their underlying ailment, as well as in the elderly. Clearly, therefore, safe agents such as probiotics would be a welcome addition to the limited means available in preventing this disorder.

Unfortunately, there are only less than a handful of RCTs that evaluated probiotics for this purpose, and they yield somewhat conflicting results. In a double-blind RCT published in 1994,[10] 55 infants aged 5 to 24 months, who were admitted to a chronic-care hospital, received either a standard infant formula supplemented with *B. bifidum* Bb12 and *S. thermophilus* or an identical formula without probiotics. The prevalence of nosocomial diarrhea was significantly reduced in the probiotic-fed infants, compared with placebo (7% vs 31%, $P < .05$). The risk of rotavirus gastroenteritis was also significantly lower in those receiving the probiotic-supplemented formula. Of note, the infants fed the probiotic-enriched formula had a significantly shorter duration of rotavirus shedding, an important observation in terms of containment of the rotavirus spreading in hospitals.

Two subsequent trials were conducted with LGG. The first[11] involved 81 children in the first 3 years of life hospitalized for reasons other than diarrhea. LGG (6×10^6 CFU) administered orally twice per day significantly reduced the risk of nosocomial diarrhea when compared with placebo (6.7% vs 33.3%, $P = .002$). Rotavirus was the predominant etiologic agent of all nosocomial gastroenteritis; although the prevalence of the infection per se did not differ between the probiotic-treated and the control group, children in the LGG group had significantly fewer episodes of rotavirus diarrhea (2.2% vs 16.7%, $P = .02$).

In the second RCT utilizing LGG,[12] Mastretta et al studied 220 children in the first 18 months of life enrolled in a single study center in Italy and compared LGG with placebo in breastfed and nonbreastfed infants. Although breastfeeding was effective, LGG (10^{10} CFU once per day) did not prevent the occurrence of nosocomial rotavirus infections as compared with placebo (25% vs 30%, $P = .4$). Symptomatic rotavirus infections were fewer in the LGG group but not significantly so (13% for LGG vs 21% for placebo, $P = .13$).

Thus, it is quite possible that probiotics may indeed have a role in protecting inpatients from clinically manifest rotavirus-induced (and possibly C. difficile) diarrhea, but the evidence is obviously not there yet. There is, therefore, little doubt that this area is worthy of further exploration, with studies adequately powered and with proper comparison of different doses and various strains.

Traveler's Diarrhea

Traveler's diarrhea is a common health complaint, which can affect 5% to 50% of travelers, both children and more commonly (also due to their prevailing number) adults, mostly depending on the destination. Although the diarrhea is usually self-limited, it has been reported that up to 10% of travelers who suffer from this problem would go on to develop persistent diarrhea and about 10% of them eventually evolve to suffer from postinfectious IBS. Again, probiotics looked from the beginning as a promising tool to prevent this bothersome event and were tried in many studies. In a recent meta-analysis of numerous studies that eventually included 12 of them, McFarland[13] determined, on the basis of the pooled relative risk, that probiotics were significantly able to prevent traveler's diarrhea (RR = 0.85, 95% CI 0.79, 0.91; $P < .001$). When analyzing the effect of single strains, it was evident that S. boulardii and a mixture of L. acidophilus and B. bifidum had significant efficacy. Also of note, no serious adverse reactions were reported in any of the 12 trials. All considered, and especially in light of possible prevention of postinfectious IBS, it appears that the preventive use of either one of the mentioned probiotics could be helpful in reducing the risk of developing traveler's diarrhea.

TREATMENT OF ACUTE DIARRHEA

Probiotics have one of their most logical applications in the treatment of infectious diarrheas. In fact, approximately 100 studies have been published since the mid-1990s, and several excellent reviews, some strictly evidence-based, have been published, especially in the past few years. The probiotic strains most studied have been LGG (16 clinical trials at the time of this writing,[14-29] mostly randomized and placebo-controlled), S. boulardii (6 RCTs),[16,30-34] and L. reuteri (5 studies),[35-39] while other species such as E. coli

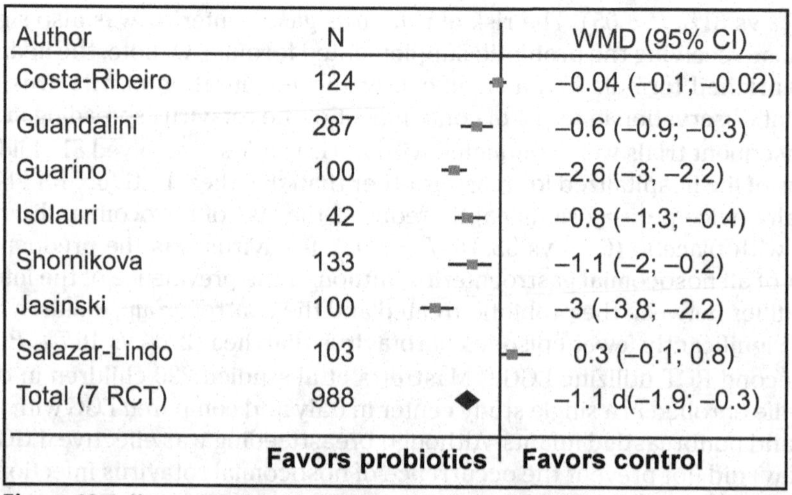

Author	N		WMD (95% CI)
Costa-Ribeiro	124		−0.04 (−0.1; −0.02)
Guandalini	287		−0.6 (−0.9; −0.3)
Guarino	100		−2.6 (−3; −2.2)
Isolauri	42		−0.8 (−1.3; −0.4)
Shornikova	133		−1.1 (−2; −0.2)
Jasinski	100		−3 (−3.8; −2.2)
Salazar-Lindo	103		0.3 (−0.1; 0.8)
Total (7 RCT)	988		−1.1 d(−1.9; −0.3)
		Favors probiotics	**Favors control**

Figure 13-1. Meta-analysis of published RCTs assessing the efficacy of LGG on the duration of diarrhea (in days). Modified from Szajewska H, Skorka A, Ruszczynski M, et al. Meta-analysis: *Lactobacillus* GG for treating acute diarrhoea in children. *Aliment Pharmacol Ther.* 2007;25(8):871-881.

Nissle 1917,[40,41] the heat-killed *L. acidophilus* LB,[42,43] and the probiotic mixture VSL#3[44] have also been investigated, but so far have received much less attention. Several meta-analyses that assess the efficacy of such probiotics, including a Cochrane Review of 2004,[45] are available.

LGG use allowed a significant reduction in the duration of diarrhea. Data extracted in a recent meta-analysis of RCTs from 7 studies including almost 1000 infants and young children[46] showed, in fact, an average reduction of 1.1 days with a 95% CI of 1.9 to 0.3 (Figure 13-1). There is also strong evidence that LGG is most effective for rotavirus diarrhea, where it induced an average reduction in the duration of diarrhea of 2.1 days. Additionally and, in the author's opinion, quite importantly, the risk of diarrhea running a protracted course of more than 7 days, assessed in an RCT involving 287 patients,[18] was also found to be significantly reduced by LGG (RR: 0.25; 95% CI: 0.09 to 0.75). The duration of hospitalization was evaluated in 3 RCTs for a total of 535 patients and was found to be, on average, reduced by approximately 1 day. Of interest, 2 open-label trials[17,19] showed efficacy in reducing the duration of rotavirus shedding due to LGG use, an observation that has obvious positive epidemiological significance. Thus, overall, these data provide rather robust evidence of efficacy for LGG in the treatment of acute diarrhea. One should, however, note that LGG does not seem effective in bacterial diarrhea. It is also of importance to point out that correctly dosing this probiotic is crucial for its efficacy: only doses above 5 billion (5×10^9 CFU) per day have shown efficacy.

As for *S. boulardii*, the bulk of the evidence from the available investigations supports an efficacy very similar to that of LGG. In a recent reassessment[47] of a previously published meta-analysis,[48] Vandenplas et al, analyzing data from the pooled results of 6 RCTs involving 756 children, concluded that *S. boulardii*, compared to placebo or no intervention, reduced the duration of diarrhea by almost 1 day (Figure 13-2). The yeast also showed an efficacy similar to LGG in preventing a protracted course of diarrhea.

L. reuteri was studied alone[38,39] or in combination with *L. rhamnosus* 19070-2[36,37] for its capacity of reducing the duration of acute-onset diarrhea in children hospitalized or having diarrhea while in daycare. In all circumstances the probiotic appeared to be able to reduce the duration of diarrhea, especially by rotavirus, and also to shorten its shedding.[36] However, only 2 groups of investigators have published results for this strain, so that general conclusions cannot be safely drawn at this stage.

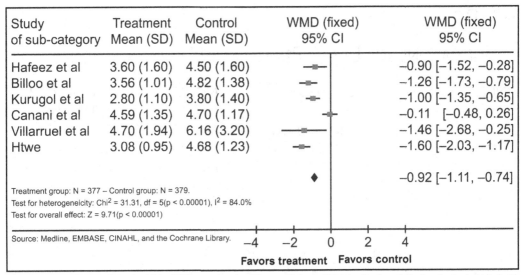

Study of sub-category	Treatment Mean (SD)	Control Mean (SD)	WMD (fixed) 95% CI	WMD (fixed) 95% CI
Hafeez et al	3.60 (1.60)	4.50 (1.60)		−0.90 [−1.52, −0.28]
Billoo et al	3.56 (1.01)	4.82 (1.38)		−1.26 [−1.73, −0.79]
Kurugol et al	2.80 (1.10)	3.80 (1.40)		−1.00 [−1.35, −0.65]
Canani et al	4.59 (1.35)	4.70 (1.17)		−0.11 [−0.48, 0.26]
Villarruel et al	4.70 (1.94)	6.16 (3.20)		−1.46 [−2.68, −0.25]
Htwe	3.08 (0.95)	4.68 (1.23)		−1.60 [−2.03, −1.17]
				−0.92 [−1.11, −0.74]

Treatment group: N = 377 – Control group: N = 379.
Test for heterogeneicity: Chi^2 = 31.31, df = 5(p < 0.00001), I^2 = 84.0%
Test for overall effect: Z = 9.71(p < 0.00001)

Source: Medline, EMBASE, CINAHL, and the Cochrane Library.

−4   −2   0   2   4

Favors treatment   Favors control

Figure 13-2. Meta-analysis of published RCTs assessing the efficacy of *S. boulardii* on the duration of diarrhea (in days). Printed with permission from Vandenplas Y, Brunser O, Szajewska H. *Saccharomyces boulardii* in childhood. *Eur J Pediatr.* 2009;168(3):253-265.

Of interest, recently, *L. reuteri* (strain RC 14), combined with *L. rhamnosus* GR-1, was studied[35] in Nigeria in 24 adult female HIV/AIDS patients with moderate diarrhea, CD4 counts over 200, and not receiving antiretrovirals or dietary supplements. Diarrhea resolved in 12/12 probiotic-treated subjects within 2 days, compared to 2/12 receiving yogurt for 15 days. While obviously it would be extremely premature to apply these findings to clinical practice, it is exciting to see the appearance of a potential application of probiotic use in such settings.

As mentioned, *E. coli* Nissle 1917 was also studied in 2 RCTs.[40,41] Both investigations were multicenter trials in Russia and Ukraine conducted by the same group. Both studies showed a significant superiority of the probiotic compared to placebo in obtaining a faster recovery from acute-onset diarrhea in infants and toddlers[40] and a shorter duration of diarrhea lasting more than 4 days at study enrollment in young children.[41]

VLS#3, a patented preparation containing 7 different strains of probiotics, was used in an RCT conducted in India on 224 children with acute, rotavirus-induced diarrhea, which proved to be significantly better than placebo in a preliminary report.[44]

In conclusion, therefore, a few probiotic strains have shown robust evidence of efficacy in the treatment of acute-onset, generally infectious, diarrhea in children and—to a much lesser degree—in adults. This is particularly true for early administration and for rotavirus-induced diarrhea. However, the clinician must be aware of the following facts: (1) the clinical relevance of such effect is moderate because no more than 1 day of reduction of duration is to be expected; (2) only a few specific strains so far have truly evidence-based proof of efficacy—LGG and *Saccharomyces* being the best examples; (3) dosage is crucial; for both these probiotics, only doses above 5 billion (5×10^9 CFU) per day seem to be effective.

TREATMENT OF PERSISTENT DIARRHEA

Limited studies have been done to address the question of whether probiotic administration can be useful in treating children presenting with persistent diarrhea. One RCT was conducted in Argentina[49] with *S. boulardii*: 89 children (age range 6 to 24 months) received milk supplemented with *L. casei* and *L. acidophilus* strains

TABLE 13-2

INDICATIONS FOR USE OF PROBIOTICS IN DIARRHEAL DISEASES*

INDICATION	PROBIOTIC	DOSE	NOTES	LEVEL OF RECOMMENDATION[†]
Prevention of daycare-acquired diarrhea	L. casei DN-114 001	100 mL of yogurt containing 10^8 CFU/mL	Present in a commercial yogurt	B
	B. lactis Bb12	1.5×10^8 CFU/L	Present in a proprietary milk formula	B
	L. reuteri	1×10^7 CFU/g of formula		B
Prevention of traveler's diarrhea	S. boulardii	250 to 500 mg/day		B
Treatment of acute diarrhea	L. rhamnosus GG	>5 × 10^9 CFU/day, better 10^{10} to 10^{11}	Should be administered as early as possible Can be administered in ORS	A
	S. boulardii	5 × 10^9 to 10^{10} CFU (found in 250 to 500 mg)/day		A

*Not considering inflammatory bowel diseases, necrotizing enterocolitis, antibiotic-associated diarrhea and irritable bowel diseases that are dealt with in separate chapters of this book.

[†]Based on definitions agreed upon during the "Advances in Clinical Use of Probiotics" Workshop, held at Yale University in November 2007.

CERELA 10^{10} to 10^{12} CFU/g, or *S. boulardii* 10^{10} to 10^{12} CFU/g ($n = 30$) twice a day for 5 days, while a third group received a placebo milk. Both *Lactobacillus* and *S. boulardii* significantly reduced the number of stools per day ($P < .001$) and diarrheal duration ($P < .005$). Similarly, both probiotics significantly ($P < .002$) reduced vomiting compared to placebo.

A second RCT[50] was performed with LGG in 235 Indian children, most of whom were malnourished, hospitalized for a diarrhea lasting more than 14 days. The study showed the mean duration of diarrhea to be significantly lower in the cases than in controls

(5.3 vs 9.2 days, $P < .05$). Also, the duration of hospitalization was greatly reduced in children on LGG (from 15.5 to 7.3 days, $P < .05$).

Clearly, no conclusions can be drawn on the basis of only 2 trials. However, it is encouraging for future research to notice that not only do probiotics appear to help, as we have seen earlier, in preventing diarrhea from running a prolonged course, but also there is preliminary evidence that they could help in abbreviating the course of an already persistent diarrhea—clearly a major problem especially in developing countries where malnutrition is still widespread.

CONCLUSION

What practical indications can be confidently given to physicians regarding the use of probiotics in diarrheal diseases? The following recommendations (see also Table 13-2 for doses) are based on the evidence reviewed above, as well as on personal, experience-based, opinion.

- *Prevention of community-acquired diarrhea*: No indications for probiotic use.

- *Prevention of daycare-acquired diarrhea*: Inconsistent results. Strains showing some efficacy (of minor clinical significance) are *L. casei*, *B. lactis* Bb12, and *L. reuteri*. Administration of any of such strains for prophylactic use should probably be limited to young children already known to experience recurrent episodes of diarrhea.

- *Prevention of nosocomial diarrhea*: No indications for use of probiotics. This area, however, is in dire need of further studies!

- *Prevention of traveler's diarrhea*: Probiotics can be helpful. The probiotic with the strongest evidence: *S. boulardii*.

- *Treatment of acute diarrhea*: Robust evidence of moderate efficacy well established for two species, *Lactobacillus* GG and *S. boulardii*.

- *Treatment of persistent diarrhea*: No indications possible at this time.

REFERENCES

1. Oberhelman RA, Gilman RH, Sheen P, et al. A placebo-controlled trial of *Lactobacillus* GG to prevent diarrhea in undernourished Peruvian children. *J Pediatr.* 1999;134(1):15-20.
2. Pereg D, Kimhi O, Tirosh A, Orr N, Kayouf R, Lishner M. The effect of fermented yogurt on the prevention of diarrhea in a healthy adult population. *Am J Infect Control.* 2005;33(2):122-125.
3. Pedone CA, Arnaud CC, Postaire ER, Bouley CF, Reinert P. Multicentric study of the effect of milk fermented by *Lactobacillus casei* on the incidence of diarrhoea. *Int J Clin Pract.* 2000;54(9):568-571.
4. Hatakka K, Savilahti E, Ponka A, et al. Effect of long term consumption of probiotic milk on infections in children attending day care centres: double blind, randomised trial. *BMJ.* 2001;322(7298):1327.
5. Thibault H, Aubert-Jacquin C, Goulet O. Effects of long-term consumption of a fermented infant formula (with *Bifidobacterium breve* c50 and *Streptococcus thermophilus* 065) on acute diarrhea in healthy infants. *J Pediatr Gastroenterol Nutr.* 2004;39(2):147-152.
6. Chouraqui JP, Van Egroo LD, Fichot MC. Acidified milk formula supplemented with *Bifidobacterium lactis*: impact on infant diarrhea in residential care settings. *J Pediatr Gastroenterol Nutr.* 2004;38(3): 288-292.
7. Saavedra JM, Abi-Hanna A, Moore N, Yolken RH. Long-term consumption of infant formulas containing live probiotic bacteria: tolerance and safety. *Am J Clin Nutr.* 2004;79(2):261-267.
8. Weizman Z, Asli G, Alsheikh A. Effect of a probiotic infant formula on infections in child care centers: comparison of two probiotic agents. *Pediatrics.* 2005;115(1):5-9.

9. Binns CW, Lee AH, Harding H, Gracey M, Barclay DV. The CUPDAY Study: prebiotic-probiotic milk product in 1-3-year-old children attending childcare centres. *Acta Paediatr.* 2007;96(11):1646-1650.

10. Saavedra JM, Bauman NA, Oung I, Perman JA, Yolken RH. Feeding of *Bifidobacterium bifidum* and *Streptococcus thermophilus* to infants in hospital for prevention of diarrhoea and shedding of rotavirus. *Lancet.* 1994;344(8929):1046-1049.

11. Szajewska H, Kotowska M, Mrukowicz JZ, Armanska M, Mikołajczyk W. Efficacy of *Lactobacillus* GG in prevention of nosocomial diarrhea in infants. *J Pediatr.* 2001;138(3):361-365.

12. Mastretta E, Longo P, Laccisaglia A, et al. Effect of *Lactobacillus* GG and breast-feeding in the prevention of rotavirus nosocomial infection. *J Pediatr Gastroenterol Nutr.* 2002;35(4):527-531.

13. McFarland LV. Meta-analysis of probiotics for the prevention of traveler's diarrhea. *Travel Med Infect Dis.* 2007;5(2):97-105.

14. Basu S, Chatterjee M, Ganguly S, Chandra PK. Efficacy of *Lactobacillus rhamnosus* GG in acute watery diarrhoea of Indian children: a randomised controlled trial. *J Paediatr Child Health.* 2007;43(12):837-842.

15. Basu S, Paul DK, Ganguly S, et al. Efficacy of high-dose *Lactobacillus rhamnosus* GG in controlling acute watery diarrhea in Indian children: a randomized controlled trial. *J Clin Gastroenterol.* 2009;43(3):208-213.

16. Canani RB, Cirillo P, Terrin G, et al. Probiotics for treatment of acute diarrhoea in children: randomised clinical trial of five different preparations. *BMJ.* 2007;335(7615):340.

17. Fang SB, Lee HC, Hu JJ, et al. Dose-dependent effect of *Lactobacillus* GG on quantitative reduction of faecal rotavirus shedding in children. *J Trop Pediatr.* 2009;55:297-301.

18. Guandalini S, Pensabene L, Zikri MA, et al. *Lactobacillus* GG administered in oral rehydration solution to children with acute diarrhea: a multicenter European trial. *J Pediatr Gastroenterol Nutr.* 2000;30(1):54-60.

19. Guarino A, Canani RB, Spagnuolo MI, Albano F, Di Benedetto L. Oral bacterial therapy reduces the duration of symptoms and of viral excretion in children with mild diarrhea. *J Pediatr Gastroenterol Nutr.* 1997;25(5):516-519.

20. Isolauri E, Juntunen M, Rautanen T, Sillanaukee P, Koivula T. A human *Lactobacillus* strain (*Lactobacillus casei* sp strain GG) promotes recovery from acute diarrhea in children. *Pediatrics.* 1991;88(1):90-97.

21. Isolauri E, Kaila M, Mykkänen H, Ling WH, Salminen S. Oral bacteriotherapy for viral gastroenteritis. *Dig Dis Sci.* 1994;39(12):2595-2600.

22. Kaila M, Isolauri E, Saxelin M, et al. Viable vs inactivated *Lactobacillus* strain GG in acute rotavirus diarrhoea. *Arch Dis Child.* 1995;72(1):51-53.

23. Kaila M, Isolauri E, Soppi E, Virtanen E, Laine S, Arvilommi H. Enhancement of the circulating antibody secreting cell response in human diarrhea by a human *Lactobacillus* strain. *Pediatr Res.* 1992;32(2):141-144.

24. Majamaa H, Isolauri E, Saxelin M, Vesikari T. Lactic acid bacteria in the treatment of acute rotavirus gastroenteritis. *J Pediatr Gastroenterol Nutr.* 1995;20(3):333-338.

25. Pant AR, Graham SM, Allen SJ, et al. *Lactobacillus* GG and acute diarrhoea in young children in the tropics. *J Trop Pediatr.* 1996;42(3):162-165.

26. Rautanen T, Isolauri E, Salo E, et al. Management of acute diarrhoea with low osmolarity oral rehydration solutions and *Lactobacillus* strain GG. *Arch Dis Child.* 1998;79(2):157-160.

27. Raza S, Graham SM, Allen SJ, Sultana S, Cuevas L, Hart CA. *Lactobacillus* GG promotes recovery from acute nonbloody diarrhea in Pakistan. *Pediatr Infect Dis J.* 1995;14(2):107-111.

28. Raza S, Graham SM, Allen SJ, et al. *Lactobacillus* GG in acute diarrhea. *Indian Pediatr.* 1995;32(10):1140-1142.

29. Shornikova AV, Isolauri E, Burkanova L, Lukovnikova S, Vesikari T. A trial in the Karelian Republic of oral rehydration and *Lactobacillus* GG for treatment of acute diarrhoea. *Acta Paediatr.* 1997;86(5):460-465.

30. Billoo AG, Memon MA, Khaskheli SA, et al. Role of a probiotic (*Saccharomyces boulardii*) in management and prevention of diarrhoea. *World J Gastroenterol.* 2006;12(28):4557-4560.

31. Htwe K, Yee KS, Tin M, Vandenplas Y. Effect of *Saccharomyces boulardii* in the treatment of acute watery diarrhea in Myanmar children: a randomized controlled study. *Am J Trop Med Hyg.* 2008;78(2):214-216.

32. Kurugol Z, Koturoglu G. Effects of *Saccharomyces boulardii* in children with acute diarrhoea. *Acta Paediatr.* 2005;94(1):44-47.

33. Ozkan TB, Sahin E, Erdemir G, Budak F. Effect of *Saccharomyces boulardii* in children with acute gastroenteritis and its relationship to the immune response. *J Int Med Res.* 2007;35(2):201-212.

34. Villarruel G, Rubio DM, Lopez F, et al. *Saccharomyces boulardii* in acute childhood diarrhoea: a randomized, placebo-controlled study. *Acta Paediatr.* 2007;96(4):538-541.

35. Anukam KC, Osazuwa EO, Osadolor HB, Bruce AW, Reid G. Yogurt containing probiotic *Lactobacillus rhamnosus* GR-1 and *L. reuteri* RC-14 helps resolve moderate diarrhea and increases CD4 count in HIV/ AIDS patients. *J Clin Gastroenterol.* 2008;42(3):239-243.
36. Rosenfeldt V, Michaelsen KF, Jakobsen M, et al. Effect of probiotic *Lactobacillus* strains in young children hospitalized with acute diarrhea. *Pediatr Infect Dis J.* 2002;21(5):411-416.
37. Rosenfeldt V, Michaelsen KF, Jakobsen M, et al. Effect of probiotic *Lactobacillus* strains on acute diarrhea in a cohort of nonhospitalized children attending day-care centers. *Pediatr Infect Dis J.* 2002;21(5):417-419.
38. Shornikova AV, Casas IA, Isolauri E, Mykkänen H, Vesikari T. *Lactobacillus reuteri* as a therapeutic agent in acute diarrhea in young children. *J Pediatr Gastroenterol Nutr.* 1997;24(4):399-404.
39. Shornikova AV, Casas IA, Mykkänen H, Salo E, Vesikari T. Bacteriotherapy with *Lactobacillus reuteri* in rotavirus gastroenteritis. *Pediatr Infect Dis J.* 1997;16(12):1103-1107.
40. Henker J, Laass M, Blokhin BM, et al. The probiotic *Escherichia coli* strain Nissle 1917 (EcN) stops acute diarrhoea in infants and toddlers. *Eur J Pediatr.* 2007;166(4):311-318.
41. Henker J, Laass MW, Blokhin BM, et al. Probiotic *Escherichia coli* Nissle 1917 vs placebo for treating diarrhea of greater than 4 days duration in infants and toddlers. *Pediatr Infect Dis J.* 2008;27(6):494-499.
42. Lievin-Le Moal V, Sarrazin-Davila LE, Servin AL. An experimental study and a randomized, double-blind, placebo-controlled clinical trial to evaluate the antisecretory activity of *Lactobacillus acidophilus* strain LB against nonrotavirus diarrhea. *Pediatrics.* 2007;120(4):e795-e803.
43. Salazar-Lindo E, Figueroa-Quintanilla D, Caciano MI, et al. Effectiveness and safety of *Lactobacillus* LB in the treatment of mild acute diarrhea in children. *J Pediatr Gastroenterol Nutr.* 2007;44(5):571-576.
44. Dubey AP, Rajeshwari K, Chakravarty A, Famularo G. Use of VSL#3 in the treatment of rotavirus diarrhea in children: preliminary results. *J Clin Gastroenterol.* 2008;42(Suppl 3 Pt 1):S126-S129.
45. Allen SJ, Okoko B, Martinez E, Gregorio G, Dans LF. Probiotics for treating infectious diarrhoea. *Cochrane Database Syst Rev.* 2004(2):CD003048.
46. Szajewska H, Skórka A, Ruszczynski M, Gieruszczak-Białek D.. Meta-analysis: *Lactobacillus* GG for treating acute diarrhoea in children. *Aliment Pharmacol Ther.* 2007;25(8):871-881.
47. Vandenplas Y, Brunser O, Szajewska H. *Saccharomyces boulardii* in childhood. *Eur J Pediatr.* 2009;168(3):253-265.
48. Szajewska H, Skorka A, Dylag M. Meta-analysis: *Saccharomyces boulardii* for treating acute diarrhoea in children. *Aliment Pharmacol Ther.* 2007;25(3):257-264.
49. Gaon D, Garcia H, Winter L, et al. Effect of *Lactobacillus* strains and *Saccharomyces boulardii* on persistent diarrhea in children. *Medicina (B Aires).* 2003;63(4):293-298.
50. Basu S, Chatterjee M, Ganguly S, Chandra PK. Effect of *Lactobacillus rhamnosus* GG in persistent diarrhea in Indian children: a randomized controlled trial. *J Clin Gastroenterol.* 2007;41(8):756-760.

14

Probiotics and Their Role in Antibiotic-Associated Diarrhea and *Clostridium difficile* Infection

Laurel H. Hartwell, MD and Christina M. Surawicz, MD, MACG

Diarrhea is a common side effect of antibiotic use, ranging from 10% to 30% in the outpatient setting and as high as 39% in hospitalized patients. There has been increased interest in the role of probiotics in prevention of AAD over the past 2 decades. AAD is defined as diarrhea that occurs during or shortly after antibiotic use, even up to 2 to 4 weeks after their discontinuation. Any antibiotic can cause diarrhea, but increasing use of broad-spectrum antibiotics, such as amoxicillin, ampicillin, cephalosporins, and clindamycin, has been identified as a risk factor for developing AAD.[1] Those active against anaerobes are also implicated. Some antibiotics, such as erythromycin, cause diarrhea directly through stimulation of motility receptors. Studies have shown that AAD results in longer hospital stays, a higher cost of care, and a threefold increase in mortality.[2]

Clostridium difficile infection (CDI) is the most severe complication of antibiotic use, and the increased morbidity and mortality are well known, as well as the increased cost associated with medical care.

The probiotics that have been most commonly studied are the LAB, including LGG, *L. casei*, *L. thermophilus*, and *L. bulgaricus*. Other species include *Bifidobacteria*, *C. butyricum*, *Enterococcus faecium*, as well as the nonpathogenic yeast *S. boulardii*.

At relative frequency, the AAD lends itself well to placebo-controlled trials investigating the efficacy of probiotics in prevention, and we now have many studies indicating a strong benefit with LGG and *S. boulardii*. The efficacy of probiotics in preventing *C. difficile*-associated diarrhea, on the other hand, has been more difficult to study. While there is no good evidence to support the role of probiotics in preventing or treating *C. difficile*-associated infection, there is evidence that *S. boulardii* can be useful in preventing further recurrences of *C. difficile*.

Floch MH, Kim AS, eds.
Probiotics: A Clinical Guide (pp 207-218)
© 2010 Taylor & Francis Group

MECHANISMS OF ACTION

The pathophysiology of AAD is incompletely understood, but it appears that changes in fecal flora lead to incomplete or altered carbohydrate digestion with a resulting osmotic diarrhea.[3] Bacterial overgrowth of pathogens has also been implicated. In the case of *C. difficile* diarrhea, antibiotics disrupt the normal protective barrier of colonic microflora and allow opportunistic pathogens to invade. The primary mechanisms of probiotics in AAD are likely the reestablishment of normal protective microflora, enhancement of the immune response, and direct inhibition of pathogens and their toxins. Probiotics such as *L. acidophilus*, *B. lactis,* and *Lactobacillus* F19 have been shown to prevent microflora disturbances in the natural *Bacteroides fragilis* species in patients taking clindamycin.[4] *L. plantarum* 299v has also been shown to increase the number of other lactobacilli in fecal flora of healthy subjects.[5]

L. casei and *L. acidophilus* have been shown to enhance plasma cell IgA production,[6] whereas other lactobacilli have been shown to induce IL-12, IL-18, and gamma interferon.[7]

Some studies have shown that probiotics such as *L. plantarum* 299v and LGG inhibit the attachment of pathogenic *E. coli* to intestinal epithelial cells. This is thought to work by competitive inhibition for attachment sites by mucins, which are upregulated by probiotic agents.[8]

Other studies have shown a direct effect of probiotics on pathogens. In vitro studies of *L. acidophilus* and *L. casei* in a fermented milk solution showed inhibition of *Listeria innocula* and *S. aureus* through secretion of acid in the gut and inhibition of Gram-positive bacteria (except *E. faecalis* and *S. aureus*) by bacteriocins.[9] The bacteria *Lactococcus lactis* produces a type of bacteriocin called lacticin 3147, originally isolated from Irish kefir grain, that has been shown to induce rapid lysis of *C. difficile* cells.[10] *S. boulardii* has been shown to destroy *C. difficile* toxin receptor sites.[11] *S. boulardii* protease inhibits effects of *C. difficile* toxins A and B in human colonic mucosa and reduces fecal toxin positivity in hamsters.[12]

To survive and be efficacious in the gut, these organisms must be able to successfully compete against pathogens by survival in bile and gastric acid. *S. boulardii* reaches a steady-state concentration in the intestinal tract after about 3 days of oral administration and is usually cleared from stools within 2 to 5 days of discontinuation.[13] It is usually administered as a lyophilized preparation. LGG, a unique strain isolated by Goldin et al in 1987, has the notable property of stability in both bile and gastric acid.[14] It has also been shown to produce bacteriocins.

PREVENTION OF ANTIBIOTIC-ASSOCIATED DIARRHEA

The most promising probiotic agents used in the prevention of AAD are LGG and *S. boulardii*, and there is strong evidence to support their efficacy.

Lactobacilli

The *Lactobacillus* species are perhaps the most studied of the probiotics. They are widely found in fermented dairy products and are rarely pathogenic. With the exception of one trial by Thomas et al in 2001,[15] most studies of LGG have shown efficacy in the prevention of AAD. In a randomized trial of 200 outpatient children in Nebraska, Vanderhoof et al showed that after 10 days of treatment, 25/95 (26%) patients in the placebo group had diarrhea compared to only 7/93 (7.5%) in the LGG group.[16] Arvola et al studied 119 outpatient children being treated for respiratory infections, and found that 3/61 (5%) in the LGG group developed diarrhea compared to 9/58 (15%) in the placebo group.[17] Along slightly different lines, Szajewska et al studied LGG in preventing nosocomial diarrhea in hospitalized infants. Not all subjects were taking antibiotics. They randomized 81 infants aged 1 to 36 months and found that 3/45 (16%) in the LGG group developed diarrhea compared to 12/36 (33%) in the placebo group ($P < .002$).[18]

In adults, results for LGG have been mixed. A small study of 16 patients taking erythromycin showed that patients in the LGG group had 2 days of diarrhea compared to 8 days in the placebo group ($P < .05$).[19] In contrast, in a larger randomized, placebo-controlled trial of 267 hospitalized patients, 29% in the LGG group had diarrhea compared to 30% in the placebo group.[15] (Of note, because of its date of publication, it was not included in a number of meta-analyses on probiotics and AAD.)

While the above trials used capsules to administer the probiotic therapy, many studies have used yogurt and milk preparations, often with combinations of probiotic organisms. In a recent study, 63 patients were given a milk drink containing LGG, La-5, and *B. lactis* BB-12. There were 2/46 (5.9%) patients with diarrhea in the treatment group compared to 8/41 (27.6%) in the control group.[20] The use of lactobacilli was tested in a large trial of 740 patients receiving preoperative antibiotics prior to cataract surgery in India. There was no diarrhea in the treatment group compared to 13% in the placebo group.[21] While the results appear quite promising, the authors reported the agent used only as "lactobacilli" without other specifics, and for this reason it has not been included in more recent meta-analyses.

Other studies of milk products containing probiotics include a recent trial by Beausoleil et al in Montreal.[22] They found that of 89 hospitalized patients given a fermented milk drink containing *L. acidophilus* and *L. casei* or placebo, 7/44 (15.9%) developed AAD in the probiotic group compared to 16/45 (35.6%) in the control group. Moreover, the hospital stay was reduced by 2 days in the probiotic group.

In trials of the efficacy of commercially available yogurt (containing *L. acidophilus*, *L. bulgaricus*, and *S. thermophilus*) to prevent AAD, one study of 202 hospitalized patients showed less AAD (12% vs 24%),[23] but another study in British outpatients failed to show a difference between groups consuming commercial yogurt, "bio-yogurt," and no yogurt.[24]

In a recent well-designed but moderate-sized, randomized, double-blind, placebo-controlled trial by Hickson et al, 135 hospitalized patients receiving antibiotics were given either placebo or a probiotic drink containing *L. casei*, *L. bulgaricus*, and *S. thermophilus* (commercially known as Actimel in Europe, DanActive in the United States). Of note, all patients were more than 50 years of age, with an average age of 74. They found that only 7/57 (12%) of the probiotic group developed AAD compared with 19/56 (34%) of the placebo group ($P = .007$). The calculated number-needed-to-treat (NNT) to prevent AAD was 5.[25]

Bifidobacteria

Bifidobacteria are saccharolytic bacteria found in abundance in the colons of breast-fed infants, and are thought to be protective against other pathogenic bacteria. There have been relatively fewer studies of bifidobacteria alone, and most have studied *B. longum*, *B. lactis*, or *B. infantis* in combination with *L. acidophilus* or *S. thermophilus*.

Correa et al showed that of 77 children taking antibiotics, 13/80 (16%) taking *B. lactis* BB12 and *S. thermophilus* developed diarrhea vs 24/77 (31%) in the control group.[26]

Other studies have shown reduced stool frequency in bifidobacteria groups in patients taking erythromycin[27] and also with use of *L. acidophilus* and *B. longum* in patients taking clindamycin.[28]

Enterococcus

E. faecium is part of the normal colonic flora of the healthy adult and is thought to produce lactic acid and to both resist antibiotics and inhibit pathogens. One small trial of 45 patients showed less AAD with *E. faecium* administration,[29] and another larger study in adults being treated for TB also showed reduced rates with this probiotic.[30]

C. butyricum

C. butyricum, a Gram-positive anaerobe that produces butyric acid, has been studied in patients receiving antibiotics for *H. pylori* treatment and in children receiving antibiotics for upper respiratory infections. Imase et al investigated 19 patients receiving antibiotic therapy for *H. pylori* infection and randomized patients to receive a probiotic preparation of *C. butyricum* called CBM 588, double dose of the probiotic, or placebo. They found that the rates of AAD were 3/7 (43%) in the placebo, 1/7 (14%) in the single-dose group, and 0/5 in the double-dose group. Of note, *C. difficile* toxin A was detected in the stools of 2/7 (29%) patients in the control group and 1/12 (8.3%) in the combined probiotic groups.[31]

In a study of 120 Japanese children receiving antibiotics for upper respiratory tract infections, Seki et al found that diarrhea developed in 59% of the patients in the placebo group, compared to 5% of patients receiving CBM 588 since the middle of antibiotic therapy and 9% of patients who received CBM 588 since the initiation of antibiotic therapy.[32]

S. boulardii

S. boulardii has been studied for preventing AAD. This nonpathogenic yeast has an optimum growth at 37°C and can resist gastric acid. Specific mechanisms of action identified have been particular to *C. difficile* disease (inactivation of toxin receptors, increase secretion of immunoglobulins[33,34]), but *S. boulardii* may play a role in the prevention of other AADs as well.

In a study of 269 children, Kotowska et al showed that when *S. boulardii* was given in conjunction with antibiotics for upper respiratory infections, 9/119 (8%) in the treatment group vs 29/127 (23%) in the control group developed diarrhea.[35] In adults, 5 placebo-controlled, randomized trials have shown significant reduction in AAD with *S. boulardii*.[36-40] An early French study of 388 outpatient adults demonstrated AAD in 9/119 (4.5%) patients receiving *S. boulardii* compared to 33/189 (17.5%) of the placebo group (*P* < .01).[36] In a US study of 180 adults taking various antibiotics, 11/116 (9.5%) patients receiving *S. boulardii* developed diarrhea compared to 14/64 (21.8%) of the placebo group.[37] A further study of 193 adults specifically taking beta-lactam antibiotics showed that 7/97 (7.2%) in the *S. boulardii* treatment group developed diarrhea, compared to 14/96 (14.6%) in the placebo group.[38]

In a study from Turkey, of 124 patients taking clarithromycin and amoxicillin for *H. pylori* infection, 9/62 (14.5%) of the treatment group receiving *S. boulardii* developed AAD compared to 19/62 in the placebo group (30%).[39] A smaller study of various probiotics as adjuncts in the treatment of *H. pylori* showed that 1/22 (5%) patients in the *S. boulardii* group compared to 6/21 (30%) in the control group developed diarrhea.[40]

Though all of these studies have shown some degree of benefit from *S. boulardii* in the prevention of AAD, Lewis et al found no significant difference between rates of diarrhea in a study of 69 elderly patients. In the treatment group, 7/33 (21%) patients developed diarrhea vs 5/36 in the control (13.9%).[41]

Meta-analyses

Overall, there have been 5 meta-analyses of trials investigating the efficacy of probiotics in preventing AAD, and 2 of those involved studies with only children. Additionally, there have also been 2 meta-analyses of trials of a single strain of probiotic alone. The overall effect shown is a decrease in the incidence of antibiotic diarrhea with the use of probiotics.

The meta-analyses by both D'Souza et al[42] and Cremonini et al[43] were published in 2002, and both have 5 trials in common that included LGG, *L. acidophilus*, *L. bulgaricus*, *E. faecium*, *B. longum,* and *S. boulardii.* D'Souza analyzed 9 trials and concluded that probiotics decreased the risk of AAD by two-thirds (pooled odds ratio 0.37, 95% CI 0.26 to 0.53).[42] The meta-analysis by Cremonini et al evaluated results from 7 trials, in which they found a combined relative risk of 0.39 (95% CI 0.275 to 0.571).[43] In a 2006 meta-analysis, Szajewska et al included 6 trials of probiotics in children only and reported a relative risk of 0.44 (95% CI 0.25 to 0.77) and an NNT of 7 to prevent AAD.[44]

A *Cochrane Database* review of the data on probiotics in preventing pediatric AAD was published in 2007. Ten trials were analyzed, including a total of 1986 children taking antibiotics and *Lactobacilli* spp., *Bifidobacterium* spp., *Streptococcus* spp., or *S. boulardii* alone or in combination. The per-protocol pooled analysis showed a statistically significant risk reduction of 0.29 (95% CI 0.32 to 0.74), but intention-to-treat analysis showed nonsignificant results. Of note, loss to follow-up was considered a treatment failure, and many studies had rates of loss to follow up as high as 21% to 37%. They identified LGG, *L. sporogenes*, and *S. boulardii* as the most promising probiotic strains, particularly when used in doses of 5 to 40 billion CFU/day.[45]

By far, the largest and most complete meta-analysis pooling trials of probiotics in the prevention of adult and pediatric AAD was by McFarland in 2006. Twenty-five RCTs were included, with 2810 total subjects. About half (13/25) of the studies demonstrated a significant reduction in AAD. The combined relative risk for AAD of all trials was 0.43 (95% CI 0.31 to 0.58, $P < .001$). Two single strains of probiotics showed the most efficacy for AAD preventions: *S. boulardii* (RR 0.37 from 6 trials) and LGG (RR 0.31 from 6 trials). Overall, studies in children showed more efficacy than those in adults (6/9 and 7/16, respectively). The author also found that higher daily dose of probiotics (>10^{10} CFU/day) was associated with efficacy, while longer duration of probiotic use was not.[46] Of note, the study by Hickson et al in 2007 described above was not included in any of these meta-analyses due to its later publication date.[25]

Two systematic reviews have been done on a single probiotic agent. In 2005, Szajewska and Mrukowicz published a meta-analysis of 5 trials investigating the efficacy of *S. boulardii* in the prevention of AAD, including a total of 1076 patients. They found that *S. boulardii* reduced the risk of AAD from 17.2% to 6.7% (RR 0.42, 95% CI 0.23 to 0.78), with an NNT of 10.[47] Hawrelak et al determined that they were unable to complete a meta-analysis of trials comparing the effectiveness of LGG to placebo in AAD secondary to statistical heterogeneity, although 5 of the 6 trials they included were included in McFarland's review.[48]

C. DIFFICILE INFECTION

While a single pathogen is rarely identified in the AAD trials described above, CDI (previously known as *C. difficile*-associated diarrhea) is at the most severe end of the

AAD spectrum. Although symptoms can be mild or moderate, severe disease can result in toxic megacolon, perforation, and multisystem organ failure. Initial treatment involves metronidazole or vancomycin, and most patients have improved condition after 2 weeks. The most severe cases may require prolonged courses of antibiotics, and in some rare cases colectomy is required. Although 80% of patients do respond to initial therapy, 20% will go on to develop recurrent CDI (RCDI).

Prevention of C. difficile Infection

We have limited data on the role of probiotics in preventing CDI, and what data we do have are largely from trials designed to evaluate the efficacy of probiotics in preventing AAD. In these trials, the incidence of CDI was often a secondary endpoint.

Hickson et al's study described in the previous section investigated a probiotic mixture of *L. casei*, *L. bulgaricus*, and *S. thermophilus* in the prevention of AAD. In 135 hospitalized patients with a mean age of 74, no one in the probiotic group and 9/53 in the control (17%) developed CDI ($P = .001$). They described an absolute risk reduction of 17%, and an NNT of 6 to prevent CDI. The authors estimated that a single case of CDI costs on average $3669 to treat in the United States, and based on their NNT only $120 to prevent one case of CDI.[25]

In a study designed to assess the efficacy of probiotics in CDI, Plummer et al studied 138 hospitalized patients in the United Kingdom receiving antibiotics. Patients were given either a capsule containing *L. acidophilus* and *B. bifidum* or placebo. While the rates of diarrhea were the same for the treatment and placebo group (15/69, 22%), those who received probiotics had a lower incidence of CDI than the placebo group. In the subset of patients who developed diarrhea, 2/30 (2.9%) in the probiotic group and 5/30 in the placebo group (7.25%) were positive for CDI. The authors tested the feces of all patients for *C. difficile* toxins (both those with and without diarrhea) and found that 46% of the probiotic group and 78% of the control group were positive for *C. difficile* toxins.[49]

In an AAD prevention trial of 151 patients randomized to either *S. boulardii* or placebo, Can et al found that no patients in the probiotic group developed CDI compared to 2 patients in the placebo group.[50] Likewise, a recent small study of *C. butyricum* in the prevention of AAD from *H. pylori* therapy identified *C. difficile* in 2/7 (29%) of the placebo group compared to 1/7 (14%) in the standard-dose probiotic group and 0/5 in the double-dose probiotic group.[31]

Treatment of C. difficile Infection

There is no good evidence that probiotics are efficacious either as primary therapy for CDI or as adjunct to standard antibiotic therapy. A 1994 study by McFarland et al of *S. boulardii* treatment of CDI and RCDI showed that of the 64 patients being treated with antibiotics for initial CDI, treatment failure was observed in 19.3% of patients given adjunctive *S. boulardii* compared to 24.2% of patients treated with placebo, but the difference was not significant.[51]

Meta-analysis

A recent *Cochrane Database* systematic review on the use of probiotics for treatment of *C. difficile*-associated colitis in adults concluded that there is insufficient evidence to recommend probiotics either alone or as an adjunct to antibiotics in initial infection.[52] Dendukuri et al, in their 2005 systematic review, also concluded that there is a lack of data to support probiotic use in CDI prevention or treatment.[53]

TREATMENT OF RECURRENT C. DIFFICILE INFECTION

RCDI is defined as the return of signs and symptoms of CDI along with a positive stool test within a month of a successful treatment of an initial episode. As *C. difficile* diarrhea becomes one of the most common causes of diarrhea in hospitalized adults, RCDI will be an increasing problem. Identified risk factors for CDI include continued use of non-CDI antibiotics after a diagnosis of CDI, concomitant use of antacid medications, and older age.[54]

RCDI is extremely difficult to treat, and one recurrence increases the likelihood of further recurrences. There is no single standard clinical approach, but retreatment with metronidazole or vancomycin is necessary, often in pulsed or tapered dosing. Some small studies have even shown efficacy with a 2-week course of rifaximin after standard treatment with vancomycin.[55] Other adjunctive therapies include bovine antibody-enriched whey, bile salt-binding resins, and intravenous immune globulin (IVIG), and a vaccine is currently in development. There have been small series and case reports of fecal bacteriotherapy (donor stool administered either via nasogastric tube or colonoscopy) indicating anecdotal evidence of efficacy in preventing RCDIs.[56,57] Although the microbiologic make-up of the donor stool was not reported, presumably these therapies use the same mechanism as probiotics in repopulating normal colonic flora and preventing further invasion by pathogens. Probiotics are yet another adjunctive therapy for preventing RCDI, and the best evidence for efficacy of probiotics is for *S. boulardii*.

S. boulardii

One of the largest trials of probiotics in RCDI was by McFarland et al in 1994.[51] Of 60 patients with a prior history of CDI, only 9/26 (35%) in the group given *S. boulardii* in combination with standard antibiotic therapy developed a further recurrence, compared to 22/34 (65%) in the placebo group ($P = .04$). They calculated a relative risk of 0.43 (95% CI 0.2 to 0.97) for recurrence of CDI in those given *S. boulardii* in conjunction with antibiotics. A later study found efficacy for *S. boulardii* in preventing CDI recurrence only in those taking high-dose vancomycin: 3/18 (16.7%) patients receiving high-dose vancomycin and *S. boulardii* developed CDI recurrence, compared to 7/14 (50%) receiving high-dose vancomycin alone. Those in the other groups receiving standard-dose vancomycin or metronidazole plus placebo or probiotic had similar rates of RCDI.[58]

Lactobacilli

Given its promising efficacy in AAD, LGG has been studied for use in preventing RCDI. In a few small, uncontrolled studies, LGG was shown to decrease further recurrences of RCDI, but the total combined number of patients from all 3 trials was 38.[59-61] Preliminary results from a RCT by Pochapin et al suggested possible efficacy of LGG in preventing RCDI, though the numbers again were quite small.[62] A randomized, placebo-controlled trial of LGG in 15 older adults hospitalized or living in a long-term care facility failed to show efficacy in the prevention of RCDI.[63] *L. plantarum* was shown to have some efficacy in preventing RCDI in 4/11 (36%) of the treatment group compared to 6/9 (66%) in the control group, though again the study was small and clearly underpowered.[64]

Meta-analyses

As part of a larger meta-analysis of probiotics in AAD, McFarland analyzed a subset of 6 randomized placebo-controlled trials of various probiotics for the treatment of RCDI. Of all the probiotics investigated, only *S. boulardii* was shown to be effective in RCDI.[46] A *Cochrane Database* systematic review in 2008 focused only on treatment of CDI and did not distinguish between treatment of CDI and prevention of RCDI. As discussed above, they concluded that there is insufficient evidence to support the use of probiotics as an adjunct to standard antibiotic therapy.[52]

SAFETY OF PROBIOTICS IN PREVENTION OF ANTIBIOTIC-ASSOCIATED DIARRHEA

While probiotics are widely used, especially in Europe, and generally considered safe, there is consensus that they are best avoided in the severely ill and immunocompromised. There have been case reports of LGG-associated sepsis, liver abscesses, and endocarditis, although few of the larger case series report the clinical indication for probiotic use.[65,66] *S. boulardii* can cause fungemia.[67,68] A recent review of 57 cases of *S. boulardii* fungemia did note that 3 of the patients infected were receiving probiotics as an adjunct to *C. difficile* treatment. Factors associated with a higher risk of developing *S. boulardii* fungemia appear to be enteral or parenteral nutrition, the presence of a central venous catheter, and an immunocompromised state.[69]

SUMMARY

Antibiotic diarrhea is common and encompasses a clinical spectrum from mild diarrhea to life-threatening *C. difficile* colitis. There is often no reliable way to predict who will develop diarrhea. Many probiotics have been shown to be effective in the prevention of AAD, and the best evidence is for LGG and *S. boulardii*. Probiotics have not yet been shown to be effective as an adjunct to antibiotics in *C. difficile* disease, although there have been very few studies investigating this. RCDI is difficult to treat, and many treatment options are not consistently successful. *S. boulardii* has shown its efficacy as an adjunct in the treatment of RCDI. Preliminary studies suggest that probiotics may prevent CDI, but more studies are needed.

REFERENCES

1. McFarland LV. Epidemiology of infectious and iatrogenic nosocomial diarrhea in a cohort of general medicine patients. *Am J Infect Control*. 1995;23:295-305.
2. McFarland LV. Epidemiology, risk factors and treatments for antibiotic associated diarrhea. *Dig Dis*. 1998;10:292-307.
3. Clausen RM, Bonnen H, Tvede M, Mortensen PB. Colonic fermentation to short-chain fatty acids is decreased in antibiotic-associated diarrhea. *Gastroenterology*. 1991;101:1497-1504.
4. Sullivan A, Larkholt L, Nord CE. *Lactobacillus acidophilus*, *Bifidobacterium lactis* and *Lactobacillus F19* prevent antibiotic-associated ecological disturbances of *Bacteroides fragilis* in the intestine. *J Antimicrobial Chemother*. 2003;52:308-311.

5. Goossens D, Jonkers D, Russel M, Stobberingh E, Van Den Bogaard A, StockbrUgger R. The effect of *Lactobacillus plantarum* 299v on the bacterial composition and metabolic activity in faeces of health volunteers: a placebo-controlled study on the onset and duration of effects. *Aliment Pharmacol Ther.* 2003;18:495-505.

6. Perdigon G, Alvarez S, Rachid M, Agüero G, Gobbato N. Immune system stimulation by probiotics. *J Dairy Sci.* 1995;78:1597-1606.

7. Miettinen M, Makitainen S, Vuopio-Varikla J, et al. Lactobacilli and streptococci induce interleukin-12 (IL-12), IL-18, and gamma interferon production in human peripheral blood mononuclear cells. *Infect Immun.* 1998;66:6058-6062.

8. Mack DR, Michail S, Wei S, McDougall L, Hollingsworth MA. Probiotic inhibit enteropathogenic *E. coli* adherence in vitro by inducing intestinal mucin gene expression. *Am J Physiol.* 1999;276:G941-G950.

9. Millette M, Laquet FM, Lacroix M. In vitro growth control of selected pathogens by *Lactobacillus acidophilus-* and *Lactobacillus casei*-fermented milk. *Lett Appl Microbiol.* 2007;44:314-319.

10. Rea MC, Clayton E, O'Connor PM, et al. Antimicrobial activity of lacticin 3147 against clinical *Clostridium difficile* strains. *J Med Microbiol.* 2007;56:940-946.

11. Castagliulo I, Riegler MF, Vlaenick L, LaMont JT, Pothulakis C. *S. boulardii* protease inhibits effects of *C. difficile* toxins A and B in human colonic mucosa. *Infect Immun.* 1999;67:302-307.

12. Elmer GW, McFarland LV. Suppression by *Saccharomyces boulardii* of toxigenic *Clostridium difficile* over-growth after vancomycin treatment in hamsters. *Antimicrob Agents Chemother.* 1987;31:129-131.

13. Blehaut H, Massot J, Elmer GW, Levy RM. Disposition kinetics of *Saccharomyces boulardii* in man and rat. *Biopharm Drug Dispos.* 1989;10:353-364.

14. Goldin BR, Gorbach SL, Saxelin M, Barakat S, Gualtieri L, Salminen S. Survival of Lactobacillus species (strain GG) in human gastrointestinal tract. *Dig Dis Sci.* 1992;73:121-128.

15. Thomas MR, Litin SC, Osmon DR, Corr AP, Weaver AL, Lohse CM. Lack of effect of *Lactobacillus GG* on antibiotic-associated diarrhea: a randomized, placebo-controlled trial. *Mayo Clin Proc.* 2001;76:883-889.

16. Vanderhoof JA, Whitney DB, Antonson DL, Hanner TL, Lupo JV, Young RJ. *Lactobacillus GG* in prevention of antibiotic-associated diarrhea in children. *J Pediatr.* 1999;135:564-568.

17. Arvola T, Laiho K, Torkkeli S, et al. Prophylactic *Lactobacillus GG* reduces antibiotic associated diarrhea in children with respiratory infections: a randomized study. *Pediatrics.* 1999;104:1121-1122.

18. Szajewska H, Kotowska M, Mrukowicz JZ, Armanska M, Mikołajczyk W. Efficacy of *Lactobacillus GG* in prevention of nosocomial diarrhea in infants. *J Pediatr.* 2001;138:361-365.

19. Siitonen S, Vapaatalo H, Salminen S, et al. Effect of *Lactobacillus GG* yoghurt in prevention of antibiotic associated diarrhoea. *Ann Med.* 1990;22:57-59.

20. Wenus C, Goll R, Loken EB, Biong AS, Halvorsen DS, Florholmen J. Prevention of antibiotic-associated diarrhoea by a fermented probiotic milk drink. *Eur J Clin Nutr.* 2008;62(2):299-301.

21. Ahuja MC, Khamar B. Antibiotic associated diarrhoea: a controlled study comparing plain antibiotic with those containing protected lactobacilli. *J Indian Med Assoc.* 2002;100:334-335.

22. Beausoleil M, Fortier N, Guenette S, et al. Effect of a fermented milk combining *Lactobacillus acidophilus* C11285 and *Lactobacillus casei* in the prevention of antibiotic-associated diarrhea: a randomized, double-blind, placebo-controlled trial. *Can J Gastroenterol.* 2007;21:732-736.

23. Beniwal RS, Arena VC, Thomas L, et al. A randomized trial of yogurt for prevention of antibiotic-associated diarrhea. *Dig Dis Sci.* 2003;48:2077-2082.

24. Conway S, Hart A, Clark A, Harvey I. Does eating yogurt prevent antibiotic-associated diarrhoea? A placebo-controlled randomized controlled trial in general practice. *Br J Gen Pract.* 2007;57:953-959.

25. Hickson M, D'Souza AL, Muthu N, Rogers TR, Want S, Bulpitt CJ. Use of probiotic *Lactobacillus* preparation to prevent diarrhoea associated with antibiotics: randomized double blind placebo controlled trial. *BMJ.* 2007;335:80.

26. Correa NB, Peret Filho LA, Penna FL, Lima FM, Nicoli JR. A randomized formula controlled trial of *Bifidobacterium lactis* and *Streptococcus thermophilus* for prevention antibiotic-associated diarrhea in infants. *J Clin Gastroenterol.* 2005;39:385-389.

27. Colombel JF, Cortot A, Neut C, Romond C. Yoghurt with *Bifidobacterium longum* reduces erythromycin-induced gastrointestinal effects. *Lancet.* 1987;2:43.

28. Orrhage K, Brignar B, Nord CE. Effects of supplements of *Bifidobacterium longum* and *Lactobacillus acidophilus* on the intestinal microbiota during administration of clindamycin. *Microb Ecol Health Dis.* 1994;7:17-25.

29. Wunderlich PF, Braun L, Fumagalli I, et al. Double-blind report on the efficacy of lactic acid-producing *Enterococcus* SF68 in the prevention of antibiotic-associated diarrhoea and in the treatment of acute diarrhoea. *J Int Med Res.* 1980;17:333-338.

30. Borgia M, Sepe N, Brancato V, Borgia B. A controlled clinical study on Streptococcus Faecium preparation for the prevention of side reactions during long-term antibiotic treatments. *Curr Ther Res.* 1982;31:266-271.

31. Imase K, Takahashi M, Tanaka A, Tokunaga K, et al. Efficacy of *Clostridium butyricum* preparation con-comitantly with *Helicobacter pylori* eradication therapy in relation to changes in the intestinal micro-biota. *Microbiol Immunol.* 2008;52:156-161.

32. Seki H, Shiohara M, Matsumura T, et al. Prevention of antibiotic associated diarrhea in children by *Clostridium butyricum* MIYARI. *Pediatr Int.* 2003;45:86-90.

33. Pothoulakis C, Kelly CP, Joshi MA, et al. *Saccharomyces boulardii* inhibits *Clostridium difficile* toxin A binding and enterotoxicity in rat ileum. *Gastroenterology.* 1993;104:1108-1115.

34. Qamar A, Aboudola S, Warny M, et al. *Saccharomyces boulardii* stimulates intestinal immunoglobulin A immune response to *Clostridium difficile* toxin A in mice. *Infect Immun.* 2001;69:2762-2765.

35. Kotowska M, Albrecht P, Szajewska H. *Saccharomyces boulardii* in the prevention of antibiotic-associated diarrhoea in children: a randomized double-blind placebo-controlled trial. *Aliment Pharmacol Ther.* 2005;21:583-590.

36. Adam J, Barret C, Barret-Bellet A, et al. Essais cliniques controles en double insu de l'ultra-levure lyophilisee. Etude multicentrique par 25 medecins de 388 cas. *Gazette Medicale de France.* 1977;84: 2072-2078.

37. Surawicz CM, Elmer GW, Speelman P, McFarland LV, Chinn J, van Belle G. Prevention of antibiotic-asso-ciated diarrhea by *Saccharomyces boulardii*: a prospective study. *Gastroenterology.* 1989;96:981-988.

38. McFarland LV, Surawicz CM, Greenberg RN, et al. Prevention of β-lactam-associated diarrhea by *Saccharomyces boulardii* compared with placebo. *Am J Gastroenterol.* 1995;90:439-448.

39. Cindoruk M, Erkan G, Karakan T, Dursun A, Unal S. Efficacy and safety of *Saccharomyces boulardii* in the 14-day triple anti-*Helicobacter pylori* therapy: a prospective randomized placebo-controlled double-blind study. *Helicobacter.* 2007;12:309-316.

40. Cremonini F, Di Caro S, Covino M, et al. Effect of different probiotic preparations on anti-*Helicobacter pylori* therapy-related side effects: a parallel group, triple blind, placebo controlled study. *Am J Gastroenterol.* 2002;97:2744-2749.

41. Lewis SJ, Potts LF, Barry RE. The lack of therapeutic effect of *Saccharomyces boulardii* in the prevention of antibiotic-related diarrhoea in elderly patients. *J Infect.* 1998;36:171-174.

42. D'Souza AL, Rajkumar C, Cooke J, Bulpitt CJ. Probiotics in prevention of antibiotic associated diar-rhoea: meta-analysis. *BMJ.* 2002;324:1341-1345.

43. Cremonini F, Di Caro S, Nista EC, et al. Meta-analysis: the effect of probiotic administration on antibiotic-associated diarrhoea. *Aliment Pharmacol Ther.* 2002;16:1461-1467.

44. Szajewska H, Ruszczynski M, Radzikowski A. Probiotics in the prevention of antibiotic-associated diar-rhea in children: a meta-analysis of randomized controlled trials. *J Pediatr.* 2006;149:367-372.

45. Johnston BC, Supina AL, Ospina M, Vohra S. Probiotics for the prevention of pediatric antibiotic-associated diarrhea. *Cochrane Database Syst Rev.* 2007;2:CD004827.

46. McFarland LV. Meta-analysis of probiotics for the prevention of antibiotic associated diarrhea and the treatment of *Clostridium difficile* disease. *Am J Gastroenterol.* 2006;1010:812-822.

47. Szajewska H, Mrukowicz J. Meta-analysis: Non-pathogenic yeast *Saccharomyces boulardii* in the preven-tion of antibiotic-associated diarrhea. *Aliment Pharmacol Ther.* 2005;22:365-372.

48. Hawrelak JA, Whitten DL, Myers SP. Is lactobacillus rhamonosus GG effective in preventing the onset of antibiotic-associated diarrhoea: a systematic review. *Digestion.* 2005;72:51-56.

49. Plummer S, Weaver MA, Harris JC, Dee P, Hunter J. *Clostridium difficile* pilot study: effects of probiotic supplementation on the incidence of *C. difficile* diarrhoea. *Int Microbiol.* 2004;7:59-62.

50. Can M, Besirbellioglu BA, Avci IY, Beker CM, Pahsa A. Prophylactic *Saccharomyces boulardii* in the pre-vention of antibiotic-associated diarrhea: a prospective study. *Med Sci Monit.* 2006;12:119-122.

51. McFarland LV, Surawicz CM, Greenberg RN, et al. A randomized placebo-controlled trial of *Saccharomyces boulardii* in combination with standard antibiotics for *Clostridium difficile* disease. *JAMA.* 1994;271: 1913-1918.

52. Pillai A, Nelson R. Probiotics for treatment of *Clostridium difficile*-associated colitis in adults (Review). *Cochrane Database Syst Rev.* 2008;1:CD004611:1-13.

53. Dendukuri N, Costa V, McGregor M, Brophy JM. Probiotic therapy for the prevention and treatment of *Clostridium difficile*-associated diarrhea: a systematic review. *CMAJ.* 2005;173:167-170.

54. Garey KW, Sethi S, Yadav Y, DuPont HL. Meta-analysis to assess risk factors for recurrent *Clostridium difficile* infection. *J Hosp Infect.* 2008;70:298-304.

55. Johnson S, Schriever C, Galang M, Kelly CP, Gerding DN. Interruption of recurrent *Clostridium difficile*-associated diarrhea episodes by serial therapy with vancomycin and rifaximin. *Clin Infect Dis.* 2007;44:846-848.

56. Aas J, Gessert CE, Bakken JS. Recurrent *Clostridium difficile* colitis: case series involving 18 patients treated with donor stool administered via a nasogastric tube. *Clin Infect Dis.* 2003;36:580-586.

57. Persky S, Brandt LJ. Treatment of recurrent *Clostridium difficile*-associated diarrhea by administration of donated stool directly through a colonoscope. *Am J Gastroenterol.* 2000;95:3283-3285.

58. Surawicz CM, McFarland LV, Greenberg RN, et al. The search for a better treatment for recurrent *Clostridium difficile* disease: use of high-dose vancomycin combined with *Saccharomyces boulardii*. *Clin Infect Dis*. 2000;31:1012-1017.

59. Gorbach SL, Chang T, Goldin B. Successful treatment of relapsing *Clostridium difficile* colitis with *Lactobacillus GG*. *Lancet*. 1987;2:1519.

60. Bennet RG, Laughon B, Lindsay J, et al. *Lactobacillus GG* treatment of *Clostridium difficile* infection in nursing home patients. Paper presented at: 3rd Decential International Conference on Nosocomial and Healthcare-Associated Infections; March 5-9, 2000; Atlanta, GA.

61. Biller JA, Katz AJ, Flores AF, Buie TM, Gorbach SL. Treatment of recurrent *Clostridium difficile* colitis with *L. rhamnosus GG*. *J Pediatr Gastroenterol*. 1995;21:224-226.

62. Pochapin M. The effect of probiotics on *Clostridium difficile* diarrhea. *Am J Gastroenterol*. 2000;95(suppl 1): S11-S13.

63. Lawrence SJ, Korzenik JR, Mundy LM. Probiotics for recurrent *Clostridium difficile* disease. *J Med Microbiol*. 2005;54:905-906.

64. Wullt M, Hagslatt ML, Odenhold I. *Lactobacillus plantarum* 299v for the treatment of recurrent *Clostridium difficile*-associated diarrhoea: a double-blind placebo-controlled trial. *Scand J Infect Dis*. 2003;35:365-367.

65. Salminen SJ, Rautelin H, Tynkkynen S, et al. *Lactobacillus* bacteremia, clinical significance, and patient outcome, with special focus on probiotic *L. rhamnosus* GG. *Clin Infect Dis*. 2004;38:62-69.

66. Land MH, Rouster-Stevens K, Woods CR, Cannon ML, Cnota J, Shetty AK. *Lactobacillus* sepsis associated with probiotic therapy. *Pediatrics*. 2005;115:178-181.

67. Niault M, Thomas F, Prost J, Ansari FH, Kalfon P. Fungemia due to *Saccharomyces* species in a patient treated with enteral *Saccharomyces boulardii*. *Clin Infect Dis*. 1999;28:930.

68. Riquelme A, Calvo MA, Guzman AM, et al. *Saccharomyces cerevisiae* fungemia after *Saccharomyces boulardii* treatment in immunocompromised patients. *J Clin Gastroenterol*. 2003;36:41-43.

69. Muñoz P, Bouza E, Cuenca-Estrella M, et al. *Saccharomyces cerevisiae* fungemia: an emerging infectious disease. *Clin Infect Dis*. 2005;40:1625-1634.

15

Use of Probiotics in the Treatment and Prevention of Surgical Infections

Nada Rayes, MD; Peter Neuhaus, PhD; and Daniel Seehofer, MD

During the past decades, the rate of bacterial infections following major abdominal surgery was essentially stable or even increased. Whereas infections caused by skin bacteria such as *Staphylococcus* spp. are more or less effectively controlled with single-shot antibiotic prophylaxis administered immediately before skin incision, infections from enteric bacteria are getting more and more important. We have learned from numerous animal and clinical studies that bacterial translocation from the gut into mesenteric lymph nodes, blood, liver, spleen, and other organs is one major pathogenic mechanism for these postoperative infections.[1] Therefore, the majority of bacterial infections following abdominal surgery are caused by gut-derived bacteria, such as *E. coli* and enterococci.[2] In an analysis of subphrenic abscesses, aerobic bacteria were cultivated in 13%, anaerobic bacteria in 21%, and a mixed flora in 65%, with clear predominance of *E. coli*, enterococci, *S. aureus,* and *B. fragilis*.[3] Bacterial smears of postoperative peritonitis in 355 patients showed *E. coli* in 51%, enterococci in 30%, and *B. fragilis* in 25%.[4] A recent study demonstrated that in 85% of septic patients following general surgery, intra-abdominal infections were the source of sepsis.[4]

THE ROLE OF THE GUT MICROFLORA IN SURGICAL INFECTIONS

Bacterial translocation is influenced by 3 factors: intestinal motility and small bacterial overgrowth, structural mucosal barrier function, and the immune system.[5] In healthy subjects, the so-called indigenous gut microbiota has several important functions, including prevention of colonization by pathogenic organisms, modulation of local and systemic immunity, feeding of enterocytes, and maintenance of intestinal motility and mucus secretion.[1,6,7] The intestinal mucosa is basically sterile because the mucus layer above the mucosa keeps away luminal bacteria from the mucosa. In contrast, the mucosa of patients with IBD or liver cirrhosis or patients in an intensive care unit shows a layer of adherent bacteria. This layer and bacterial translocation leads

Floch MH, Kim AS, eds.
Probiotics: A Clinical Guide (pp 219-232)
© 2010 Taylor & Francis Group

to an inflammation that is able to enhance the disturbance of the intestinal barrier.[8] The loss of the intestinal barrier function in intensive care patients is caused by such factors as stress, lack of enteral nutrition, reduced IgA-secretion, and defensin-production, as well as rupture of tight junctions between epithelial cells. Another source of bacteria causing postoperative infections is occult or overt aspirations from the upper gastrointestinal tract.

Patients scheduled for major abdominal surgery have a severely disturbed microflora and additional risk factors for bacterial translocation[9]—eg, decreased postoperative intestinal motility, jaundice, antibiotics leading to small bowel bacterial overgrowth,[10] loss of mucosal barrier function due to malnutrition, manipulation of the bowel and parenteral nutrition,[11] and suppression of the immune system by blood products and operative trauma.[12] A certain degree of bacterial translocation is physiological and occurs even after sham operations.[13] Severe bacterial overgrowth and subsequent translocation result in bacterial infections or even sepsis.[14-16]

Data from a study of 927 patients described bacterial translocation in mesenteric lymph nodes in approximately 14% of surgical patients,[8] which was independently associated with postoperative sepsis. In addition, gastric colonization in nasogastric aspirates was detected in 54% of patients and showed an association with bacterial translocation and sepsis. Risk factors for bacterial translocation were emergency procedures and total parenteral nutrition.

PREVENTION OF SURGICAL INFECTIONS

At the end of the nineteenth century, scientists believed that the indigenous microflora was potentially dangerous. At that time, a British surgeon named Lane proposed to perform a total colectomy in order to prevent intestinal toxemia.[17]

After the development of antibiotic prophylaxis, surgical infection rates, especially with Gram-positive bacteria, decreased significantly. On the other hand, the number of postoperative infections with gut-derived bacteria remained high.

One of the few double-blind, RCTs assessing the effect of antibiotic prophylaxis in surgical patients did not demonstrate a beneficial effect of intravenous antibiotics on infection of pancreatic necrosis, sepsis, or mortality in patients with acute pancreatitis.[18]

With the development of broad-spectrum antibiotics, a novel concept was designed to eliminate potential pathogenic bacteria in the gut using selective bowel decontamination (SBD) with a mixture of intravenous plus oral antibiotics and antimycotics.[19] Most studies showed that SBD was indeed able to reduce bacterial colonization of the gut, but had no impact on overall infection rates or mortality. The spectrum of isolated bacteria under SBD changed from Gram-negative to Gram-positive bacteria, especially enterococci.[20,21]

The routine use of broad-spectrum antibiotics also led to the development of resistance.[22,23] In 1980, for example, 80% of staphylococci were resistant to penicillin.[24] Recently, a survey showed that 20% of staphylococci in German hospitals and up to 60% of staphylococci in American intensive care units are already resistant to newer penicillin derivatives (MRSA).[25] Some staphylococci have even developed resistance against the next reserve antibiotic (vancomycin-resistant *S. aureus*).[26] In 2000, approximately 27% of enterococci isolated in intensive care units were not susceptible to vancomycin.[27] In contrast, the number of newly approved antibiotics has decreased during the past few years,[28] probably because pharmaceutical companies are more interested in drugs for long-term use, and therefore, there is a need for alternatives.

Certain specific probiotic strains demonstrated effects on the gastrointestinal tract, which might be useful for the prevention of bacterial translocation and gut-derived bacterial infections. Direct effects include prevention of bacterial overgrowth by secretion of antimicrobial bacteriocins and competitive growth,[29] induction of colonization resistance against pathogenic bacteria by competitive blocking of bacterial adhesion and invasion of epithelial cells,[30] upregulation of intestinal mucus production,[31] and secretion of antimicrobial peptides such as beta-defensin 2.[32] Furthermore, they help in maintaining epithelial integrity through feeding of enterocytes, production of omega-3-fatty acids,[33] inhibition of pathogenic-induced alterations of epithelial permeability, and regulation of enterocyte gene expression.[34] Indirectly, some strains are able to specifically stimulate the innate and systemic immune system. Probiotics have been shown to modulate the human DC phenotype and function,[35] reduce proinflammatory cytokines[36] and induce anti-inflammatory cytokines such as IL-10,[37] stimulate nonspecific resistance to microbial pathogens by activation of macrophages,[38] and increase systemic and mucosal IgA responses.[39]

Two animal trials were performed using probiotics in surgical models. A Japanese group showed that intraperitoneal pretreatment with *L. casei* resulted in significantly lower mortality rates, higher numbers of polymorphonuclear cells, and reduced viable bacterial growth in the peritoneal cavity in a murine model of abdominal sepsis (cecal ligation and puncture).[40]

In a rat model of combined synchronous liver resection and colonic anastomosis, oral application of a synbiotic cocktail containing 4 *Lactobacillus* spp. and 4 fibers (Synbiotic 2000, Medipharm, Kagerod, Sweden) could significantly reduce increased bacterial translocation.[41]

PROBIOTICS FOR PREVENTION OF BACTERIAL INFECTIONS IN SURGICAL PATIENTS

In total, 15 randomized, controlled clinical trials with probiotics in surgical patients have been published so far. All of these trials analyze the effect of probiotics as prophylaxis for surgical infections. Currently, no experience exists with probiotic treatment in patients who already have developed an acute bacterial infection. Risk factors for nosocomial bacterial infections in surgical patients are a high APACHE II-score, advanced age, presence of significant comorbidity, complications of operations,[42] male gender,[43] shock, poor nutritional status, multisystem organ failure, emergency procedures, and multiple procedures.[44,45]

Mixed Abdominal Surgery (Table 15-1)

Currently, 3 studies have been published that do not show a significant positive effect of probiotics in postoperative outcome. All 3 studies were performed by the same group. First, 64 patients received pre- (1 week) and postoperatively (median 5 days) 10^7 CFU *L. plantarum* 299v plus oat fiber (Proviva, Skanemejerier, Malmö, Sweden).[46] Approximately 50% of patients were operated on for colorectal cancer, another 10% for aneurysm of the aorta, and the rest for miscellaneous diseases. Compared to a control group (*n* = 65), there were no significant differences regarding bacterial infection rates (13% vs 15%) and degree of bacterial translocation in mesenteric lymph nodes (12% vs 12%). There was a trend toward a lower rate of gastric colonization with potentially pathogenic enteric spe-

TABLE 15-1

RECOMMENDATION FOR PROBIOTIC USE IN MIXED ABDOMINAL SURGERY

OPERATION	LEVEL OF RECOMMENDATION	ORGANISM	DOSE	REFERENCES
Mixed (50% colorectal)	None	L. plantarum 299v (Proviva)	1×10^7/day	46
Mixed (not specified)	None	L. acidophilus, L. bulgaricus, B. lactis, S. thermophilus (Trevis)	1×10^9/day	47
Rectum resection	None	L. acidophilus, L. bulgaricus, B. lactis, S. thermophilus (Trevis)	1×10^9/day	48
Mixed (colon, liver, pancreas, stomach)	Partially	L. plantarum 299	1×10^9/day	49

cies, but this was not statistically significant (11% vs 17%). Interestingly, gastric colonization but not bacterial translocation predisposed to postoperative sepsis in this trial.

After that, 72 patients mainly operated for gastrointestinal malignancy without precise characterization were treated with a synbiotic combination containing L. acidophilus La5, B. lactis Bb-12, S. thermophilus, L. bulgaricus (Trevis, Christen Hansen, Denmark), and oligofructose.[47] The treatment was started 2 weeks before surgery and was continued for a median of 4 days postoperatively. Here again, no significant differences could be demonstrated in comparison to placebo ($n = 65$) with regard to infectious complications (32% vs 31%), gastric colonization with enteric bacteria (44% vs 41%), and bacterial translocation (12% vs 11%). In contrast to the first study, gastric colonization was strongly associated with bacterial translocation but not with postoperative sepsis.

In a third study, 88 patients scheduled for colorectal surgery either received mechanical bowel preparation (MBP) alone, neomycin plus MBP, neomycin plus MBP plus synbiotics (Trevis, the same preparation as in the second trial), or neomycin plus synbiotics.[48] The combination of MBP, neomycin, and synbiotics significantly reduced bacterial translocation (21%, 5%, 0%, and 18%, respectively) and the amount of fecal enterobacteriaceae, but this was not associated with a reduction in serum levels of CRP and IL-6, a change in intestinal permeability measured by a triple sugar test, or septic morbidity (21%, 18%, 15%, and 14%, respectively).

Possible explanations for the lack of effectiveness of these studies and the probiotics strains are the relatively short postoperative period of administration, the oral (instead of jejunal) route of administration with unclear survival of probiotics in the stomach due to low pH, and the inhomogenous distribution of operations with a high percentage of low-risk operations (simple colectomies), resulting in low overall rates of bacterial translocation and infections.

We performed our first study with synbiotics in mixed surgical patients (colectomies, resections of liver, stomach, and pancreas).[49] Early enteral nutrition plus nasojejunal administration of one probiotic (*L. plantarum* 299) and inulin as fiber was compared with enteral nutrition plus inulin alone or parenteral nutrition without synbiotics.[49] Thirty percent in the parenteral group developed infections compared to 10% in the other two groups. Cellular immune markers were not different between the groups. Patients with parenteral nutrition and without synbiotics received antibiotics significantly longer than the other patients. Unfortunately, we did not stratify for the type of operation, and therefore operations with different risk rates for bacterial infections were not equally distributed in the three groups. Secondly, synbiotics were only administered for a short period postoperatively (5 days). In addition, the results were presumably influenced by the mode of nutrition because bacterial infection rates in both groups with enteral nutrition were lower than in the group with parenteral nutrition. However, a subgroup analysis of 26 patients following the Whipple's procedure showed that these patients had the highest infection rates under parenteral nutrition (50%) and profited most from synbiotic treatment, bringing the infection rate down to 14%.

Pancreas Resection (Table 15-2)

Patients with pancreas resection have multiple risk factors for bacterial translocation and infection. In an American study with 300 patients following pylorus-preserving pancreatoduodenectomy (PPPD), bacterial infection rates were 46% to 57%,[50] and in a recent Indian study, they were up to 61%.[51]

Nomura et al studied 64 patients scheduled for pancreatoduodenectomy.[52] Thirty patients were treated with a probiotic mixture of *Enterococcus faecalis* T-110, *Clostridium butyricum* TO-A, and *Bacillus mesentericus* TO-A (BIO-THREE, Toa Pharmaceutical, Tokyo, Japan), and 34 patients did not receive any probiotics. Treatment started 3 to 15 days before an operation, was restarted on the second postoperative day, and continued until discharge. In the probiotic group, there was a significant reduction in infectious complications (23% vs 53%), median length of hospital stay (19 days vs 24 days), and percentage of patients with delayed gastric emptying, which is a frequent complication after this operation (10% vs 20%).

In a recent double-blind study,[53] we enrolled 80 patients after PPPD. All patients received early enteral nutrition via nasojejunal route; 40 patients additionally received a synbiotic cocktail of 10^{10} CFU *L. plantarum* 2362, *L. paracasei* spp. *paracasei* F19, *Leuconostoc mesenteroides* 77:1, and *Pediacoccus pentosaceus* 5-33:3 plus betaglucan, resistant starch, inulin, and pectin (Synbiotic 2000, Medipharm, Kagerod, Sweden). The other 40 patients received the fibers only. The treatment started 1 day preoperatively and continued for 8 days postoperatively. In the group with synbiotics, the incidence of nosocomial bacterial infections was significantly lower (12.5% vs 40%), and only mild wound and urinary tract infections occurred. In addition, there was a trend toward a shorter stay on intensive care unit (2 vs 6 days) and a shorter total length of hospital stay (17 vs 22 days).

TABLE 15-2

RECOMMENDATION FOR PROBIOTIC USE IN PANCREAS RESECTION

OPERATION	LEVEL OF RECOMMENDATION	ORGANISM	DOSE	REFERENCES
PPPD	A	E. faecalis, C. butyricum, B. mesentericus (BIO-THREE)	Not said	52
	A	L. plantarum 2362, L. paracasei, L. mesenteroides, P. pentosaceus (Synbiotic 2000)	1 × 10^{10}/day	53

Our levels of recommendation will be based on the UK National Health Service categories:
- Level A: Consistent Randomized Controlled Clinical Trial, cohort study, clinical decision rule validated in different populations.
- Level B: Consistent Retrospective Cohort, Exploratory Cohort, Ecological Study, Outcomes Research, case-control study; or extrapolations from level A studies.
- Level C: Case-series study or extrapolations from level B studies.
- Level D: Expert opinion without explicit critical appraisal, or based on physiology, bench research, or first principles.

Acute Pancreatitis (Table 15-3)

A placebo-controlled study from Hungary included 45 patients with acute pancreatitis. One study group was treated with L. plantarum 299 plus oat fiber; the second group with oat fiber plus heat-inactivated L. plantarum 299 for 1 week by nasojejunal tube. In the first group, only 1 out of 22 patients developed an infected necrosis of the pancreas compared with 7/23 patients in the second group.[54] The mean length of hospital stay was 14 days in the treatment group vs 21 days in the control group (P-value not significant).

The same author compared Synbiotic 2000 administered for 1 week with only fibers in 62 patients with acute pancreatitis (double-blind, placebo-controlled trial). The total incidence of systemic inflammatory response syndrome and multiorgan failure was significantly lower in the synbiotic group (8 vs 14 patients).[55] In addition, lower incidences of multiorgan failure, septic complications, and mortality were detected in this group; however, the differences were not statistically different.

The first and, to date, the only surgical trial with serious adverse events of synbiotics was recently published by a Dutch group.[56] In this multicenter, double-blind, placebo-controlled trial, 296 patients with predicted severe acute pancreatitis received either a synbiotic preparation consisting of 10^{10} CFU L. acidophilus, L. casei, L. salivarius, L. lactis, B. bifidum, and B. lactis plus cornstarch and maltodextrins (Ecologic 641, Winclove Bio Industries, Amsterdam, The Netherlands) or placebo for 28 days together with fiber-enriched enteral nutrition. The rate of infectious complications was comparable in both groups (30% vs 28%), and the mortality rate was even higher in the synbiotic group

TABLE 15-3

RECOMMENDATION FOR PROBIOTIC USE IN ACUTE PANCREATITIS

DISEASE	LEVEL OF RECOMMENDATION	ORGANISM	DOSE	REFERENCES
Acute pancreatitis	A	L. plantarum 299	1×10^9/day	54
	A	L. plantarum 2362, L. paracasei, L. mesenteroides, P. pentosaceus (Synbiotic 2000)	1×10^{10}/day	55
	None	L. acidophilus, L. casei, L. sali-varius, L. lactis, B. bifidum, B. lactis (Ecologic 641)	1×10^{10}/day	56

(16% vs 6%). The main cause of death was bowel ischemia (8 patients). One possible explanation for these results is the fact that more patients in the synbiotic group had organ failures before or during the day of the first dose of treatment than those in the placebo group (13.2% vs 4.9%). Therefore, the groups might have differed from each other beforehand. In addition, mortality rates in patients with severe acute pancreatitis generally are very high regardless of the type of treatment. Whether there is an association between bowel ischemia and the synbiotic combination is still unclear. One could speculate that enteral feeding using high amounts of a fiber-enriched formula plus probiotics could lead to intestinal oxygen consumption and ischemia in patients with organ failure, consecutive low blood pressure, and splanchnic hypoperfusion. However, this type of complication has never been reported before. Nevertheless, this specific synbiotic combination should not be used in critically ill patients in the future.

Liver Resection (Table 15-4)

Following liver resection, approximately 30% of patients develop bacterial infections and 10% intra-abdominal sepsis mainly caused by enterogenic bacteria[57]; after extended resections, the incidence of bacterial infections is up to 45%.[58] In the case of bacteremia, the risk of liver failure increases to more than 50% and the mortality to more than 40%.[59]

Reasons for bacterial translocation and infection in liver resection are the limited hepatic clearance of lipopolysaccharides, excessive cytokine production of the liver, reduction of the function of the reticuloendothelial system, bile production, intestinal blood flow, and bowel motility.[60,61]

Intestinal microflora and liver function interact in many different ways, a connection called gut-liver axis.[62] A Japanese group investigated the impact of synbiotics on the clinical course of extended liver resection for bile duct carcinoma. For 14 days, 21

TABLE 15-4

RECOMMENDATION FOR PROBIOTIC USE IN LIVER RESECTION

OPERATION	LEVEL OF RECOMMENDATION	ORGANISM	DOSE	REFERENCES
Liver resection	A	B. breve, L. casei (Yakult BL Seichoyaku)	1×10^8/day	63
	A	B. breve, L. casei (Yakult 400)	1×10^{10}/day	64

patients received enteral nutrition plus a synbiotic combination of 10^8 B. breve Yakult and L. casei Shirota (Yacult BL Seichoyaku, Japan) as well as GOS postoperatively, and 23 patients only received enteral nutrition. In the synbiotics group, 19% had bacterial infections compared to 52% in the group without synbiotics.[63] In addition, a significant reduction of pathogenic bacteria and an increase of organic acids in the feces were observed. In a second study with 81 patients operated for bile duct carcinoma, the same synbiotics were given in a higher concentration (10^{10}) either only postoperatively or 14 days preoperatively plus postoperatively.[64] Pre- and postoperative treatment with synbiotics resulted in a significantly lower bacterial infection rate compared to only postoperative treatment (12.1% vs 30%). Moreover, in this group, an increased activity of natural killer cells, a lower concentration of interleukin-6 levels in the blood as expression of a stimulation of the immune response, and a reduction in the systemic inflammatory response were observed.

Liver Transplantation (Table 15-5)

Patients after liver transplantation also have numerous risk factors for bacterial infections: preoperative malnutrition, ascites, portal hypertension, transient loss of hepatic macrophage function that serves as a filter for Gram-negative bacteria in the mesenteric circulation, the extended operation with potential extensive blood loss and manipulation, edema of the bowel, biliary complications, and immunosuppression.[59] Therefore, sepsis is the most important cause of death in liver transplant recipients.[65] A recent analysis of 777 liver transplantations revealed that in the first year posttransplant, 37.8% of the patients developed bacterial infections. If an infection occurred, the 1-year organ survival was significantly decreased and the hospital stay prolonged for 24 days, costing an additional US $159967 per patient.[66]

We published 2 randomized studies with synbiotics in liver transplant recipients. Ninety-five patients were enrolled in the first study.[67] Study treatment consisted of early enteral nutrition plus either SBD (group 1), a synbiotic combination with L. plantarum 299 and inulin as prebiotic (group 2), or inulin only (group 3) for 12 days postoperatively. Bacterial infection rates were lower in the synbiotic group than in the other groups; the difference between group 1 and group 2 was statistically significant (48% vs 13%). Most infections were caused by enterogenic bacteria. Mean duration of

TABLE 15-5

RECOMMENDATION FOR PROBIOTIC USE IN LIVER TRANSPLANTATION

OPERATION	LEVEL OF RECOMMENDATION	ORGANISM	DOSE	REFERENCES
Liver transplantation	A	L. plantarum 299	1 × 10⁹/day	67
		L. plantarum 2362, L. paracasei, Leuc mesenteroides, P. pentosaceus (Synbiotic 2000)	1 × 10¹⁰/day	68

antibiotic therapy (7 vs 12 days), mean hospital stay (35 vs 39 days), and stay on intensive care unit (12 vs 16 days) were shorter in the patients receiving probiotics, but the differences did not reach statistical significance.

In the second study, 66 liver transplant recipients either received a synbiotic combination with 4 probiotics and prebiotics (Synbiotic 2000, as previously mentioned) or only the prebiotics starting 1 day before operation and for 2 weeks postoperatively.[68] In the synbiotic group, only 1 patient (3%) had a bacterial infection compared to 48% in the other group. In addition, duration of antibiotic therapy was significantly shorter (0.1 day vs 3.8 days). No severe side effects were observed in the studies, especially no infections were caused by the probiotics.

Trauma Patients (Table 15-6)

Recently, 2 studies have been performed in trauma patients—a patient group in whom bacterial infection rates have been reported to be around 51%.[69] A Greek group randomized 65 multiple trauma patients for treatment with a synbiotic formula (Synbiotic 2000 forte) or maltodextrin as placebo for 15 days.[70] Synbiotic therapy resulted in a significantly lower infection rate (49% vs 77%), severe sepsis rate (17% vs 40%), and a reduced number of days on ICU (28 days vs 41 days) and on mechanical ventilation (17 days vs 30 days). Mortality was also lower (14% vs 30%), but this difference was not statistically significant ($P = .12$).

Spindler-Vesel et al used the same synbiotic cocktail in a study of 113 multiple-injured patients.[71] Patients either received an enteral formula enriched with glutamine (group 1), fermentable fiber (group 2), a peptide diet (group 3), or a standard formula plus Synbiotic 2000 (group 4) for a nonspecified time. Mortality was very low and comparable in the 4 groups. Significantly fewer patients in group 4 developed infections than in the other 3 groups (19% vs 50%, 59%, and 50%, respectively). This positive effect was accompanied by a decrease in the lactulose-mannitol index as a parameter for intestinal permeability in the synbiotic group.

TABLE 15-6

RECOMMENDATION FOR PROBIOTIC USE IN TRAUMA PATIENTS

DISEASE	LEVEL OF RECOMMENDATION	ORGANISM	DOSE	REFERENCES
Multiple trauma patients	A	L. plantarum 2362, L. paracasei, Leuc mesenteroides, P. pentosaceus (Synbiotic 2000 forte)	1×10^{11}/day	70
Multiple injured patients	A	L. plantarum 2362, L. paracasei, Leuc mesenteroides, P. pentosaceus (Synbiotic 2000 forte)	1×10^{11}/day	71

CONCLUSION

Only 15 RCTs in surgical patients have been published so far. All of them were designed to analyze the effect of probiotic prophylaxis in the prevention of postoperative bacterial infections. Unfortunately, many of them differ in the most relevant parameters, especially type of probiotics, length and mode of administration, kind of disease and operation, as well as type of nutrition. Three studies do not show any benefit, and 1 study even revealed serious adverse events. The remaining 11 trials consistently demonstrate a reduction in postoperative bacterial infections in the patients who received probiotic preparations. The effect of synbiotics depends on several factors. One main factor is the type of preparation and the concentration of the probiotics. In addition, the time of probiotic therapy should be sufficiently long, especially postoperatively. Patients with a high risk of bacterial infections, for example, following operations of the pancreas or liver, and multiple trauma patients profited most from probiotic treatment. Although serious adverse events were reported from only one study, the probiotic preparations should be carefully tested before using them in critically ill patients.

REFERENCES

1. Guarner F, Malagelada JR. Gut flora in health and disease. *Lancet.* 2003;361:512-519.
2. Rüden H, Daschner F, Schumacher M. Nosokomiale Infektionen in Deutschland-Erfassung und Prävention (NIDEP Studie), Teil 1. Prävalenz nosokomialer Infektionen, Qualitätssicherung in der Krankenhaushygiene, Bd 56. Schriftenreihe des Bundesministeriums für Gesundheit. Nomos, Baden-Baden; 1995.
3. Brook I, Frazier EH. Microbiology of subphrenic abscesses: a 14-year experience. *Am Surg.* 1999;65: 1049-1053.
4. Barie PS, Williams MD, McCollam JS, et al; The PROWESS Surgical Evaluation Committee. Benefit/risk profile of drotrecogin alfa (activated) in surgical patients with severe sepsis. *Am J Surg.* 2004;188:212-220.

5. Besselink MGH, Timmermann HM, van Minnen LP, Akkermans LMA, Gooszen HG. Prevention of infectious complications in surgical patients: potential role of probiotics. *Dig Surg.* 2005;22:234-244.
6. Hooper LV, Gordon JL. Commensal host-bacterial relationships in the gut. *Science.* 2001;292:1115-1118.
7. Bäckhed F, Ley RE, Sonnenburg JL, Peterson DA, Gordon JI. Host-bacterial mutualism in the human intestine. *Science.* 2005;307:1915-1919.
8. Swidsinski A, Ladhoff A, Pernthaler A, et al. Mucosal flora in inflammatory bowel disease. *Gastroenterology.* 2002;122(1):44-54.
9. MacFie J, Reddy BS, Gatt M, Jain PK, Sowdi R, Mitchell CJ. Bacterial translocation studied in 927 patients over 13 years. *Br J Surg.* 2006;93(1):87-93.
10. Nieuwenhuijs VB, Verheem A, Duijvenbode-Beumer H, et al. The role of interdigestive small bowel motility in the regulation of gut microflora, bacterial overgrowth, and bacterial translocation in rats. *Ann Surg.* 1998;228:188-193.
11. Deitch EA, Dazhong X, Naruhn MB, Deitch DC, Qi L, Marino AA. Elemental diet and iv-TPN-induced bacterial translocation is associated with loss of intestinal mucosal barrier function against bacteria. *Ann Surg.* 1995;221:299-307.
12. Bengmark S. Gut environment and immune function. *Curr Opin Clin Nutr Metab Care.* 1999;2:83-85.
13. Seehofer D, Rayes N, Schiller R, et al. Probiotics partly reverse increased bacterial translocation after simultaneous liver resection and colonic anastomosis in rats. *J Surg Res.* 2004;117:262-271.
14. Naaber P, Smidt I, Tamme K, et al. Translocation of indigenous microflora in an experimental model of sepsis. *J Med Microbiol.* 2000;49:431-439.
15. Runkel NSF, Moody FG, Smith GS, Rodriguez LF, LaRocco MT, Miller TA. The role of the gut in the development of sepsis in acute pancreatitis. *J Surg Res.* 1991;51:18-23.
16. Tran DD, Cuesta MA, van Leeuwen PA, Nauta JJ, Wesdorp RI. Risk factors for multiple organ system failure and death in critically injured patients. *Surgery.* 1993;114:21-30.
17. Lane WA. Results of the operative treatment of chronic constipation. *Br Med J.* 1908;1:126.
18. Isenmann R, Runzi M, Kron M, et al. Prophylactic antibiotic treatment in patients with predicted severe acute pancreatitis: a placebo-controlled double-blind trial. *Gastroenterology.* 2004;126:997-1004.
19. Mulder JG, Wiersma WE, Welling GW, van der Waaij D. Low dose oral tobramycin treatment for selective decontamination of the digestive tract: a study in human volunteers. *J Antimicrob Chemother.* 1984;13(5):495-504.
20. Hellinger WC, Yao JD, Alvarez S, et al. A randomized, prospective, double-blind evaluation of selective bowel decontamination. *Tranplantation.* 2002;73(12):1904-1909.
21. Zwaveling JH, Maring JK, Klompmaker IJ, et al. Selective decontamination of the digestive tract to prevent postoperative infection: a randomized placebo-controlled trial in liver transplant recipients. *Crit Care Med.* 2002;30(6):1204-1209.
22. Bonten MJ, Mascini EM. The hidden faces of the epidemiology of antibiotic resistance. *Intensive Care Med.* 2003;29:1-2.
23. Imahara SD, Nathens AB. Antimicrobial strategies in surgical critical care. *Curr Opin Crit Care.* 2003;9:286-291.
24. O'May GA, Reynolds N, Smith AR, Kennedy A, Macfarlane GT. Effect of pH and antibiotics on microbial overgrowth in the stomachs and duodena of patients undergoing percutaneous endoscopic gastrostomy feeding. *J Clin Microbiol.* 2005;43(7):3059-3065.
25. Meyer E, Schwab F, Gastmeier P, Rueden H, Daschner FD. Surveillance of antimicrobial use and antimicrobial resistance in German intensive care units (SARI): a summary of the data from 2001 through 2004. *Infection.* 2006;34(6):303-309.
26. Sievert DM, Rudrik JT, Patel JB, McDonald LC, Wilkins MJ, Hageman JC. Vancomycin-resistant *Staphylococcus aureus* in the United States, 2002-2006. *Clin Infect Dis.* 2008;46(5):668-674.
27. Murray BE. Vancomycin-resistant enterococcal infections. *N Engl J Med.* 2000;342:710-721.
28. Shlaes DM, Projan SJ, Edwards JE. Antibiotic discovery: state of the state. *ASM News.* 2004;70:275-281.
29. Servin AL. Antagonistic activities of lactobacilli and bifidobacteria against microbial pathogens. *FEMS Microbial Rev.* 2004;28:405-440.
30. Marco ML, Pavan S, Kleerezebem M. Towards understanding molecular modes of probiotic action. *Curr Opin Biotechnol.* 2006;17:204-210.
31. Mack DR, Michail S, Wel S, et al. Probiotics inhibit enteropathogenic *E. coli* adherence in vitro by inducing intestinal mucin gene expression. *Am J Physiol.* 1999;276:G941-G950.
32. Schlee M, Harder J, Köten B, Stange EF, Wehkamp J, Fellermann A. Probiotic lactobacilli and VSL#3 induce enterocyte beta-defensin 2. *Clin Exp Immunol.* 2008;151(3):528-535.
33. Bengmark S. Bioecological control of the gastrointestinal tract: the role of flora and supplemented probiotics and synbiotics. *Gastroenterol Clin North Am.* 2005;34:413-436.
34. Otte JM, Podolsky DK. Functional modulation of enterocytes by gram-positive and gram-negative microorganisms. *Am J Physiol Gastrointest Liver Physiol.* 2004;286:613-626.

35. Hart AL, Lammers K, Brigidi P, et al. Modulation of human dendritic cell phenotype and function by probiotic bacteria. *Gut.* 2004;53:1602-1609.

36. Sheih YH, Chiang BL, Wang LH, Liao CK, Gill HS. Systemic immunity-enhancing effects in healthy subjects following dietary consumption of the lactic acid bacterium *Lactobacillus rhamnosus HN001. J Am Coll Nutr.* 2001;20:149-156.

37. Niers LE, Timmermann HM, Rijkers GT, van Bleek GM, van Uden NO, Knol EF. Identification of strong interleukin-10 inducing lactic acid bacteria which down-regulate T helper type 2 cytokines. *Clin Exp Allergy.* 2005;35:1481-1489.

38. Perdigon G, Nader de Macias ME, Alvarez S, et al. Systemic augmentation of the immune response in mice by feeding fermented milks with *Lactobacillus casei* and *Lactobacillus acidophilus. Immunology.* 1988;63:17-23.

39. Kaila M, Isolauri E, Soppi E, et al. Enhancement of the circulating antibody secreting cell response in human diarrhoea by a human *Lactobacillus* strain. *Pediatr Res.* 1992;32:141-144.

40. Tsunoda A, Shibusawa M, Tsunoda Y, Watanabe M, Nomoto K, Kusano M. Effect of *Lactobacillus casei* on a novel murine model of abdominal sepsis. *J Surg Res.* 2002;107(1):37-43.

41. Seehofer D, Rayes N, Schiller RA, et al. Probiotics partly reverse increased bacterial translocation after simultaneous liver resection and colonic anastomosis in the rat. *J Surg Res.* 2004;117:262-271.

42. Wacha H, Hau T, Dittmer R, Ohmann C. Risk factors associated with intraabdominal infections: a prospective multicenter study. *Langenbeck's Arch Surg.* 1999;384:24-32.

43. Sawyer RG, Raymond DP, Pelletier SJ, et al. Implications of 2457 consecutive surgical infections entering year 2000. *Ann Surg.* 2001;233:867-874.

44. Farinas-Alvarez C, Farinas MC, Fernandez-Mazarrasa C, et al. Analysis of risk factors for nosocomial sepsis in surgical patients. *Br J Surg.* 2000;87:1076-1081.

45. Wilson SE, Faulkner K. Impact of anatomical site on bacteriological and clinical outcome in the management of intra-abdominal infections. *Am Surg.* 1998;64:402-407.

46. McNaught CE, Woodcock NP, MacFie J, Mitchell CJ. A prospective randomised study of the probiotic *Lactobacillus plantarum* 299v on indices of gut barrier function in elective surgical patients. *Gut.* 2002;51:827-831.

47. Anderson ADG, McNaught CE, Jain PK, MacFie J. Randomised clinical trial of synbiotic therapy in elective surgical patients. *Gut.* 2004;53:241-245.

48. Reddy BS, MacFie J, Gatt M, Larsen CN, Jensen SS, Leser TD. Randomized clinical trial of effect of synbiotics, neomycin and mechanical bowel preparation on intestinal barrier function in patients undergoing colectomy. *Br J Surg.* 2007;94:546-554.

49. Rayes N, Hansen S, Seehofer D, et al. Early enteral supply of fiber and lactobacilli versus conventional nutrition: a controlled trial in patients with major abdominal surgery. *Nutrition.* 2002;18:609-615.

50. Pisters PW, Hudec WA, Hess KR, et al. Effect of preoperative biliary decompression on pancreaticoduodenectomy-associated morbidity in 300 consecutive cases. *Ann Surg.* 2001;234(1):47-55.

51. Jagannath P, Dhir V, Shrikande S, Shah RC, Mullerpatan P, Mohandas KM. Effect of preoperative biliary stenting on immediate outcome after pancreatoduodenectomy. *Br J Surg.* 2005;92:356-361.

52. Nomura T, Tsuchiya Y, Nashimoto A, et al. Probiotics reduce infectious complications after pancreaticoduodenectomy. *Hepato-Gastroenterology.* 2007;54:661-663.

53. Rayes N, Seehofer D, Theruvath T, et al. Effect of enteral nutrition and synbiotics on bacterial infection rates after pylorus-preserving pancreatoduodenectomy. *Ann Surg.* 2007;246:36-41.

54. Olah A, Belagyi T, Issekutz A, Gamal ME, Bengmark S. Randomized clinical trial of specific *Lactobacillus* and fibre supplement to early enteral nutrition in patients with acute pancreatitis. *Br J Surg.* 2002;89:1103-1107.

55. Oláh A, Belágyi T, Pótó L, Romics L Jr, Bengmark S. Synbiotic control of inflammation and infection in severe acute pancreatitis: a prospective, randomized, double-blind study. *Hepatogastroenterology.* 2007;54:590-594.

56. Besselink MGH, van Santvoort HC, Buskens E, et al. Probiotic prophylaxis in predicted severe acute pancreatitis: a randomised, double-blind, placebo-controlled trial. *Lancet.* 2008;371:651-659.

57. Shigata H, Nagino M, Kamiya J, et al. Bacteremia after hepatectomy: an analysis of a single-center, 10-year experience with 407 patients. *Langenbecks Arch Surg.* 2002;387:117-124.

58. Togo S, Matsuo K, Tanaka K, et al. Perioperative infection control and its effectiveness in hepatectomy patients. *J Gastroenterol Hepatol.* 2007;22(11):1942-1948.

59. Rolando N, Philpott-Howard J, Williams R, et al. Bacterial and fungal infection in acute liver failure. *Semin Liver Dis.* 1996;16:389-402.

60. Wang X, Andersson R, Soltesz V, Wang L, Bengmark S. Effect of portal hypertension on bacterial translocation induced by major liver resection in rats. *Eur J Surg.* 1993;159:343-350.

61. Wang X, Guo WD, Wang Q, et al. The association between enteric bacterial overgrowth and gastrointestinal motility after subtotal resection or portal vein obstruction in rats. *Eur J Surg.* 1994;160:153-160.

62. Zeuzem S. Gut-liver axis. *Int J Colorectal Dis.* 2000;15(2):59-82.
63. Kanazawa H, Nagino M, Kamiya S, et al. Synbiotics reduce postoperative infectious complications: a randomized controlled trial in biliary cancer patients undergoing hepatectomy. *Langenbeck's Arch Surg.* 2005;390:104-113.
64. Sugawara G, Nagino M, Nishio H, et al. Perioperative synbiotic treatment to prevent postoperative infectious complications in biliary cancer surgery. A randomized controlled trial. *Ann Surg.* 2006;244:706-714.
65. Rayes N, Bechstein WO, Keck H, Blumhardt G, Lohmann R, Neuhaus P. Todesursachen nach Lebertransplantation: eine Analyse von 41 Fällen bei 382 Patienten. *Zentralbl Chir.* 1995;120:435-438.
66. Hollenbaek CS, Alfrey EJ, Souba WW. The effect of surgical site infection on outcomes and resource utilization after liver transplantation. *Surgery.* 2001;130:388-395.
67. Rayes N, Seehofer D, Hansen S, et al. Early enteral supply of Lactobacillus and fiber versus selective bowel decontamination: a controlled trial in liver transplant recipients. *Transplantation.* 2002;74(1):123-128.
68. Rayes N, Seehofer D, Theruvath T, Schiller RA, Langrehr JM, Jonas S, Bengmark S, Neuhaus P. Supply of pre- and probiotics reduces bacterial infection rates after liver transplantation- a randomized, double-blind trial. *Am J Transplant.* 2005;5(1):125-130.
69. Hammond JM, Potgieter PD, Saunders GL. Selective decontamination of the digestive tract in multiple trauma patients: is there a role? Results of a prospective, double-blind, randomized trial. *Crit Care Med.* 1994;22(1):33-39.
70. Kotzampassi K, Giamarellos-Bourboulis EJ, Voudouris A, Kazamias P, Eleftheriadis E. Benefits of a synbiotic formula (Synbiotic 2000Forte) in critically ill trauma patients: early results of a randomized controlled trial. *World J Surg.* 2006;30:1848-1855.
71. Spindler-Vesel A, Bengmark S, Vovk I, Cerovic O, Kompan L. Synbiotics, prebiotics, glutamine, or peptide in early enteral nutrition: a randomized study in trauma patients. *J Parent Enteral Nutr.* 2007;31(2):119-126.

16

Allergic Diseases

Shira Doron, MD and Sherwood L. Gorbach, MD

The most prevalent allergic diseases are atopic dermatitis, allergic asthma, allergic rhinitis, and food allergies. These diseases affect 17%, 8.5%, 40% and 8% of US children, respectively[1,2] and substantial percentages of adults as well. These prevalences are increasing at a rapid rate. Over a third of children in many countries have symptoms of asthma, eczema, or allergic rhinitis,[3] and a twofold increase in peanut allergy has been reported in the United States and the United Kingdom.[4] Allergic disease has reached pandemic proportions in the industrialized world. The predominant theory for its cause is that with improved hygiene, exposure to infectious pathogens has decreased, and this has created an imbalance in the normal immune response for many individuals. Because of this epidemic of allergic disorders, both preventive strategies as well as effective therapies are crucial.

Allergic sensitization has been linked to reduced exposure to various microbial pathogens such as hepatitis A, helminths, and measles.[5-7] Children with more exposure to microbes in their environment, such as those who attend daycare centers or live on farms, have a lower prevalence of allergic disease.[8-11] The protective effects of these exposures against the development of allergies may be greatest in the very earliest stages of life.

In a prospective study, children who later developed atopic sensitization had fewer bifidobacteria, more clostridia, and significantly different bacterial cellular fatty acid profiles in stool in the first few weeks of life.[12] Additional studies have correlated fecal bifidobacteria levels as well as the predominant strains and their adhesion properties to presence or severity of eczema and allergies.[13-15] Probiotics may provide the microbial stimulation of the gut immune system that is lacking in today's hygienic environment and may counteract some of the microbiologic imbalances that lead to allergic disease.

CURRENT TREATMENTS

Prevention strategies for allergic disease can be categorized as primary, secondary, and tertiary. Primary prevention involves avoidance of initial immune sensitization and consequent development of allergen-specific IgE antibody response. Secondary

Floch MH, Kim AS, eds.
Probiotics: A Clinical Guide (pp 233-242)
© 2010 Taylor & Francis Group

prevention consists of reduction in symptom triggers after sensitization, and tertiary prevention is equivalent to treatment of allergic manifestations.

Primary Prevention

For children at high risk of developing allergic disease, specifically those with at least one afflicted first-degree relative, some clinicians recommend avoidance of allergens (such as cow's milk, eggs, and peanuts) early in life, or even in utero, through dietary interventions undertaken in pregnancy or during breastfeeding. Neither the American Academy of Pediatrics nor the European pediatric societies' guidelines support this practice because the preponderance of evidence is that long-term benefits are lacking. A number of clinical trials have explored the efficacy of prenatal omega-3 fatty acids, known to have potent in vitro anti-inflammatory effects, for the prevention of allergic sensitization.[16-18] Results are conflicting, but one study using a particularly high dose of omega-3 fatty acids did manage to demonstrate a reduction in egg sensitization and severe eczema in offspring at 1 year of age.[16,17] There is confusion about whether breastfeeding increases or decreases the likelihood of developing allergic disease, particularly if the mother suffers from allergic disease herself, with some studies showing that infants are more likely to become sensitized to allergens if exposed to the breast milk of an allergic mother and others showing that breastfeeding is protective.

Secondary Prevention

Five major categories of allergens trigger allergic symptoms: pollens, insects (such as house dust mites and cockroaches), animal allergens, molds, and foods. Individuals with sensitivities to one or more of these are advised to avoid them through often difficult lifestyle modification.

Tertiary Prevention: Treatment of Allergic Manifestations

Atopic Dermatitis

Atopic dermatitis (also known as eczema or atopic eczema) is generally treated by eliminating exacerbating factors, hydration of the skin, and improving the skin's barrier function. Topical corticosteroids, tar, tacrolimus, and pimecrolimus may be recommended. Dietary exclusions are generally not helpful in treating eczema.

Allergic Asthma

Pharmacologic treatment of allergic asthma depends on the severity of the disease. Approved medications include inhaled and systemic steroids, inhaled beta-2-selective adrenergic agonists, leukotriene receptor antagonists, cromoglycates, theophylline, and anti-IgE therapy where the recombinant human monoclonal antibody omalizumab is used to bind circulating IgE and prevent its interaction with the mast cell receptors.

Allergic Rhinitis

Allergic rhinitis is generally treated with topical intranasal glucocorticoids or antihistamines with or without decongestants. Cromolyn sodium and ipratropium bromide nasal sprays and oral montelukast can also be used. Allergen injection immunotherapy is a very safe and effective treatment for this condition. New therapies include sublingual immunotherapy (similar to injection immunotherapy, but the allergen is administered in higher doses and under the tongue) and omalizumab.

Food Allergies

Food allergies are treated like any allergic reaction: antihistamines are given for early signs of a reaction and epinephrine is administered for progressive or life-threatening symptoms.

PROBIOTICS FOR ALLERGIC DISEASE

Dietary antigens can cause intestinal inflammation in individuals predisposed to allergy. Inflammatory mediators are released, and intestinal permeability increases. The intestinal microflora is a key component of the gut mucosal barrier. In germ-free mice with no intestinal microflora, antigen transport is increased.[19] The induction of oral tolerance may be disrupted by derangements in this complex interaction. Changes in intestinal flora, intestinal inflammation, and increased permeability have all been implicated in the pathogenesis of atopic dermatitis and asthma even in the absence of food allergy.[20-22] Though early probiotic research typically demonstrated stimulation of the immune response after consumption of probiotics,[23-25] it is now believed that probiotics may actually have bidirectional immunomodulatory effects. In one study, milk protein consumption increased expression of complement and antibody receptors on the leukocytes of milk-hypersensitive adults, while normal volunteers showed no such response. When these same groups of subjects were given a probiotic strain known as LGG, expression of receptors was stimulated in the normal subjects and attenuated in the milk hypersensitive group, demonstrating that the probiotic was able to down-regulate the milk-induced immunoinflammatory response in the allergic subjects and enhance the normal immune response of healthy subjects.[26] Probiotics have also been shown to reverse the increased intestinal permeability, which would facilitate intestinal absorption of large molecules and allergens in animal models of allergy and in atopic patients.[27,28] Probiotics can also enhance immune responses beneficial to atopic individuals such as the gut-specific IgA responses, TGFβ, and IL10.[29] LGG has been shown to produce enzymes that generate peptides from bovine caseins with suppressive effects on lymphocyte proliferation[30] and to downregulate IL-4 production by peripheral blood mononuclear cells.[31]

Probiotics for Prevention of Allergic Disease

The most impressive data on the use of probiotics for allergic disease comes from trials on prevention of atopic disease. In a study by Erika Isolauri's group published in the *Lancet* in 2001, 132 pregnant women with a family history of atopic disease (eczema, allergic rhinitis, or asthma) were randomized to receive 2 LGG or placebo capsules daily for 2 to 4 weeks prior to expected delivery. These women then either continued the study treatment while breastfeeding or administered the LGG or placebo directly to their babies for 6 months. At 2 years of age, the frequency of atopic eczema in the children in the probiotic group was half that of the children in the placebo group (23% vs 46%, $P = .008$).[32] There were no differences between the groups in circulating IgE or skin-prick responses, suggesting that probiotics affect only non-IgE-mediated responses. Interestingly, even among infants never directly given probiotics for the first 3 months, whose mothers exclusively breastfed, there was a significant reduction in the rate of atopic eczema (15% in the probiotic group vs 47% in the placebo group, $P = .0098$). In fact, the relative risk reduction for breastfed babies whose mothers received LGG was twice that of formula-fed babies receiving their LGG directly, suggesting the possibility of an enhancement of the effect of LGG supplementation by exclusive breastfeeding. Breast milk concentration of TGF-β2 in the milk was significantly higher in those mothers who were taking probiotics compared to those taking placebo (2885 pg/mL vs 1340 pg/mL, $P = .018$). TGF-β2 is a regulatory cytokine that suppresses intestinal inflammation in some instances. In this case, it may be providing the downregulation of intestinal allergic inflammation and thus an immunoprotective effect that could contribute to the prevention of eczema. This concept needs further study. The study has been criticized for its failure to define the method of allocation concealment, conduct an intention-to-treat analysis, and specifically define atopic eczema.[33] However, none of these shortcomings are likely to invalidate the study. In a follow-up study of these children at the age of 4 years, the preventive effects of probiotics on the development of atopic eczema were maintained. Of note, the mean concentration of exhaled nitric oxide, a marker of bronchial inflammation, was significantly higher in the placebo group, suggesting a possible effect of probiotics on subclinical respiratory allergic disease (an IgE-mediated disease) as well.[34] The findings from this cohort should not be generalized to those without a positive family history of atopy.

Another study conducted by Abrahamsson et al in Sweden in 2007 suggested that IgE-mediated disease may in fact be modulated by probiotics.[35] In this double-blind, placebo-controlled multicenter study, 232 families with allergic disease were randomized to *L. reuteri* or placebo taken by the mother during pregnancy, starting 4 weeks before term and administered to the infant until 12 months of age. There was no difference in the incidence of eczema between the 2 groups. IgE-associated eczema, however, defined as eczema in an infant who was also "sensitized" (at least 1 positive skin prick test and/or detectable circulating allergen-specific IgE antibodies), was less common in the probiotic-treated group. This difference was only statistically significant in the second year of life (8% vs 20%, $P = .02$) and remained so even after adjustment for potential confounders. The cumulative incidence of any positive skin-prick test and the rate of sensitization at 2 years of age were also lower in the probiotic-treated group. When analyzing only infants of mothers with allergic disease, these differences became more pronounced. A similar reduction in IgE-mediated atopic disease was demonstrated in a very large study by Kukkonen et al, in which a probiotic mixture was administered starting before birth and continuing to 6 months of age.[36]

A 2007 review published in the *Cochrane Database of Systematic Reviews* evaluated 6 randomized controlled clinical trials enrolling 2080 infant participants given probiotics vs placebo for the prevention of allergic disease and/or food allergy. There was a significant reduction in development of eczema, but not food hypersensitivity, asthma, or allergic rhinitis. Due to the significant heterogeneity between studies reporting on eczema as an outcome, the authors could not make a strong recommendation to add probiotics to infant feeds to prevent this condition. LGG and *B. lactis* seem to be the most promising probiotics for this indication. Adverse events were measured in most of the studies included in the review, and probiotics were found to be safe in this population.[37]

Further study is needed to determine the importance of prenatal administration of probiotics as compared to early neonatal administration alone. Further, the difference between direct administration to infants vs administration to breastfeeding mothers needs to be elucidated. Probiotics administered during pregnancy do appear to result in changes in breast milk composition. In one study, TGF-β2 levels were higher in the colostrum of mothers given probiotics vs placebo. A low level of TGF-β2 in this study was associated with a positive skin-prick test result in the infant.[38]

Probiotics for Treatment of Allergic Disease

Eczema

Attempts to treat allergic disease once manifested using probiotics have been somewhat less successful than prevention efforts. A 2008 review published in the *Cochrane Database of Systematic Reviews* evaluated 12 randomized controlled clinical trials with 781 pediatric participants treated with probiotics for eczema and concluded that there was no significant difference favoring probiotic therapy in participant- or parent-rated symptom scores, participant- or parent-rated eczema severity, investigator-rated eczema severity, or the well-validated Severity Scoring of Atopic Dermatitis (SCORAD) score. There was significant heterogeneity between studies that may represent the differences in the strains' effects. No subgroup (age, severity, comorbid allergic conditions) was found to demonstrate more of an effect than others. Only 5 studies reported on adverse events, and there were no differences in the adverse event rates between the probiotic and placebo groups.[39] It is likely that treatments intended to counteract the allergic tendencies of the immune system must take place in infancy and preferably at the time of early encounters with allergens. Majamaa and Isolauri conducted a study on 31 very young infants, 2.5 to 15.7 months old, with atopic eczema and a clinical history suggestive of cow's milk allergy. The subjects were randomized to receive extensively hydrolyzed whey formula with or without LGG for 1 month. The study was double blind. There was a significant improvement in SCORAD score in the infants treated with LGG but not in those given formula without LGG. Markers of inflammation were compared between the 2 groups and with a group of healthy controls. Fecal concentrations of α-1-antitrypsin and TNF-α were higher in atopic infants than healthy controls, and decreased significantly in the group treated with LGG but not the group treated with formula alone.[40] These results suggest that probiotics may be useful for the treatment of atopic disease if the right strain is given at an early enough age.

Food Allergy

The use of probiotics to treat food allergy has not been formally studied. There is evidence that LGG administration reduces the levels of fecal inflammatory markers[40] and decreases intestinal permeability,[27,28] both of which might be of benefit in the patient with food allergies. In addition, a decrease in gastrointestinal symptoms in the LGG-treated group was observed in one very large study of probiotics for children with moderate to severe eczema, a population with a high rate of concomitant food allergies.[27]

Allergic Rhinitis

Evidence for the use of probiotics to treat allergic rhinitis is not encouraging. In a study of LGG vs placebo given to adults with birch pollen allergy throughout birch pollen season, no differences in outcome measures were seen.[41] In another study of children with dust mite allergy given milk fermented with the starter cultures *S. thermophilus* and *L. bulgaricus* with or without the addition of the probiotic *L. paracasei*-33, improvements in both groups were seen.[42] Other studies looked at live vs heat-killed starter cultures in yogurt for the treatment of allergic rhinitis, but were methodologically flawed.[43,44] In one small trial, investigators randomized 20 patients with seasonal allergic rhinitis to receive *L. casei* Shirota or placebo daily for 2 weeks just prior to pollen season. They reported significant reductions in levels of antigen-induced IL-5, IL-6, and IFN-γ production in the probiotic-supplemented group as well as increased levels of pollen-specific IgG and decreased pollen-specific IgE. These changes suggest the need for future studies that should include measurement of rhinitis symptoms.[45]

TABLE 16-1

RECOMMENDATION FOR PROBIOTIC USE IN ALLERGY

ALLERGY	LEVEL OF RECOMMENDATION	ORGANISM	DOSE	REFERENCES
Eczema prevention	A*	LGG†	Varied	32,34-38,46,47
Eczema treatment	B	LGG‡	Varied	39,40,48-50
Asthma prevention	Insufficient evidence to recommend			37
Asthma treatment	Insufficient evidence to recommend			51
Allergic rhinitis prevention	Insufficient evidence to recommend			37
Allergic rhinitis treatment	Insufficient evidence to recommend			45
Food allergy prevention	Insufficient evidence to recommend			37
Food allergy treatment	Insufficient evidence to recommend			26

LGG = *Lactobacillus* GG; CFU = colony forming units.

*Although the *Cochrane Systematic Review* did not make a recommendation in favor of the use of probiotics for prevention or treatment of allergic disease due to inconsistency of results between studies, we feel that it is inappropriate to combine, as they did, the results of studies using different probiotic strains into one analysis. Several clinical trials using LGG and other probiotic strains have yielded positive results with narrow confidence intervals.

†LGG is the most well-studied probiotic for eczema prevention. Other probiotics studied with favorable results have included *B. lactis, B. bifidum, L. lactis* and *L. reuteri.*

‡LGG is the most well-studied probiotic for eczema treatment. Other probiotics studied with favorable results have included *B. lactis* and *L. reuteri.*

Allergic Asthma

Few studies have been done evaluating the effectiveness of probiotics for the treatment of asthma. In a crossover study, 15 adolescents and adults were given a placebo treatment of yogurt containing the starter cultures *S. thermophilus* and *L. bulgaricus* and an active treatment of the same yogurt with the addition of the probiotic *L. acidophilus.* No differences in clinical outcomes or laboratory markers of inflammation were seen between the treatments.[51]

SUMMARY

The strongest evidence for the use of probiotics in allergic disease comes from the literature on eczema prevention and treatment (see Table 16-1). Not all probiotics have the same effects, just as not all allergic responses stem from the same pathogenesis. A clinical effect attributed to a particular strain of probiotic may not be exhibited by other strains, even within the same species. Individuals probably vary in their response to probiotics, possibly due to genetic polymorphisms in microbial recognition pathways. Environmental factors likely contribute to differences in both colonization and immune development, making meta-analyses in this field especially fraught with error. While it is premature to conclude from the existing literature that a recommendation should be made to treat or prevent allergic disease using probiotics, they are generally safe for most individuals. It should be noted that some probiotic strains are grown on whey-based media and could result in allergic reactions in people with severe milk protein allergy.

REFERENCES

1. US Department of Health and Human Services AHRQ. Management of allergic and nonallergic rhinitis. Boston, MA: US Department of Health and Human Services; 2002.
2. National Center for Health Statistics. US Department of Health and Human Services. Centers for Disease Control and Prevention. Data from National Health Interview Survey; 2003, 2005.
3. Worldwide variation in prevalence of symptoms of asthma, allergic rhinoconjunctivitis, and atopic eczema: ISAAC. The International Study of Asthma and Allergies in Childhood (ISAAC) Steering Committee. *Lancet.* 1998;351:1225-1232.
4. Grundy J, Matthews S, Bateman B, Dean T, Arshad SH. Rising prevalence of allergy to peanut in children: data from 2 sequential cohorts. *J Allergy Clin Immunol.* 2002;110:784-789.
5. Matricardi PM, Rosmini F, Ferrigno L, et al. Cross-sectional retrospective study of prevalence of atopy among Italian military students with antibodies against hepatitis A virus. *BMJ.* 1997;314:999-1003.
6. Lynch NR, Hagel I, Perez M, Di Prisco MC, Lopez R, Alvarez N. Effect of anthelmintic treatment on the allergic reactivity of children in a tropical slum. *J Allergy Clin Immunol.* 1993;92:404-411.
7. Shaheen SO, Aaby P, Hall AJ, et al. Measles and atopy in Guinea-Bissau. *Lancet.* 1996;347:1792-1796.
8. Krämer U, Heinrich J, Wjst M, Wichmann HE. Age of entry to day nursery and allergy in later childhood. *Lancet.* 1999;353:450-454.
9. Ball TM, Castro-Rodriguez JA, Griffith KA, Holberg CJ, Martinez FD, Wright AL. Siblings, day-care attendance, and the risk of asthma and wheezing during childhood. *N Engl J Med.* 2000;343:538-543.
10. Braun-Fahrlander C, Gassner M, Grize L, et al. Prevalence of hay fever and allergic sensitization in farmer's children and their peers living in the same rural community. SCARPOL team. Swiss Study on Childhood Allergy and Respiratory Symptoms with Respect to Air Pollution. *Clin Exp Allergy.* 1999;29:28-34.
11. Riedler J, Braun-Fahrlander C, Eder W, et al. Exposure to farming in early life and development of asthma and allergy: a cross-sectional survey. *Lancet.* 2001;358:1129-1133.
12. Kalliomäki M, Kirjavainen P, Eerola E, Kero P, Salminen S, Isolauri E. Distinct patterns of neonatal gut microflora in infants in whom atopy was and was not developing. *J Allergy Clin Immunol.* 2001;107:129-134.
13. Björkstén B, Sepp E, Julge K, Voor T, Mikelsaar M. Allergy development and the intestinal microflora during the first year of life. *J Allergy Clin Immunol.* 2001;108:516-520.
14. Watanabe S, Narisawa Y, Arase S, et al. Differences in fecal microflora between patients with atopic dermatitis and healthy control subjects. *J Allergy Clin Immunol.* 2003;111:587-591.
15. Ouwehand AC, Isolauri E, He F, Hashimoto H, Benno Y, Salminen S. Differences in *Bifidobacterium* flora composition in allergic and healthy infants. *J Allergy Clin Immunol.* 2001;108:144-145.
16. Dunstan JA, Mori TA, Barden A, et al. Fish oil supplementation in pregnancy modifies neonatal allergen-specific immune responses and clinical outcomes in infants at high risk of atopy: a randomized, controlled trial. *J Allergy Clin Immunol.* 2003;112:1178-1184.
17. Dunstan JA, Mori TA, Barden A, et al. Maternal fish oil supplementation in pregnancy reduces interleukin-13 levels in cord blood of infants at high risk of atopy. *Clin Exp Allergy.* 2003;33:442-448.
18. Peat JK, Mihrshahi S, Kemp AS, et al. Three-year outcomes of dietary fatty acid modification and house dust mite reduction in the Childhood Asthma Prevention Study. *J Allergy Clin Immunol.* 2004;114:807-813.

19. Heyman M, Corthier G, Petit A, Meslin JC, Moreau C, Desjeux JF. Intestinal absorption of macromolecules during viral enteritis: an experimental study on rotavirus-infected conventional and germ-free mice. *Pediatr Res.* 1987;22:72-78.

20. Wold AE. The hygiene hypothesis revised. Is the rising frequency of allergy due to changes in the intestinal flora? *Allergy.* 1999;83:20-25.

21. Majamaa H, Miettinen A, Laine S, Isolauri E. Intestinal inflammation in children with atopic eczema: faecal eosinophil cationic protein and tumour necrosis factor-alpha as non-invasive indicators of food allergy. *Clin Exp Allergy.* 1996;26:181-187.

22. Majamaa H, Isolauri E. Evaluation of the gut mucosal barrier: evidence for increased antigen transfer in children with atopic eczema. *J Allergy Clin Immunol.* 1996;97:985-990.

23. Fukushima Y, Kawata Y, Hara H, Terada A, Mitsuoka T. Effect of a probiotic formula on intestinal immunoglobulin A production in healthy children. *Int J Food Microbiol.* 1998;42:39-44.

24. Link-Amster H, Rochat F, Saudan KY, Mignot O, Aeschlimann JM. Modulation of a specific humoral immune response and changes in intestinal flora mediated through fermented milk intake. *FEMS Immunol Med Microbiol.* 1994;10:55-63.

25. Isolauri E, Joensuu J, Suomalainen H, Luomala M, Vesikari T. Improved immunogenicity of oral D x RRV reassortant rotavirus vaccine by *Lactobacillus casei* GG. *Vaccine.* 1995;13:310-312.

26. Pelto L, Isolauri E, Lilius EM, Nuutila J, Salminen S. Probiotic bacteria down-regulate the milk-induced inflammatory response in milk-hypersensitive subjects but have an immunostimulatory effect in healthy subjects. *Clin Exp Allergy.* 1998;28(12):1474-1479.

27. Rosenfeldt V, Benfeldt E, Valerius NH, Paerregaard A, Michaelsen KF. Effect of probiotics on gastrointestinal symptoms and small intestinal permeability in children with atopic dermatitis. *J Pediatr.* 2004;145:612-616.

28. Isolauri E, Majamaa H, Arvola T, Rantala I, Virtanen E, Arvilommi H. *Lactobacillus casei* strain GG reverses increased intestinal permeability induced by cow milk in suckling rats. *Gastroenterology.* 1993;105(6):1643-1650.

29. Pessi T, Sütas Y, Hurme M, Isolauri E. Interleukin-10 generation in atopic children following oral *Lactobacillus rhamnosus* GG. *Clin Exp Allergy.* 2000;30:1804-1808.

30. Sutas Y, Soppi E, Korhonen H, et al. Suppression of lymphocyte proliferation in vitro by bovine caseins hydrolyzed with *Lactobacillus casei* GG-derived enzymes. *J Allergy Clin Immunol.* 1996;98:216-224.

31. Sutas Y, Hurme M, Isolauri E. Down-regulation of anti-CD3 antibody-induced IL-4 production by bovine caseins hydrolysed with *Lactobacillus* GG-derived enzymes. *Scand J Immunol.* 1996;43:687-689.

32. Kalliomäki M, Salminen S, Arvilommi H, Kero P, Koskinen P, Isolauri E. Probiotics in primary prevention of atopic disease: a randomised placebo-controlled trial. *Lancet.* 2001;357:1076-1079.

33. Williams HC. Pre- and postnatal administration of *Lactobacillus* GG reduced the occurrence of atopic disease in offspring. *ACP J Club.* 2001;135:106-108.

34. Kalliomäki M, Salminen S, Poussa T, Arvilommi H, Isolauri E. Probiotics and prevention of atopic disease: 4-year follow-up of a randomised placebo-controlled trial [see comment]. *Lancet.* 2003;361(9372):1869-1871.

35. Abrahamsson TR, Jakobsson T, Bottcher MF, et al. Probiotics in prevention of IgE-associated eczema: a double-blind, randomized, placebo-controlled trial. *J Allergy Clin Immunol.* 2007;119:1174-1180.

36. Kukkonen K, Savilahti E, Haahtela T, et al. Probiotics and prebiotic galacto-oligosaccharides in the prevention of allergic diseases: a randomized, double-blind, placebo-controlled trial. *J Allergy Clin Immunol.* 2007;119:192-198.

37. Osborn DA, Sinn JK. Probiotics in infants for prevention of allergic disease and food hypersensitivity. *Cochrane Database Syst Rev.* 2007:CD006475.

38. Huurre A, Laitinen K, Rautava S, Korkeamäki M, Isolauri E. Impact of maternal atopy and probiotic supplementation during pregnancy on infant sensitization: a double-blind placebo-controlled study. *Clin Exp Allergy.* 2008;38:1342-1348.

39. Boyle RJ, Bath-Hextall FJ, Leonardi-Bee J, Murrell DF, Tang ML. Probiotics for treating eczema. *Cochrane Database Syst Rev.* 2008:CD006135.

40. Majamaa H, Isolauri E. Probiotics: a novel approach in the management of food allergy. *J Allergy Clin Immunol.* 1997;99:179-185.

41. Helin T, Haahtela S, Haahtela T. No effect of oral treatment with an intestinal bacterial strain, *Lactobacillus rhamnosus* (ATCC 53103), on birch-pollen allergy: a placebo-controlled double-blind study. *Allergy.* 2002;57:243-246.

42. Wang MF, Lin HC, Wang YY, Hsu CH. Treatment of perennial allergic rhinitis with lactic acid bacteria. *Pediatr Allergy Immunol.* 2004;15:152-158.

43. Trapp CL, Chang CC, Halpern GM, et al. The influence of chronic yogurt consumption on populations of young and elderly adults. *Int J Immunother.* 1993;9:53-64.

44. Van de WJ, Keen CL, Gershwin ME. The influence of chronic yogurt consumption on immunity. *J Nutr.* 1999;129(suppl):1492S-1495S.
45. Ivory K, Chambers SJ, Pin C, Prieto E, Arqués JL, Nicoletti C. Oral delivery of *Lactobacillus casei* Shirota modifies allergen-induced immune responses in allergic rhinitis. *Clin Exp Allergy.* 2008;38:1282-1289.
46. Rautava S, Kalliomaki M, Isolauri E. Probiotics during pregnancy and breast-feeding might confer immunomodulatory protection against atopic disease in the infant. *J Allergy Clin Immunol.* 2002;109: 119-121.
47. Kalliomäki M, Salminen S, Poussa T, Isolauri E. Probiotics during the first 7 years of life: a cumulative risk reduction of eczema in a randomized, placebo-controlled trial. *J Allergy Clin Immunol.* 2007;119:1019-1021.
48. Isolauri E, Arvola T, Sütas Y, Moilanen E, Salminen S. Probiotics in the management of atopic eczema. *Clin Exp Allergy.* 2000;30:1604-1610.
49. Rosenfeldt V, Benfeldt E, Nielsen SD, et al. Effect of probiotic *Lactobacillus* strains in children with atopic dermatitis. *J Allergy Clin Immunol.* 2003;111:389-395.
50. Weston S, Halbert A, Richmond P, Prescott SL. Effects of probiotics on atopic dermatitis: a randomised controlled trial. *Arch Dis Child.* 2005;90:892-897.
51. Wheeler JG, Shema SJ, Bogle ML, et al. Immune and clinical impact of *Lactobacillus acidophilus* on asthma. *Ann Allergy Asthma Immunol.* 1997;79:229-233.

17

Treatment of Ulcerative Colitis

Karen Kroeker, MD, FRCP(C) and Levinus A. Dieleman, MD, PhD

Ulcerative colitis (UC) is a chronic inflammatory disease that is limited to the large intestine. It was first described by Dr Samuel Wilks in 1859 as "idiopathic colitis." Its diagnosis is distinct from CD in its distal distribution and continuous inflammation confined to the mucosa of the large intestine. Symptoms include rectal bleeding, diarrhea, urgency, incontinence, tenesmus, and abdominal pain. Complications include toxic megacolon, medication side effects, need for colectomy, and colorectal cancer. Histologically, it is characterized by crypt architectural distortion, crypt atrophy, gland dropout, and a diffuse chronic inflammatory infiltrate without granuloma formation. The etiology is likely multifactorial and a result of a complex interplay between genetic susceptibility, host immunity, and the environment.[1]

Treatment of UC has several goals: induction of remission, maintenance of remission, and improving quality of life. Medical treatment of UC is directed against the exaggerated proinflammatory immune response and includes 5-aminosalicylic acid (5-ASA) compounds, corticosteroids, immunosuppressives (including azathioprine/6-mercaptopurine and cyclosporine), and, more recently, biologics such as antitumor necrosis factor-α (anti-TNF-α). Surgical treatment is usually reserved for medically refractory disease or for colon dysplasia and malignancy.[1] In recent years, alteration of the intestinal microflora has been studied as an alternative option to standard drugs to prevent or even treat mild to moderately active UC.

Probiotics have been defined as a "preparation of or a product containing viable, defined microorganisms in sufficient numbers, which alter the intestinal microflora (by implantation or colonization) in a compartment of the host and by that exert beneficial health effects in this host."[2] A prebiotic is a nondigestible food ingredient that beneficially affects the host by selectively stimulating the growth and/or activity of one or a limited number of bacteria in the colon, and thus improves host health.[3] The term synbiotic is used when a product contains both probiotics and prebiotics, and should be used only when the probiotics and prebiotics are known to work together.[2]

Floch MH, Kim AS, eds.
Probiotics: A Clinical Guide (pp 243-252)
© 2010 Taylor & Francis Group

RATIONALE FOR PROBIOTICS IN ULCERATIVE COLITIS

The altered immune response to intestinal bacteria in genetically susceptible individuals leads to the development of chronic IBD. Probiotics have been shown to impact the development or remission of UC through several protective mechanisms. First, probiotics are able to inhibit the pathogenic effects of specific gut microflora.[4,5] Some *Lactobacillus* strains produce small antimicrobial peptides, called bacteriocins, that are able to interfere with the essential enzyme activity of other bacteria by making pores in the cell membrane.[4] Furthermore, probiotics are able to competitively bind to carbohydrate binding sites on intestinal epithelial cells and thereby displace and inhibit binding by pathogenic organisms. In addition, probiotics can exert their effects through the regulation of the immune response of the host. This is achieved though enhancement of host innate immunity as well as the modulation of the adaptive immune response—eg, by increasing anti-inflammatory and decreasing proinflammatory cytokines.[6] Probiotics are also able to regulate the function of intestinal epithelial cells, such as improving the intestinal epithelial barrier through changes in tight junction proteins. The production of β-defensin (an antimicrobial peptide produced by Paneth cells) is upregulated by *E. coli* Nissle 1917 via NF-κB and AP-1 transcription, allowing cells to prevent bacterial adherence and invasion.[7] LGG has been shown to prevent cytokine-induced apoptosis via activation of Akt (anti-apoptotic) and inhibiting p38/MAPK activation, which is pro-apoptotic.[8] These protective mechanisms of probiotics will be discussed in more detail elsewhere.

CLINICAL STUDIES

Antibiotics are of little benefit as a therapeutic for UC, but they continue to be used in the treatment of severe UC, mostly to prevent bacterial translocation and sepsis. Probiotics are another way to change the enteric microflora and impact the course of disease. In 1918, Alfred Nissle published the benefits of the use of a nonpathogenic strain of *E. coli* in the treatment of gastrointestinal illness.[9] This strain was called *E. coli* 1917 and is one of the probiotics that has been studied in the treatment of UC. During the past decade, a number of other probiotics and prebiotics have been studied in the treatment of UC. Table 17-1 outlines the overall recommendations for the use of probiotics in the treatment of UC. The results of these peer-reviewed studies, divided into induction and maintenance of remission, are detailed in the following subsections.

Induction of Remission

The medical therapies used to induce remission of UC include 5-ASA, corticosteroids, and more recently anti-TNF-α medications. A summary of the various probiotics studied to induce remission in UC is shown in Table 17-2.

The first randomized controlled trial using probiotics to induce remission in patients with UC was published in 1999 by Rembacken et al.[10] In this study, 120 patients with active UC were randomized to either Asacol (800 mg tid) or *E. coli* Nissle (Mutaflor 2.5 × 10^{10} viable bacteria/capsule; Ardeypharm GmbH, Herdecke, Germany) (2 capsules bid) for up to 3 months. Patients were also treated with a 1-week course of oral gentamicin to suppress native *E. coli* at the start of the study. In addition, remission was induced using corticosteroids (hydrocortisone enemas for proctitis or prednisolone 30 to 60 mg/day for more extensive disease). Remission was achieved in 75% of patients

TABLE 17-1

RECOMMENDATION FOR PROBIOTIC USE IN ULCERATIVE COLITIS

ULCERATIVE COLITIS	LEVEL OF RECOMMENDATION	ORGANISM	DAILY DOSE	REFERENCES
Inducing remission	B	*E. coli* Nissle 1917	10×10^{10} CFU	[10]
	B	VSL#3	0.9 to 3.6×10^{12} CFU	[11-13]
	C	Yakult	1×10^{10} CFU	[14]
	C	*B. longum* plus oligofructose-enriched inulin	2×10^{11} CFU plus 12 g	[15]
	C	*S. boulardii*	750 mg	[16]
Maintenance of remission	B	*E. coli* Nissle 1917	5×10^{10} CFU/day	[10,17,18]
	C	LGG	18×10^9 CFU/day	[19]
	C	Yakult	10^{10} CFU/d	[20]
	B	VSL#3	0.45 to 1.8×10^{12} CFU	[13]

Levels of recommendation based on definitions agreed upon during the "Advances in Clinical Use of Probiotics" Workshop, held at Yale University in November 2007.[24]
Level A: Strong, positive, well-conducted, controlled studies in the primary literature, not abstract form.
Level B: Positive, controlled studies but some negative studies are present.
Level C: Positive studies but clearly inadequate amount of work to establish level A or B.

treated with mesalazine and in 68% treated with *E. coli* Nissle ($P = .0508$). The mean time to remission requiring 44 days and 42 days for the mesalazine and *E. coli* Nissle, respectively, was found to be statistically different ($P = .0092$).[10] However, a difference of 2 days is arguably not clinically significant. However, a drawback of this study is the subtherapeutic dose of Asacol.

In 2003, Guslandi et al published an open-label pilot study studying the addition of *S. boulardii* (250 mg tid) for the induction of remission in 25 patients with UC flares while on high-dose mesalazine (1 g tid).[16] They found a 68% remission rate at 4 weeks with a statistically significant reduction in clinical index score.

VSL#3 is a commercially available probiotic mixture that has been studied by several investigators in the treatment of mild to moderate UC. VSL#3 contains 4 strains of *Lactobacillus* (*L. casei*, *L. plantarum*, *L. acidophilus*, and *L. delbrueckii*), 3 strains of *Bifidobacterium* (*B. longum*, *B. breve*, *B infantis*), and one strain of *Streptococcus* spp. (*S. thermophilus*). In 2004, Tursi et al used VSL#3 in combina-

TABLE 17-2

Clinical Studies Examining the Use of Probiotics in the Induction of Remission in Ulcerative Colitis

REFERENCE	DESIGN DURATION	PROBIOTIC	COMPARATOR	CONCOMITANT THERAPY	RESULTS
Rembacken et al[10]	Randomized, double-blind; 12 wks	E. coli Nissle 1917 (10 × 10¹⁰ CFU/day, then 5 × 10¹⁰ CFU/day); n = 57	Asacol (2.4 g/day); n = 59	Induction with corticosteroids (PO or rectal); gentamicin × 1 week	NSD between the groups in induction of remission
Guslandi et al[16]	Open label; 1 month	S. boulardii (250 mg tid); n = 25	None	Mesalazine 1 g tid	Reduction in clinical index score; 68% remission
Tursi et al[11]	Randomized; 8 weeks	VSL#3 (9 × 10¹¹ CFU/day) plus balsalazide (2.25 g/day); n = 30	Balsalazide (4.5 g/day), n = 30; or mesalazine (2.4 g/day), n = 30	Unknown	Higher remission rates in VSL#3 group (P < .02)
Kato et al[14]	Randomized; 12 weeks	Yakult 1 × 10¹⁰ CFU/day; n = 10	Placebo; n = 10	Salazosulfapyridine or 5-ASA	Lower CAI scores, NSD in endoscopic score, SCFA concentrations
Bibiloni et al[12]	Open label; 6 weeks	VSL#3; 3.6 × 10¹² CFU/day; n = 32	None	Mesalamine, corticosteroids, 6-MP, azathioprine were allowed	Remission in 53%, response in 24%
Furrie et al[5]	Randomized, double-blind; 4 weeks	B. longum; 2 × 10¹¹/day plus oligofructose-enriched inulin (12 g/day); n = 9	Placebo; n = 9	Steroids, 5-ASA, immunosuppressants	Reduction in inflammation; trend to reduced sigmoidoscopy score
Suzuki et al[21]	Open label; 4 weeks	Bifidogenic growth stimulator (4.5 g/day); n = 12	None	5-ASA, sulfasalazine, corticosteroids were allowed	Reduction in CAI, endoscopic score; increase in stool SCFA concentrations

tion with balsalazide in the treatment of patients with mild to moderate UC.[11] In this study, 90 patients were equally randomized to 3 groups: VSL#3/balsalazide, balsalazide (4.5 g/day), and mesalazine (2.4 g/day). At 8 weeks, the VSL#3/balsalazide group had a higher rate of remission than other groups per protocol (85.71% vs 80% vs 72.73%) as well as intention to treat (80.77% vs 77% vs 53.33%; $P < .02$) analysis. In 2005, Bibiloni et al performed an open-label study using VSL#3 in 32 mild to moderately active UC patients who did not respond to conventional treatment. Patients received oral VSL#3 (1.8×10^{12} bacteria bid) for 6 weeks.[12] Patients were then assessed using the Ulcerative Colitis Disease Activity Score (UCDAI). Fifty-three percent achieved remission after 6 weeks (UCDAI ≤ 3), whereas 28% of the patients showed a clinical response (decrease by ≥ 3; final score >3). These beneficial effects using VSL#3 in adults were confirmed in pediatric UC patients. In a recent prospective placebo-controlled 1-year study, 29 children with newly diagnosed mild to moderate UC were randomized to receive either VSL#3 or placebo in conjunction with concomitant steroids and mesalamine maintenance treatment. Remission was achieved in 92.8% treated with VSL#3 vs only 36.4% in the placebo group. In addition, the 1-year relapse rate was 21.4% in patients treated with VSL#3 vs 73.3% in the placebo group ($P = .014$).[13]

Bifidogenic growth stimulator (BGS) selectively stimulates the growth of bifidobacteria. In a small open-label study, BGS was used to induce remission in 12 patients with mild to moderate UC.[21] Patients were treated with BGS (Meiji Dairies Co., Tokyo, Japan) 4.5 g/day for weeks and were then evaluated for clinical and endoscopic response. Patients were permitted to remain on stable doses of 5-ASA, sulfasalazine, and/or low-dose prednisolone (doses not specified). After 4 weeks of treatment, there was a statistically significant reduction in a clinical activity score, previously described by Lichtiger et al,[22] from 7.4 ± 2.8 to 4.7 ± 1.5 ($P < .01$), whereas the endoscopic index score decreased from 4.4 ± 1.7 to 3.0 ± 1.3 ($P < .05$). The authors also found a trend toward increased stool SCFA concentration, but only with butyrate reaching statistical significance.

Kato et al conducted a small randomized placebo-controlled trial comparing the addition of bifidobacteria-fermented milk (BFM) to standard treatment with 5-ASA (2.25 to 3 g/day) or sulfasalazine (3 to 4 g/day) to induce remission in 20 patients with mild to moderate UC.[14] Patients were treated for 12 weeks with 100 mL/day BFM, containing at least 10 billion bacteria consisting of *B. breve, B. bifidum*, and *L. acidophilus* YIT 0168. At the end of the study, the clinical activity index (CAI) scores were significantly lower in both BFM and placebo groups; however, the BFM-treated patients had a significantly lower CAI score compared to placebo (3.7 ± 0.4 vs 5.8 ± 0.8; $P < .05$). Endoscopic and histological scores improved in the BFM group, but not the placebo group; however, this difference did not reach statistical significance.

More recently, both synbiotics and prebiotics have been studied in randomized trials to induce remission in patients with mild to moderate UC. In 2005, Furrie et al conducted the first RCT using synbiotics in only 18 active UC patients, studying the effects of 4 weeks of synbiotic treatment (2×10^{11} CFU *B. longum* plus 12 g of the prebiotic combination of inulin and oligofructose) on sigmoidoscopy scores and inflammatory markers.[15] There was a significant decrease in the mRNA expression of human beta defensins (hBD2, hBD3, hBD4) and the proinflammatory cytokines TNF-α and IL-1α ($P < .05$) after use of synbiotics, although these levels were not significantly different from placebo. There was a trend toward a reduction in sigmoidoscopy scores; however, this parameter was not statistically different ($P = .06$).

In a small, prospective, randomized study using prebiotics by Casellas et al, 12 patients with mild to moderate UC were treated with mesalazine (3 g/day) plus 12 g of oligofructose-enriched inulin or placebo for only 2 weeks.[23] Although the Rachmilewitz disease activity score was significantly lower in both groups, the concentration of the inflammatory stool marker fecal calprotectin was statistically lower in the prebiotic-treated group vs the controls both at 7 and 14 days (day 0: 4377 ± 659 µg/g; day 7: 1033 ± 393 µg/g; day 14: 1211 ± 449 µg/g, $P < .05$ vs day 0).

Maintenance of Remission

After the induction of remission, medical therapies including 5-ASA products, immunosuppressives, and biologics are used to maintain remission of UC. Table 17-3 summarizes the studies in which various probiotics are used in the maintenance of remission induced by either probiotics or standard medical therapies.

The first randomized controlled study investigating the use of probiotics to maintain remission in patients with UC was published in 1997 by Kruis et al.[17] This study compared E. coli Nissle to mesalazine in a randomized, double-blind, double-dummy study for 12 weeks in patients with remission of UC. At the time of study entry, patients needed to have a CAI ≤ 4. However, it is important to know that 20% and 34% of patients in the E. coli Nissle and mesalazine groups, respectively, had only proctitis. Patients were randomized to either E. coli Nissle (serotype O6:K5:H1) 5×10^{10} viable bacteria (Ardeypharm GmbH, Herdecke, Germany) or mesalazine (Salofalk) 500 mg tid with dummy controls. No significant difference in CAI score was observed after 12 weeks of treatment between the 2 groups ($P = .12$), indicating equal efficacy of the compared treatment modalities.

Rembacken et al followed the 39 and 44 patients in which they had induced remission with E. coli Nissle or mesalamine, respectively, for up to 1 year.[10] Following induction of remission, these patients were confirmed to have quiescent colitis during sigmoidoscopy. Subsequently, these patients were placed on maintenance doses of either mesalazine (1.2 g/day) or E. coli Nissle (5×10^{10} CFU/day). The mean duration of remission was slightly longer in the probiotic group (221 days vs 206 days, $P = .0174$), suggesting that E. coli Nissle had an equivalent effect to mesalazine in the maintenance of remission at 1 year.

In 2004, Kruis et al conducted a large multicenter, randomized, double-blind, double-dummy study to determine whether E. coli Nissle was equivalent to mesalazine in maintaining remission in patients with UC.[18] Patients were treated with E. coli Nissle (serotype O6:K5:H1) 2.5 to 25×10^9 viable bacteria (Mutaflor 100 mg; Ardeypharm GmbH, Herdecke, Germany) or mesalazine (1.5 g/day) for 12 months. In this study, designed to determine noninferiority, E. coli Nissle was found to be equivalent to 1.5 g daily of mesalazine in terms of relapse at 12 months per protocol (36.4% vs 33.9% relapse, $P = .003$) as well as per intention to treat (45.1% vs 37% relapse, $P = .013$) analysis in the E. coli Nissle and mesalazine groups, respectively.

Several other probiotic preparations have been used to try to maintain remission in patients with UC. A small randomized controlled study ($n = 11$, controls = 10) by Ishikawa et al found that patients treated with Yakult 100 mL/day showed less UC relapses compared to controls.[20] Patients were treated with BFM, which contains strains of B. breve, B. bifidum, and L. acidophilus YIT 0168 in at least 10 billion per 100 mL. Patients and controls were treated with salazosulfapyridine, mesalamine, or steroids as clinically indicated. Clinical relapses were assessed through patient interviews in terms of abdominal pain, stool frequency, or change in blood or mucus. In this open-label study, 3/11 BFM-treated patients had relapses vs 9/10 control patients ($P = .0075$); patients treated with BFM had fewer exacerbations compared to controls ($P = .009$).

TABLE 17-3

PROBIOTIC STUDIES OF THE MAINTENANCE OF REMISSION IN ULCERATIVE COLITIS

REFERENCE	STUDY DESIGN, DURATION	PROBIOTIC	COMPARATOR	CONCOMITANT THERAPY	RESULTS
Kruis et al[17]	Randomized, double-blind; 12 weeks	E. coli Nissle 1917; (25 × 10⁹ CFU); n = 50	Mesalazine (1.5 g); n = 53	None	NSD in CAI scores or relapse rates (16% vs 11.3%)
Rembacken et al[10]	Randomized, double-blind; 12 months	E. coli Nissle 1917 (5 × 10¹⁰ CFU); n = 59	Asacol (1.2 g/day); n = 57	Induction with corticosteroids (PO or rectal); gentamicin × 1 week	NSD between the groups in maintenance
Ishikawa et al[20]	Randomized; 12 months	Yakult; 10¹⁰ CFU/day; n = 11	No addition; n = 10	Prednisolone, mesalazine, salazosulfapyridine allowed	Less exacerbation in the Yakult group
Kruis et al[18]	Randomized, double-blind; 12 months	E. coli Nissle 1917 (2.5 to 25 × 10⁹ CFU); n = 162	Mesalazine (1.5 g); n = 165	None	Equivalence in terms of relapse (36.4% vs 33.9%) (P = .003)
Zocco et al[19]	Randomized, open label; 12 months	LGG (18 × 10⁹ CFU/day); n = 65	Mesalazine (2.4 g); n = 60; or combination; n = 62	N/A	NSD in relapse at 6, 12 months
Miele et al[13]	Randomized, double-blind; 12 months	VSL#3 (0.45 to 1.8 × 10¹² CFU/day); n = 14	Mesalazine (50 mg/ kg/day); n = 15	Induction with corticosteroids (PO)	Relapse at 12 months 21% with VSL#3 vs 73% in placebo (P = .014)

In a prospective open-label study using 180 patients, Zocco et al examined the efficacy of using LGG in maintaining remission in patients with UC.[19] Patients were randomized to LGG (18 × 10^9 CFU/day) (Giflorex, Errekappa, Euroterapici) with mesalazine 2.4 g/day, LGG alone, or mesalazine alone. Primary endpoint was the maintenance of remission. No difference was found between the 3 groups at 6 and 12 months. No statistically significant difference was seen in clinical, endoscopic, or histological scores. There was a trend toward a decrease in the odds for relapse in the groups treated with LGG, but this was not statistically different.

CONCLUSION

Currently, the use of probiotics has a B-level evidence for the induction and maintenance of remission of UC.[24] The studies for probiotics to date are emerging as a first-line adjunct treatment of active UC. *E. coli* Nissle and lately the probiotic cocktail VSL#3 are showing benefit in controlled induction studies for active UC, and also for maintenance of remission. Unfortunately, other induction studies lack sufficient numbers and/or are uncontrolled. The various protective mechanisms of probiotics hold promise for their application to this chronic inflammatory condition. Due to the diversity in currently available probiotics, their specific bacteria-host interactions, and the study of various doses, it remains difficult to assess which preparation is the best for the individual UC patient.

REFERENCES

1. So C, Lichtenstein GR. Ulcerative colitis. In: Feldman M, Friedman LS, Brandt LJ, Sleisenger MS, eds. *Sleisenger and Fordtran's Gastrointestinal and Liver Disease.* 8th ed. Philadelphia, PA: Saunders Elsevier; 2006:2499-2538.
2. Schrezenmeier J, de Vrese M. Probiotics, prebiotics, and synbiotics: approaching a definition. *Am J Clin Nutr.* 2001;73:361S-364S.
3. Gibson GR, Roberfroid MB. Dietary modulation of the human colonic microbiota: introducing the concept of prebiotics. *J Nutr.* 1995;125:1401-1412.
4. Vanderpool C, Yan F, Polk DB. Mechanisms of probiotic action: implications for therapeutic applications in inflammatory bowel diseases. *Inflamm Bowel Dis.* 2008;14:1585-1596.
5. Ewaschuk JB, Dieleman LA. Probiotics and prebiotics in chronic inflammatory bowel diseases. *World J Gastroenterol.* 2006;12:5941-5950.
6. Vanderpool C, Yan F, Polk DB. Mechanisms of probiotic action: implications for therapeutic applications in inflammatory bowel diseases. *Inflamm Bowel Dis.* 2008;14:1585-1596.
7. Wehkamp J, Harder J, Wehkamp K, et al. NF-κB- and AP-1-mediated induction of human beta defensin-2 in intestinal epithelial cells by *Escherichia coli* Nissle 1917: a novel effect of a probiotic bacterium. *Infect Immun.* 2004;72:5750-5758.
8. Yan F, Polk DB. Probiotic bacterium prevents cytokine-induced apoptosis in intestinal epithelial cells. *J Biol Chem.* 2002;277:50959-50965.
9. Nissle A. Die antagonistische Behandlung chronischer Darmstoerungen mit Colibakterien [The antagonistic therapy of chronic intestinal disturbances]. *Med Klinik.* 1918;2:29-30.
10. Rembacken BJ, Snelling AM, Hawkey PH, Chalmers DM, Axon ATR. Non-pathogenic *Escherichia coli* versus mesalazine for the treatment of ulcerative colitis: a randomized trial. *Lancet.* 1999;354:635-639.
11. Tursi A, Brandimarte G, Giorgetti GM, Forti G, Modeo ME, Gigliobianco A. Low-dose balsalazide plus a high-potency probiotic combination is more effective that balsalazide alone or mesalazine in the treatment of acute mild-to-moderate ulcerative colitis. *Med Sci Monit.* 2004;10:126-131.
12. Bibiloni R, Fedorak RN, Tannock GW, et al. VSL#3 probiotic-mixture induces remission in patients with active ulcerative colitis. *Am J Gastroenterol.* 2005;100:1539-1546.
13. Miele E, Pascarella F, Giannetti E, Quaglietta L, Baldassano RN, Staiano A. Effect of a probiotic preparation (VSL#3) on induction and maintenance of remission in children with ulcerative colitis. *Am J Gastroenterol.* 2009;104:437-443.

14. Kato K, Mizuno S, Umesaki Y, et al. Randomized placebo-controlled trial assessing the effect of bifidobacteria-fermented mild on active ulcerative colitis. *Aliment Pharmacol Ther.* 2004;20:1133-1141.
15. Furrie E, Macfarlane S, Kennedy A, et al. Synbiotic therapy (*Bifidobacterium longum*/Synergy 1) initiates resolution of inflammation in patients with active ulcerative colitis: a randomised controlled pilot trial. *Gut.* 2005;54;242-249.
16. Guslandi M, Giollo P, Testoni PA. A pilot trial of *Saccharomyces boulardii* in ulcerative colitis. *Eur J Gastro Hepatol.* 2003;15:697-698.
17. Kruis W, Schutz E, Fric P, Fixa B, Judmaier G, Stolte M. Double-blind comparison of an oral *Escherichia coli* preparation and mesalazine in maintaining remission of ulcerative colitis. *Aliment Pharmacol Ther.* 1997;11:853-858.
18. Kruis W, Fric P, Pokrotneiks J, et al. Maintaining remission of ulcerative colitis with the probiotic *Escherichia coli* Nissle 1917 is as effective as with standard mesalazine. *Gut.* 2004;53:1617-1623.
19. Zocco MA, Zileri Dal Verme L, Cremonini F, et al. Efficacy of *Lactobacillus* GG in maintaining remission of ulcerative colitis. *Aliment Pharmacol Ther.* 2006;23:1597-1574.
20. Ishikawa H, Akedo I, Umesaki Y, Tanaka R, Imaoka MS, Otani T. Randomized controlled trial of the effect of bifidobacteria-fermented milk on ulcerative colitis. *J Am Coll Nutr.* 2003;22:56-63.
21. Suzuki A, Mitsuyama K, Koga H, et al. Bifidogenic growth stimulator for the treatment of active ulcerative colitis: a pilot study. *Nutrition.* 2006;22:76-81.
22. Lichtiger S, Present DH, Kornbluth A, et al. Cyclosporine in severe ulcerative colitis refractory to steroid therapy. *N Engl J Med.* 1994;330:1841-1845.
23. Casellas F, Borruel N, Torrejo A, et al. Oral oligofructose-enriched inulin supplementation in acute ulcerative colitis is well tolerated and associated with lowered faecal calprotectin. *Aliment Pharmacol Ther.* 2007;25:1061-1067.
24. Floch MH, Walker WA, Guandalini S, Hibbert P, Gorbach S, Surawicz C. Recommendations for probiotic use: 2008. *J Clin Gastroenterol.* 2008;42:S104-S108.

18

Probiotic Treatment in Crohn's Disease

Karen Kroeker, MD, FRCP(C) and Richard N. Fedorak, MD, FRCP(C)

Crohn's disease (CD) is chronic inflammatory disease characterized by aphthous ulcers, transmural inflammation, skip lesions, and granuloma formation. Pathogenesis of CD is the result of a complex interplay between genetic susceptibility, the environment, enteric microflora, and the host immune response. Traditionally, treatment of CD has focused on attempted modification of the host immune response and surgical resection of diseased areas. Antibiotics, to alter intestinal flora, have been used to treat abscesses and perianal fistula and prevent postoperative recurrence.

Over the millennium, food probiotics have been used to promote health and wellness and a broad range of folk and traditional medicinal remedies. However, only recently have they been considered as potential mainstream therapeutics for modern medicine. This transition is a result of recent, well-designed clinical trials and investigations at the cellular and subcellular levels in experimental systems and animal models. Because of this, anecdotal observations in support of probiotic therapies for IBD are being slowly replaced by experimental insight into the complex interactions of probiotics with the endemic gut microflora, the epithelia, and the host's mucosal and systemic immune system. Taken together, this mechanistic understanding is building the foundation to support the level 1 randomized controlled clinical trials that are needed for probiotics to enter mainstream medical therapy algorithms.

RATIONALE FOR USING PROBIOTICS IN CROHN'S DISEASE

Recent studies have identified several mechanisms by which probiotics can have a direct effect on epithelial cell function and intestinal health, including enhancing epithelial barrier function, modulating epithelial cytokine secretion into an anti-inflammatory dominant profile, altering mucus production, changing bacterial luminal flora, modifying the innate and systemic immune system, and inducing regulatory T-cell effects (Figure 18-1). This research has been facilitated by the development of molecular methods for identifying and analyzing complex bacterial communities within the mammalian intestine. A series of review articles have been published outlining the

Floch MH, Kim AS, eds.
Probiotics: A Clinical Guide (pp 253-266)
© 2010 Taylor & Francis Group

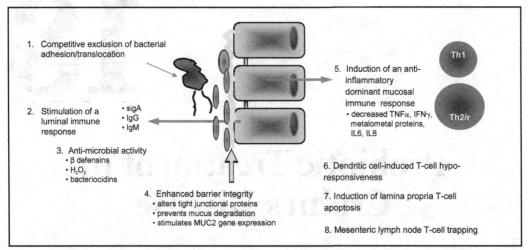

Figure 18-1. Schematic illustration of the various mechanisms by which probiotics exert therapeutic effects at the cellular level in the intestinal tract.[1,2]

efficacy of probiotics in human health.[3-14] The production of antibacterial substances by probiotics inhibits the growth of pathogens. Lactobacilli lower the pH by the production of acetic, lactic, and propionic acid, which can inhibit the growth of Gram-negative bacteria.[15] Lactic acid produced by LGG has been identified as a primary antimicrobial compound in the inhibition of growth of *Salmonella typhimurium*.[16] Bacteriocin-like compounds produced by Gram-positive bacteria including bifidobacteria are toxic to Gram-positive and Gram-negative bacteria.[17] The action of bacteriocins is the formation of pores in the cytoplasmic membrane of certain bacteria.[13] Probiotics also play a role in the inhibition of pathogenic bacteria through competition via decreasing adhesion of bacteria and their toxins. Strains of *Lactobacillus* and bifidobacteria have been shown to bind to intestinal mucus and inhibit and displace the adhesion of *Bacteroides*, *Clostridium*, *Staphylococcus*, and *Enterobacter*.[18] The demonstration that immune and epithelial cells can discriminate between different microbial species has extended the known mechanism(s) of action of probiotics beyond simple barrier and antimicrobial effects.[1]

Aligning the mechanism of action of the individual probiotics with pathogenic mechanisms of the diseases, including CD, will assist clinicians in understanding the action of probiotics, test these hypotheses in randomized controlled clinical trials, and, eventually, develop a therapeutic algorithm for their effective use in IBD and other disorders.

The Microbial-Related Pathogenesis of Crohn's Disease

Although closer than ever to understanding the pathogenesis of CD, it is acutely apparent that there is a myriad of complex associations between an individual's genetics and the luminal microbial environment of the genetics. New concepts, developed out of this appreciation, suggest the involvement of dysfunctional mucosal and systemic immune cells that (1) are unable to detect and/or eradicate potentially injurious microbes and/or (2) help in detecting normal enteric flora as "foreign" and setting up an inflammatory response that cannot be shut down and/or (3) alter the enteric microbiota composition, thereby disrupting the otherwise platonic relationship with the host's tissues.[19] Appreciation for the transmetabolic functioning of the human intestinal tract is a relatively new concept. Bacterial strain ratios in otherwise healthy humans are being linked to a range of whole-body manifestations, most notably obesity.[20] With respect to IBD, recent studies have identified significant strain variations between healthy and diseased individuals. For instance, Kotlowski et al determined that patients with either CD or UC had 3 to 4 logs greater amounts of enterobacteriaceae in their tissues compared to healthy individuals ($P = .05$).[21] A recent study has found significant differences regarding both the number and genetic composition of bacteria associated with intestinal biopsies between UC and CD patients.[22] As well, it was found that patients with CD had more bacteria from bacteroidetes phylum than those with UC. In another study, inflamed and noninflamed ileal mucosa from CD patients were assessed. No significant differences regarding bacteria composition or numbers were found, suggesting that the systemic gut's biome is altered as opposed to a localized response.[23] Conversely, a difference in both the leukocyte count and the concentration of *Faecalibacterium prausnitzii* have been identified, and the stability of variance is such that it could be considered as a noninvasive marker to identify IBD and help discriminate between CD and UC.[24] Furthermore, *F. prausnitzii* has been found to be markedly reduced in CD patients who have rapid recurrence following surgical resection, again implying a strong bacterial association between disease and health.[25]

Increased intestinal permeability may have an important role in the pathogenesis of CD. Recently, Garcia Vilela et al have demonstrated that 31 patients with CD in remission have an increased intestinal permeability, measured by lactulose/mannitol ratio, as compared to healthy controls.[26] Administration of *S. boulardii* (4×10^8 CFU q8h) resulted in improved intestinal permeability over the 3-month study period.[26]

Currently, the exact roles of bacteria within the pathogenesis of CD are unknown, but emerging evidence confirms that the gut's biome of patients is measurably distinct from that of healthy individuals. Assuming that IBD occurs as a consequence of an altered response to the mucosal microflora, it is conceivable that the introduction of probiotic organisms as therapeutic agents will change the luminal microflora and/or enhance epithelial barrier function or mollify the response of the mucosal and systemic immune systems in such a way as to attenuate the intestinal inflammatory response.

Probiotics and Animal Models of Inflammatory Bowel Disease

In order to understand biological processes, it is essential to develop both experimental systems and animal models. Such models have been proven invaluable in the overall advancement of our understanding of IBD. Recently, they have been essential to advance the study of probiotics both at the cellular and subcellular levels as well as to identify their localized and systemic effects. As early as 1992, a murine model was used to examine the effect of *Bifidobacterium breve* on antibody production.[27] Since then, other animal models have been used including rats, pigs, and cats. The development of models of animals that are deficient in key proteins that have been associated with IBD has enhanced the research options, enabling an increased understanding of the physiology. The first such study explored the ameliorating effect of *L. reuteri* enemas administered to interleukin (IL)-10 gene-deficient mice that, when raised under nonsterile conditions, normally develop colitis similar to CD.[28] Since then, multiple other gene knockout and transgenic animal models have been used for the study of probiotics.

In studying probiotics for the treatment of IBD, the murine model is the most popular, evidenced by the fact that it was used by 7 well-designed studies in 2007. The majority of these studies assessed the effect of probiotic therapy on various inflammatory markers in animals with colitis induced using either trinitrobenzenesulphonic acid or dextran sulfate sodium. Mucosal integrity was enhanced by *E. coli* Nissle 1917 via upregulating the junction-associated protein, zonula occludens 1 (ZO-1), in intestinal epithelial cells.[29] In IL-10-deficient mice, secreted bioactive factors from *B. infantis* have been shown to attenuate inflammation, normalize colonic permeability, and decrease IFN-γ secretion.[30] The commercial probiotic mixture, VSL#3, ameliorated colitis through immune modulation involving colonic inhibitory κβ-α, IL-1β, and myeloperoxidase.

Optimum dosing of the probiotic mixture to attenuate colitis was also explored; this was also a concern in previous human trials as dose-finding studies with probiotics is very limited.[31] Kim et al presented convincing evidence that *B. bifidum* BGN4 suppressed cytokine production in colitis-induced mice, concluding that it should help restore dysfunctional immune responses in intestinal tissues.[32] In a comparative study, *L. casei*, *L. acidophilus*, and *B. lactis* yielded similar therapeutic benefits in colitis-induced rats, but each species had its own anti-inflammatory profile.[33] With respect to *L. casei*, Chung et al found that this probiotic modulates the expression of inflammatory cytokines and is dependent on the signaling of the Toll-like receptor (TLR)-4 complex determined by using TLR-4 mutant mice.[34] The effect of 2 putative probiotics on ameliorating inflammation in colitis-induced murine models was investigated. *Enterococcus durans*, isolated from healthy human feces, decreased the colonic cDNA concentration of IL-1β and TNF-α, suggesting that further trials are warranted to explore possible therapeutic benefits for UC patients.[33] A comparison of the anti-inflammatory properties of a previously studied probiotic, *L. reuteri*, and *L. fermentum* (both of which were isolated from breast milk) concluded that the ability of *L. fermentum* to significantly lower TNF-α relative to *L. reuteri* suggests that it possesses immunomodulatory properties beneficial to humans and merits additional study.[35]

PROBIOTIC AGENTS IN THE TREATMENT OF CROHN'S DISEASE

An overview of the recommendations for the use of probiotics in the treatment of CD is summarized in Table 18-1. The individual results of both open-label and randomized controlled clinical trials investigating probiotic use in treating humans with CD are discussed hereafter and are summarized in Table 18-2.

Induction of Crohn's Disease Remission

There is a paucity of data available on the treatment of active CD with probiotics. To date, there have been only 4 open-label studies published that included a paucity of only 50 patients. A recent, open-label trial examined the effect of synbiotic therapy in 10 CD patients with active disease, primarily diarrhea and abdominal pain, refractory to aminosalicylates and prednisolone.[36] After 13 months (±4.5), 2 of the 6 responders successfully discontinued steroid therapy while 4 were able to decrease their dosages. Values for both the CD activity index (CDAI) and the International Organization for the Study of Inflammatory Bowel Disease (IOIBD) index were significantly reduced (255 to 136, $P = .009$ and 3.5 to 2.1, $P = .03$, respectively). Concomitant therapy with prednisolone, aminosalicylate, and home enteral nutrition was allowed.

In a small, double-blinded trial of 11 patients, Schultz et al treated CD patients with antibiotics and a tapering course of glucocorticoids.[37] When the antibiotics were stopped at 2 weeks, the subjects were randomized to receive either LGG (2×10^9 CFU/day) or placebo. The study found no difference in remission rates between the groups (4/5 LGG vs 5/6 placebo).

(text continued on page 261)

TABLE 18-1

RECOMMENDATION FOR PROBIOTIC USE IN CROHN'S DISEASE

	LEVEL OF RECOMMENDATION	ORGANISM	DOSE (DAILY)	REFERENCES
Induction of remission	C	Synbiotic mixture:		36
		B. breve	3×10^{10} CFU	
		B. longum	1.5×10^{10} CFU	
		L. casei	3×10^{10} CFU	
	C	L. salivarius	1×10^{10} CFU	38
	C	LGG	2×10^{10} CFU	39
Maintenance of medically induced remission	Not recommended (B)	LGG	4×10^{10} CFU	40
	B	S. boulardii (with mesalamine 2 g/day)	1 g	41
	Not recommended (B)	E. coli Nissle 1917	5×10^{10} CFU	42
Maintenance of surgically induced remission	A	VSL#3*	1 sachet BID (3×10^{11} CFU)	43,44
	Not recommended (B)	L. johnsonii LA1, Nestle	2×10^{9} to 1×10^{10} CFU	45,46
	Not recommended (B)	Synbiotic 2000†	Single dose	47

Levels of Recommendation are based on the UK National Health Service categories:

- Level A: Consistent randomized controlled clinical trial, cohort study, clinical decision rule validated in different populations.
- Level B: Consistent retrospective cohort, exploratory cohort, ecological study, outcomes research, case-control study, or extrapolations from level A studies.
- Level C: Case-series study or extrapolations from level B studies.
- Level D: Expert opinion without explicit critical appraisal or based on physiology, bench research, or first principles.

*VSL#3, commercial product containing B. longum, B. infantis, B. breve, L. acidophilus, L. casei, L. delbrueckii ssp. bulgaricus, L. plantarum, and Streptococcus salivarius ssp. thermophilus.

†Synbiotic 2000, commercial product containing 1×10^{10} CFU each of Pediacoccus pentosaceus, L. raffinolactis, L. paracasei ssp. paracasei 19, L. plantarum 2362 and fermentable fibers (prebiotic component) consisting of 2.5 g of each of β-glucans, inulin, pectin, resistant starch.

TABLE 18-2

SUMMARY OF STUDIES INVESTIGATING THE EFFECT OF PROBIOTIC TREATMENT ON THE INDUCTION AND MAINTENANCE OF REMISSION IN CROHN'S DISEASE

REFERENCE	DESIGN/ DURATION	DOSE/DAY PROBIOTIC	COMPARATOR	CONCOMITANT THERAPY	RESULTS
Induction of remission					
Fujimori et al[36]	O; 13 ± 4.5 months	B. breve (3 × 10^10 CFU), L. casei (3 × 10^10 CFU), B. longum (1.5 × 10^10 CFU), Psyllium (9.9 g); n = 10	None	Aminosalicylate, prednisolone, home enteral nutrition	Improved CDAI and IOIBD scores compared with baseline (255 to 136, P = .009 and 3.5 to 2.1, P = .03, respectively). 60% (6/10) achieved remission
Schultz et al[37]	DB, R, C; 6 months	LGG (2 × 10^9 CFU); n = 5	Placebo; n = 6	Ciprofloxacin, metronidazole, corticosteroids	No difference in remission rates
McCarthy et al[38]	O; 6 weeks	LGG (1 × 10^10 CFU); n = 25	None	Not listed	Reduced disease activity compared with baseline
Gupta et al[39]	O; 6 months	LGG (2 × 10^10 CFU); n = 4	None	Prednisone, immunomodulatory agents, metronidazole	Improvement in CDAI scores compared with baseline (P < .05)
Maintenance of medically induced remission					
Bousvaros et al[40]	DB, R, C; 2 years	LGG (4 × 10^10 CFU); n = 39	Placebo; n = 36	Aminosalicylates, 6-MP, azathioprine, corticosteroids	NSD in relapse rate or time to relapse

(continued)

TABLE 18-2 (continued)

REFERENCE	DESIGN/ DURATION	DOSE/DAY PROBIOTIC	COMPARATOR	CONCOMITANT THERAPY	RESULTS
Guslandi et al[41]	R, C; 6 months	S. boulardii (1 g/day) + mesalamine (2 g); n = 16	Mesalamine (3 g/day); n = 16	Not listed	Significant prolongation of remission (P < .05)
Malchow et al[42]	DB, R, C; 1 year	E. coli Nissle 1917 (5 × 10¹⁰ CFU); n = 16	Placebo; n = 12	Prednisolone	No difference in remission rates
Maintenance of surgically induced remission					
Madsen et al[43]	DB, R, C; 90 days	VSL#3; n = 58	Placebo; n = 62	None	less severe endoscopic recurrence (P = .04) Reduced Il-1β, TNFα, IFNγ and increased TGFβ (P < .05)
Chermesh et al[47]	DB, R, C; 2 years	Synbiotic 2000 (single dose); n = 7	Placebo; n = 2	Not indicated	NSD regarding postoperative recurrence of CD • High drop-out rate (n = 21)
Van Gossum et al[46]	DB, R, C; 12 weeks	L. johnsonii LA1, Nestle (1 × 10¹⁰ CFU); n = 27	Placebo; n = 22	None	NSD for endoscopic score post ileocaecal resection • High drop-out rate/ violations (n = 21)

(continued)

TABLE 18-2 (continued)

SUMMARY OF STUDIES INVESTIGATING THE EFFECT OF PROBIOTIC TREATMENT ON THE INDUCTION AND MAINTENANCE OF REMISSION IN CROHN'S DISEASE

REFERENCE	DESIGN/DURATION	DOSE/DAY PROBIOTIC	COMPARATOR	CONCOMITANT THERAPY	RESULTS
Marteau et al[45]	DB, R, C; 6 months	L. johnsonii LA1, Nestle (2 × 10⁹ CFU); n = 43	Placebo; n = 47	Loperamide, cholestyramine, corticosteroids tapered to nil by week 3	NSD for endoscopic scores • Drop-out rate (n = 8)
Prantera et al[48]	DB, R, C; 1 year	LGG (1.2 × 10¹⁰ CFU); n = 23	Placebo; n = 22	Loperamide, cholestyramine	No significant difference in remission`
Campieri et al[44]	R, C; 1 year	VSL#3 (3 × 10¹¹ CFU); n = 20	Mesalamine (4 g/day); n = 20	None listed	Equivalent to mesalamine in preventing recurrence

C = controlled trial; CDAI = Crohn's disease activity index; CFU = colony-forming units; DB = double blind; IOIBD = International Organization for the Study of Inflammatory Bowel Disease; NSD = no significant difference; O = open label; R = randomized.

(text continued from page 256)

However, in an open-label uncontrolled trial of 25 patients with mild/moderately active CD taking 5-ASA, McCarthy et al showed that oral administration of *L. salivarius* UCC118 (1×10^{10} CFU/day for 6 weeks) caused a significant drop in disease activity (217 vs 150 at the end of the trial; $P < .05$) and kept 70% of the study group off of steroids for 3 months.[38]

Gupta et al conducted a 6-month open-label trial using LGG (2×10^{10} CFU/day for 6 months) to treat 4 children with mild to moderate CD.[39] All patients were also receiving concomitant prednisone and immunomodulatory agent therapy. A significant improvement in pediatric CDAI scores ($P < .05$) were noted as early as 1 week after starting therapy. This improvement was sustained throughout the study, and for 3 patients it was possible to taper their dose of steroids.

Maintenance of Crohn's Disease Remission

Since 1997, there have been 6 RCTs reported examining the efficacy of single- or dual-agent probiotic therapy to maintain remission. Although there is considerable variation in the probiotics and concomitant therapy, the evidence with respect to trial size, duration, and results strongly suggest that probiotics examined had negligible impact on the duration of maintenance for patients with CD. Two recent meta-analyses by independent groups also arrived at the same conclusion for these single- or dual-agent probiotic therapies.[49,50]

Nevertheless, it important to recognize that not all probiotics are the same. In this regard, a recently conducted postoperative prevention trial with a combination of 8 probiotics did demonstrate prevention of recurrence when the probioitic was administered immediately after surgery, but not when it was administered later.[43] This study implies that probiotics do not have class effect therapeutics and must be individualized to the therapeutic requirement.

Maintenance of Medically Induced Remission

In 2005, Bousvaros and colleagues completed a 2-year trial in which pediatric CD patients in remission (PCDAI < 10) were randomly assigned to receive either LGG ($n = 39$) or placebo ($n = 36$).[40] Concomitant medications (5-ASA, azathioprine, 6-MP, corticosteroids <0.5 mg/kg every other day) were permitted throughout the study. There were no significant differences between the groups with respect to the median time to relapse (9.8 vs 11.0 months for the LGG and placebo groups, respectively) or the number of patients who relapsed (12/39 vs 6/36, respectively).

The only study to demonstrate a statistically significant prolongation of medically induced remission in CD was that of Guslandi et al, who investigated *S. boulardii* and mesalamine treatment (1 g/day + 2 g/day mesalamine, 6 months) vs mesalamine treatment alone (3 g/day, 6 months).[41] Clinical relapses were observed in 37.5% of patients receiving mesalamine alone and in 6.25% of patients in the group treated with mesalamine plus *S. boulardii* ($P = .04$).

In a randomized, double-blind, placebo controlled study, Malchow et al demonstrated that *E. coli* Nissle 1917 (5×10^{10} CFU/day for 1 year) reduced disease relapse rates in a group of 28 patients with active colonic CD for whom remission had been induced by corticosteroid treatment (70% still in remission in the probiotic group at 1 year vs 30% placebo); however, these results did not achieve statistical significance.[42]

Maintenance of Surgically Induced Remission

Recently, an encouraging study demonstrated that probiotic therapy with a combination product significantly reduced CD postoperative recurrence when the probiotic was administered immediately after surgery but not when administered some months after surgery. In this study 120 patients were randomly assigned to receive 1 sachet of VSL#3 (900 billion bacteria) or matching placebo twice daily within 30 days postresection. After 90 days of randomized treatment, all patients demonstrating either no or mild endoscopic recurrence could receive VSL#3 until Day 365. Colonoscopy was performed at Days 90 and 365 to evaluate the neoterminal ileum for disease recurrence and obtain mucosal biopsies for cytokine analysis. The primary outcome was the proportion of patients with severe endoscopic recurrence (Rutgeerts Grades 3 or 4). At Day 90 the proportion of patients with severe lesions was numerically lower for those taking VSL#3 (10.0%) relative to placebo (17.4%) ($P = .36$). However, the 90-day recurrence rate was markedly lower than predicted, leading to statistical underpowering. Nevertheless, at Day 365 the proportion of patients with severe endoscopic recurrence was significantly lower in patients who received VSL#3 immediately after surgery (11.5%) compared to those who received placebo immediately after surgery followed by VSL#3 from Days 90 to 365 (36.6%), ($P = .01$). Patients receiving VSL#3 had significantly reduced levels of ileal mucosal proinflammatory cytokine levels ($P < .05$).[43]

In 2007, Chermesh and colleagues conducted a small trial to examine the efficacy of Synbiotic 2000 (a commercial mixture containing 4 probiotics and 4 prebiotics) to extend the duration of remission following surgery for CD.[47] A total of 30 subjects were randomized 2:1 into either the active treatment group or the placebo group. During the 2-year study, a total of 21 subjects dropped out for various reasons, some of which were unrelated to the study (eg, pregnancy). When considering the data that was collected, there were no significant differences with respect to either endoscopic or clinical relapses. It is noteworthy to mention that the majority of subjects had the fistulizing form of CD and their response to the active treatment may differ substantially than those who have the inflammatory disease form.

In 2006, Marteau et al conducted a larger trial ($n = 98$) over 6 months to investigate the efficacy of a single probiotic strain (*L. johnsonii*, LA1, Nestle) to prolong the time to relapse in CD patients.[45] Eligibility required that the individual had undergone resection of less than 1 m of the intestinal tract within the previous 21 days, in which all macroscopic lesions had been removed and were in a state of disease remission. At the conclusion of the 6 months, a total of 8 subjects had dropped out of the study in both the active treatment and placebo groups. Nevertheless, the per-protocol analysis confirmed that there was no significant difference between the 2 cohorts regarding endoscopic recurrence of disease at 6 months or the distribution of the endoscopic score.

Similarly, Van Gossum et al[46] examined the efficacy of *L. johnsonii*, LA1, Nestle, to prolong the time to relapse following elective ileocaecal resection to alleviate CD symptoms. Subjects were randomly assigned to either the active treatment ($n = 34$) or placebo ($n = 36$) cohorts. At the conclusion of the 12-week study, 7 and 14 subjects had dropped out of the respective groups for various reasons, rendering the study slightly underpowered. The intention-to-treat analyses showed that there were no significant differences between the groups with respect to the endoscopic recurrence of CD at 12 weeks following ileocaecal resection. Although hampered by high dropout rates, the evidence indicated that *L. johnsonii* is ineffective for preventing postoperative recurrence in CD patients.

In a randomized, double-blind trial by Prantera et al, 40 patients received either LGG (dose not listed) or placebo following surgical resection for their CD.[48] After 52 weeks of treatment, there were no significant differences in clinical or endoscopic remission between the 2 groups.

Campieri et al reported that a combination of antibiotic and VSL#3 was more effective in preventing postoperative recurrence of CD than was mesalamine.[44] In that study,

40 patients were randomized to receive either rifaximin (1.8 g/day) for 3 months followed by VSL#3 (3×10^{11} CFU /day) for 9 months or mesalamine for 12 months. After 1 year, the antibiotic/VSL#3 group had an endoscopic remission rate of 80% compared to 60% in the mesalamine group.

CONCLUSION

Probiotic research is maturing. This is evidenced by the increasing number of well-designed trials that are supported by bench research investigating the cellular and subcellular mechanisms of how probiotics produce a therapeutic effect. Results from metagenomic research initiatives begun in the past 2 years by independent study groups[51-53] will further expand the knowledge regarding the gut's biome through the identification of unculturable organisms that are estimated to range from 15,000 to 36,000, depending on the conservatism of species classification.[54] The continued use of animal models and development of new mutant lines will provide an efficient, reliable method by which to study these new and putative probiotic organisms.

For probiotics to have a therapeutic role in the management of CD, their therapeutic mechanism of action must be aligned with the pathogenic mechanism of action of the disease. In this regard, the role of probiotics for the clinical treatment of CD is emerging, as both the mechanisms and pathogenesis are being unraveled. Working in concert, results from the bench and animal models will better inform which probiotics should graduate to clinical trials. Also, the variety of immunomodulatory mechanisms used by probiotic species is being exploited to provide new drug delivery systems for conventional drugs. An example of this is the IL-10-producing *Lactococcus lactis* for CD that has successfully completed Phase I trials.[55]

It remains clear that probiotics are able to reduce gastrointestinal inflammation by exerting positive effects on epithelial cell and mucosal immune dysfunction. Currently, the evidence for use of probiotics in the treatment of CD is limited. The majority of studies show no significant difference in the induction or maintenance of remission of CD; however, the recent beneficial effects of the probiotic mixture, VSL#3, from a randomized controlled clinical trial in the maintenance of postoperative remission suggests a role of probiotics in preventing disease recurrence. Future research will strive to align individual probiotics and their unique mechanism(s) of action with specific IBD populations. Not all probiotics will have equal efficacy or similar therapeutic value, and thus, incorporation of probiotics into the physicians' therapeutic armamentarium will need to be tempered by appropriately designed RCTs.

REFERENCES

1. Boirivant M, Strober W. The mechanism of action of probiotics. *Curr Opin Gastroenterol.* 2007;23(6):679-692.
2. Llopis M, Antolin M, Guarner F, Ahrne S, Molin G, Malagelada JR. Downregulation of TNF-alpha gene expression in human intestinal mucosa by non-adherent probiotic bacteria. *Gastroenterology.* 2006;130(4, suppl 2):A369-A370.
3. Bengmark S. Use of some pre-, pro- and synbiotics in critically ill patients. *Best Pract Res Clin Gastroenterol.* 2003;17(5):833-848.
4. Ewaschuk JB, Dieleman LA. Probiotics and prebiotics in chronic inflammatory bowel diseases. *World J Gastroenterol.* 2006;12(37):5941-5950.
5. Gionchetti P, Amadini C, Rizzello F, Venturi A, Poggioli G, Campieri M. Probiotics for the treatment of postoperative complications following intestinal surgery. *Best Pract Res Clin Gastroenterol.* 2003;17(5):821-831.

6. Kruis W. Review article: antibiotics and probiotics in inflammatory bowel disease. *Aliment Pharmacol Ther.* 2004;20(suppl 4):75-78.

7. Marteau P, Seksik P, Jian R. Probiotics and intestinal health effects: a clinical perspective. *Br J Nutr.* 2002;88(suppl 1):S51-S57.

8. O'Hara AM, Shanahan F. Mechanisms of action of probiotics in intestinal diseases. *Sci World J.* 2007;7:31-46.

9. Quigley EM, Flourie B. Probiotics and irritable bowel syndrome: a rationale for their use and an assessment of the evidence to date. *Neurogastroenterol Motil.* 2007;19(3):166-172.

10. Sazawal S, Hiremath G, Dhingra U, Malik P, Deb S, Black RE. Efficacy of probiotics in prevention of acute diarrhoea: a meta-analysis of masked, randomised, placebo-controlled trials. *Lancet Infect Dis.* 2006;6(6):374-382.

11. Shanahan F. Probiotics in inflammatory bowel disease—therapeutic rationale and role. *Adv Drug Deliv Rev.* 2004;56(6):809-818.

12. Tuohy KM, Rouzaud GC, Bruck WM, Gibson GR. Modulation of the human gut microflora towards improved health using prebiotics: assessment of efficacy. *Curr Pharm Des.* 2005;11(1):75-90.

13. Zigra PI, Maipa VE, Alamanos YP. Probiotics and remission of ulcerative colitis: a systematic review. *Neth J Med.* 2007;65(11):411-418.

14. Isaacs K, Herfarth H. Role of probiotic therapy in IBD. *Inflamm Bowel Dis.* 2008;14(11):1597-1605.

15. Vanderpool C, Yan F, Polk DB. Mechanisms of probiotic action: implications for therapeutic applications in inflammatory bowel diseases. *Inflamm Bowel Dis.* 2008;14(2):1585-1596.

16. De Keersmaecker SCJ, Verhoeven TLA, Desair J, Marchal K, Vanderleyden J, Nagy I. Strong antimicrobial activity of *Lactobacillus rhamnosus* GG against *Salmonella typhimuriumis* due to accumulation of lactic acid. *FEMS Microbiol Lett.* 2006;259(1):89-96.

17. Collado MC, Hernandez M, Sanz Y. Production of bacteriocin-like compounds by human fecal *Bifidobacterium* strains. *J Food Prot.* 2005;68(5):1034-1040.

18. Collado MC, Meriluoto J, Salminen S. Role of commercial probiotic strains against human pathogen adhesion to intestinal mucus. *Lett Appl Microbiol.* 2007;45(4):454-460.

19. Sartor RB, Muehlbauer M. Microbial host interactions in IBD: implications for pathogenesis and therapy. *Curr Gastroenterol Rep.* 2007;9(6):497-507.

20. Cani PD, Bibiloni R, Knauf C, et al. Changes in gut microbiota control metabolic endotoxemia-induced inflammation in high-fat diet-induced obesity and diabetes in mice. *Diabetes.* 2008;57(6):1470-1481.

21. Kotlowski R, Bernstein CN, Sepehri S, Krause DO. High prevalence of *Escherichia coli* belonging to the B2+D phylogenetic group in inflammatory bowel disease. *Gut.* 2007;56(5):669-675.

22. Bibiloni R, Mangold M, Madsen KL, Fedorak RN, Tannock GW. The bacteriology of biopsies differs between newly diagnosed, untreated, Crohn's disease and ulcerative colitis patients. *J Med Microbiol.* 2006;55(pt 8):1141-1149.

23. Vasquez N, Mangin I, Lepage P, et al. Patchy distribution of mucosal lesions in ileal Crohn's disease is not linked to differences in the dominant mucosa-associated bacteria: a study using fluorescence in situ hybridization and temporal temperature gradient gel electrophoresis. *Inflamm Bowel Dis.* 2007;13(6):684-692.

24. Swidsinski A, Loening-Baucke V, Theissig F, et al. Comparative study of the intestinal mucus barrier in normal and inflamed colon. *Gut.* 2007;56(3):343-350.

25. Sokol H, Pigneur B, Watterlot L, et al. *Faecalibacterium prausnitzii* is an anti-inflammatory commensal bacterium identified by gut microbiota analysis of Crohn disease patients. *Proc Natl Acad Sci U S A.* 2008;105(43):16731-16736.

26. Garcia Vilela E, De Lourdes De Abreu Ferrari M, Oswaldo Da Gama Torres H, et al. Influence of *Saccharomyces boulardii* on the intestinal permeability of patients with Crohn's disease in remission. *Scand J Gastroenterol.* 2008;43(7):842-848.

27. Kaila M, Isolauri E, Soppi E, Virtanen E, Laine S, Arvilommi H. Enhancement of the circulating antibody secreting cell response in human diarrhea by a human *Lactobacillus* strain. *Pediatr Res.* 1992;32(2):141-144.

28. Madsen KL, Doyle JS, Jewell LD, Tavernini MM, Fedorak RN. *Lactobacillus* species prevents colitis in interleukin 10 gene-deficient mice. *Gastroenterology.* 1999;116(5):1107-1114.

29. Ukena SN, Singh A, Dringenberg U, et al. Probiotic *Escherichia coli* Nissle 1917 inhibits leaky gut by enhancing mucosal integrity. *PLoS ONE.* 2007;2(12):e1308.

30. Ewaschuk JB, Daiz H, Meddings L, et al. Secreted bioactive factors from *Bifidobacterium infantis* enhance epithelial cell function. *Am J Physiol Gastrointest Liver Physiol.* 2008;295(5):G1025-G1034.

31. Matthes H, Krummener T, Giensch M, Wolff C, Schulze J. Treatment of mild to moderate acute attacks of distal ulcerative colitis with rectally-administered *E. coli* Nissle 1917: dose-dependent efficacy (#812). *Gastroenterology.* 2006;30(4, suppl 2):A-119.

32. Kim N, Kunisawa J, Kweon MN, Eog JG, Kiyono H. Oral feeding of *Bifidobacterium bifidum* (BGN4) prevents CD4(+) CD45RB(high) T cell-mediated inflammatory bowel disease by inhibition of disordered T cell activation. *Clin Immunol.* 2007;123(1):30-39.

33. Peran L, Camuesco D, Comalada M, et al. A comparative study of the preventative effects exerted by three probiotics, *Bifidobacterium lactis*, *Lactobacillus casei* and *Lactobacillus acidophilus*, in the TNBS model of rat colitis. *J Appl Microbiol.* 2007;103(4):836-844.

34. Chung YW, Choi JH, Oh T-Y, Eun CS, Han DS. *Lactobacillus casei* prevents the development of dextran sulphate sodium-induced colitis in Toll-like receptor 4 mutant mice. *Clin Exp Immunol.* 2007;151:182-189.

35. Raz I, Gollop N, Polak-Charcon S, Schwartz B. Isolation and characterisation of new putative probiotic bacteria from human colonic flora. *Br J Nutr.* 2007;97(4):725-734.

36. Fujimori S, Tatsuguchi A, Gudis K, et al. High dose probiotic and prebiotic cotherapy for remission induction of active Crohn's disease. *J Gastroenterol Hepatol.* 2007;22(8):1199-1204.

37. Schultz M, Timmer A, Herfarth HH, et al. *Lactobacillus* GG in inducing and maintaining remission of Crohn's disease. *BMC Gastroenterol.* 2004;4:5.

38. McCarthy J, O'Mahony L, Dunne C. An open trial of a novel probiotic as an alternative to steroids in mild/moderately active Crohn's disease. *Gut.* 2001;49(suppl III):A2447.

39. Gupta P, Andrew H, Kirschner BS, Guandalini S. Is *Lactobacillus* GG helpful in children with Crohn's disease? Results of a preliminary, open-label study. *J Pediatr Gastroenterol Nutr.* 2000;31:453-457.

40. Bousvaros A, Guandalini S, Baldassano RN, et al. A randomized, double-blind trial of *Lactobacillus* GG versus placebo in addition to standard maintenance therapy for children with Crohn's disease. *Inflamm Bowel Dis.* 2005;11(9):833-839.

41. Guslandi M, Mezzi G, Sorghi M, Testoni PA. *Saccharomyces boulardii* in maintenance treatment of Crohn's disease. *Dig Dis Sci.* 2000;45:1462-1464.

42. Malchow HA. Crohn's disease and *Escherichia coli.* A new approach in therapy to maintain remission of colonic Crohn's disease? *J Clin Gastroenterol.* 1997;25:653-658.

43. Madsen K, Backer JL, Leddin D, et al. A randomized controlled trial of VSL#3 for the prevention of endoscopic recurrence following surgery for Crohn's disease. *Gastroenterology.* 2008;134(4, suppl 1):M1207.

44. Campieri M, Rizzello F, Venturi A. Combination of antibiotic and probiotic treatment is efficacious in prophylaxis of post-operative recurrence of Crohn's disease: a randomised controlled trial with *Lactobacillus* GG. *Gastroenterology.* 2000;118:A781.

45. Marteau P, Lemann M, Seksik P, et al. Ineffectiveness of *Lactobacillus johnsonii* LA1 for prophylaxis of postoperative recurrence in Crohn's disease: a randomised, double blind, placebo controlled GETAID trial. *Gut.* 2006;55(6):842-847.

46 Van Gossum A, Dewit O, Louis E, et al. Multicenter randomized-controlled clinical trial of probiotics (*Lactobacillus johnsonii*, LA1) on early endoscopic recurrence of Crohn's disease after illeo-caecal resection. *Inflamm Bowel Dis.* 2007;13(2):135-142.

47. Chermesh I, Tamir A, Reshef R, et al. Failure of Synbiotic 2000 to prevent postoperative recurrence of Crohn's disease. *Dig Dis Sci.* 2007;52(2):385-389.

48. Prantera C, Scribano ML, Falasco G, Andreoli A, Luzi C. Ineffectiveness of probiotics in preventing recurrence after curative resection for Crohn's disease: a randomised controlled trial with *Lactobacillus* GG. *Gut.* 2002;51:405-409.

49. Rolfe VE, Fortun PJ, Hawkey CJ, Bath-Hextall F. Probiotics for maintenance of remission in Crohn's disease. *Cochrane Database Syst Rev.* 2006;(4):CD004826.

50. Rahimi R, Nikfar S, Rahimi F, et al. A meta-analysis on the efficacy of probiotics for maintenance of remission and prevention of clinical and endoscopic relapse in Crohn's disease. *Dig Dis Sci.* 2008;53(9):2524-2531.

51. Office of Portfolio Analysis and Strategic Initiatives. Roadmap 1.5 Update. National Institutes of Health. 1-30-2008. http://nihroadmap.nih.gov/roadmap15update.asp. Accessed February 4, 2010.

52. Metagenome.jp. Human Metagenome Consortium, Japan (HMGJ). Metagenome.jp. 2007. http://metagenome.jp/microbes/data.html. Accessed February 4, 2010.

53. INRA. Sequencing the human intestinal flora: launching of the European project MetaHIT coordinated by INRA. http://www.international.inra.fr/partnerships/with_the_private_sector/live_from_the_labs/project_metahit. Accessed February 4, 2010.

54. Frank DN, St Amand AL, Feldman RA, Boedeker EC, Harpaz N, Pace NR. Molecular-phylogenetic characterization of microbial community imbalances in human inflammatory bowel diseases. *Proc Natl Acad Sci U S A.* 2007;104(34):13780-13785.

55. Yuvaraj S, Peppelenbosch MP, Bos NA. Transgenic probiotica as drug delivery systems: the golden bullet? *Expert Opin Drug Deliv.* 2007;4(1):1-3.

19

Probiotics and Pouchitis

Mario Guslandi, MD, FACG

Restorative proctocolectomy with ileal pouch-anal anastomosis (IPAA) is the surgical treatment of choice for patients with refractory UC, dysplasia complicating UC, or familial adenomatous polyposis (FAP).[1,2]

The most common long-term complication after IPAA for UC—but not FAP—is inflammation of the ileal reservoir, called pouchitis,[2-4] occurring in 24% to 60% of cases.[2,4-6] About 60% of patients undergo 1 or more recurrences and 5% to 32% of them develop chronic pouchitis, which in turn may require pouch excision in 10% of the cases.[2,3,5,7]

Pouchitis is characterized by increased stool frequency, rectal bleeding, urgency, tenesmus, incontinence, and abdominal pain with systemic symptoms such as fever, fatigue, arthralgia, and erythema nodosum.[4,8]

Clinical diagnosis needs to be confirmed by endoscopy, which shows mucosal reddening, contact bleeding, petechial lesions, erosions, or ulcerations, and by the histological finding of inflammatory infiltrate with crypt hyperplasia and/or abscesses and villous atrophy. In order to define and grade pouchitis, a Pouchitis Disease Activity Index (PDAI), based on clinical symptoms as well as endoscopic and histological findings, has been developed by Sandborn et al.[9]

Although the exact etiology of pouchitis is unknown, the fact that it occurs only after the diverting ileostomy is closed and the rapid response to antibiotic treatment suggest a key role for the microbial flora. According to some authors, bacterial flora, which seems to be normal in the healthy pouch, appears to be altered in pouchitis, with a decrease in anaerobes, bifidobacteria, and lactobacilli, high levels of *Clostridium perfringens*,[10,11] and a rise in local pH, which would make the protective mucus layer of the reservoir more prone to bacterial degradation.[10] Others were either unable to detect changes in the bacterial population in pouchitis,[12] or found low bacterial and high fungal diversity.[13]

Floch MH, Kim AS, eds.
Probiotics: A Clinical Guide (pp 267-272)
© 2010 Taylor & Francis Group

STANDARD TREATMENT

Antibiotics

The use of antibiotics in the treatment of pouchitis is well established, in spite of a striking paucity of controlled clinical trials. A controlled, double-blind, crossover study vs placebo carried out in a small number of patients (13, of whom only 11 completed the study) has shown that a 2-week course of therapy with metronidazole 400 mg tid is significantly effective in promoting clinical improvement of acute pouchitis, but not in ameliorating the endoscopic and histological features.[14] On the other hand, more than 50% of patients experienced side effects such as nausea, vomiting, metallic taste, abdominal discomfort, and skin rash.

The risk of developing peripheral neuropathy is a further reason of concern, especially in long-term metronidazole administration. Systemic side effects could be avoided if metronidazole is administered topically, but after the encouraging results observed years ago in a small-sized pilot study,[15] no further similar experiences have been reported.

Metronidazole 20 mg/kg/day and ciprofloxacin 1 g/daily have been compared in a small, randomized trial in acute pouchitis.[16] Both drugs were effective in promoting clinical, endoscopic, and histological improvement, and a consequent reduction in PDAI scores, with ciprofloxacin inducing a greater therapeutic effect and being better tolerated.

In an open trial, 18 patients with active pouchitis unresponsive to a 4-week standard treatment with either metronidazole or ciprofloxacin were given a combined treatment with rifaximin 2 g/day plus ciprofloxacin 1 g/day for 15 days.[17] In 88% of the cases, either improvement or remission was obtained, with a statistically significant reduction in the PDAI score.

Similarly, combined treatment with metronidazole 800 to 1000 mg/day and ciprofloxacin 1 g/day for 4 weeks promoted remission of refractory pouchitis with a significant decrease in the median PDAI score and improvement in the patient's quality of life, as assessed by the Inflammatory Bowel Disease Questionnaire.[18]

A recent open-label trial in 51 cases of antibiotic-dependent pouchitis examined the effect of long-term maintenance treatment with rifaximin in doses ranging from 200 to 1800 mg/day for up to 24 months.[19] At 3 months, 65% of patients were still in remission. Of these patients, 65% maintained remission at 6 months and 58% at 12 months. In view of the excellent tolerability of rifaximin, further controlled studies are warranted to confirm these preliminary data and better define the optimal maintenance dose.

Other Therapies

Although antibiotic treatment remains the most commonly employed pharmacological approach to pouchitis, other therapeutic avenues have been explored. A double-blind, double-dummy 6-week controlled trial has compared the efficacy of budesonide enemas (2 mg/100 mL bedtime) and oral metronidazole (500 mg bid).[20] The 2 treatments were equally effective in promoting clinical and endoscopic improvement and a decrease in the PDAI score, with budesonide enemas being responsible for fewer side effects.

Oral budesonide 9 mg/day for 8 weeks has been administered in an open study to 20 patients with antibiotic-resistant pouchitis.[21] Seventy-five percent of patients achieved remission, showing a highly significant decrease in the median values of PDAI.

Pilot, uncontrolled studies have suggested, but not proven, a possible therapeutic benefit by cyclosporine enemas,[22] butyrate suppositories,[23] and oral or rectal bismuth.[24,25]

Probiotics

The rationale for employing probiotics in the management of pouchitis relies upon the various mechanisms of action of those agents: modulation of barrier function, inhibitory activity against pathogenic bacteria, anti-inflammatory effect through modulation of cytokine production, and decreased gut permeability.[26] Furthermore, the reduced amount of lactobacilli and the high pH values observed in the pouch[10] suggest a possible benefit by the administration of probiotic products containing strains of lactobacilli, which are also known to attenuate spontaneous colitis in interleukin (IL)-10 knockout mice as well as experimentally induced colitis.[27-30]

In particular, lactobacilli-containing probiotics have been found to reduce the expression of proinflammatory cytokines IL-1β and IL-8, as well as tissue influx of polymorphonuclear cells in subjects given the product to prevent the onset of pouchitis.[31]

The efficacy of probiotics in pouchitis has been clinically tested in a number of trials carried out under different conditions.

Induction of Remission

A randomized, double-blind, placebo-controlled trial investigated the effects of *L. rhamnosus* GG supplementation for 3 months in 20 patients with active pouchitis.[32] The treatment, although capable of changing the pouch intestinal flora by increasing the ratio of total fecal lactobacilli to total fecal anaerobes, failed to promote clinical and endoscopic improvement, as assessed by means of the PDAI index.

A fermented milk product (Cultura) containing lactobacilli and bifidobacteria was given for 4 weeks to UC patients with either IPAA or ileorectal anastomosis and IPAA patients with FAP.[33] IPPA/UC patients experienced a significant improvement in both clinical and endoscopic scores.

Anecdotal benefit by *E. coli* strain Nissle 1917 in inducing and maintaining remission of pouchitis has been also reported.[34] More recently, following the favorable results obtained in the prevention and maintenance of treatment of pouchitis (see below), the probiotic cocktail VSL#3 has been tested as a possible therapeutic tool to induce remission in mildly active pouchitis in a small, uncontrolled trial.[35] When administered in high doses (2 sachets bid, ie, 3600 billion bacteria/day) for 4 weeks, the product significantly ($P < .01$) decreased the median PDAI values, inducing remission in 69% of cases. Subsequent maintenance treatment with VSL#3 (1 sachet bid) for 6 months maintained remission in all healed subjects.[35]

Maintenance of Remission

The efficacy of VSL#3 in maintaining remission of pouchitis after successful antibiotic treatment has been investigated in 3 clinical studies.[36-38] Forty patients in clinical and endoscopic remission after 1 month of ciprofloxacin 1 g/day plus rifaximin 2 g/day were randomized to VSL#3 (1 sachet bid; 1800 billion bacteria/day) or placebo for 9 months. All patients in the placebo group relapsed, whereas 85% of probiotic-treated patients remained in remission.

Similarly, in a placebo-controlled, randomized study, 36 patients who had achieved remission after 4 weeks of combined treatment with metronidazole 500 mg bid plus ciprofloxacin 500 mg bid received a single, high daily dose of VSL#3 (1800 billion bacteria/day) for 12 months.[37] Remission was maintained in 85% of patients with the probiotic cocktail and in 6% of patients in the placebo group ($P < .0001$).

In contrast, an open-label clinical trial employing VSL as a maintenance treatment for 8 months after remission of pouchitis induced by a 2-week therapy with ciprofloxacin 1 g/day reported that the majority of patients (80.6%) discontinued probiotic

TABLE 19-1

RECOMMENDATION FOR PROBIOTIC USE IN POUCHITIS

POUCHITIS	LEVEL OF RECOMMENDATION	ORGANISM	DOSE	REFERENCES
Inducing	B	VSL#3	12 g/day	35
remission	B	Cultura milk	500 mL/day	33
	C	E. Coli Nissle 1917	2.5 × 10^10 bid	34
Maintenance	A	VSL#3	6 g/day	36,37
Prevention	A	VSL#3	3 g/day	40
		L. rhamnosus GG	1.4 × 10^10 CFU/day	39

treatment due to either recurrence of symptoms while on treatment or development of side effects.[38] The reasons for this discrepancy may be the differences in type and duration of initial antibiotic therapy and in criteria for defining remission, concomitant NSAID use in the US trial, and possible limited adherence to therapy of the patient because of the cost of the probiotic medication.[38]

Prevention

In an open-label study, the incidence of pouchitis after IPAA in patients receiving *L. rhamnosus* GG was compared with that of a historical control group.[39] The incidence of pouchitis at 3 years was 7% and 29%, respectively ($P = .011$).

VSL#3 (1 sachet/day; 900 billion bacteria/day) was employed in a double-blind, placebo-controlled trial involving 40 patients who had undergone IPPA[40] for 1 year. Pouchitis developed in only 10% of patients on probiotic treatment, compared to 40% in the placebo group ($P < .05$). Furthermore, patients on VSL#3 experienced a significant improvement in the quality of life as assessed by the IBDQ score.

Meta-Analysis

A recent meta-analysis on the use of probiotics in the management of pouchitis, pooling the results observed in clinical trials where probiotic agents were employed either for achieving or maintaining remission or for preventing the outset of pouchitis, yielded an odds ratio of 0.04 with a 95% CI of 0.01 to 0.14 ($P < .0001$) in favor of the treatment group vs placebo.[41]

CONCLUSION

Only a limited number of studies are available concerning the use of probiotics in the management of pouchitis. The level of recommendation of the various probiotics is summarized in Table 19-1. The most extensively examined product is the probiotic cocktail VSL#3, which was found in placebo-controlled trials to significantly prevent the development of pouchitis in IPAA patients and maintain antibiotic-induced remission for up to 12 months.

A possible efficacy of probiotic administration in inducing remission of active pouchitis has been suggested for products such as VSL#3 and Cultura (fermented milk with lactobacilli + bifidobacteria), but evidence from controlled studies is still lacking. Clearly, much more work in this area has to be done, but in view of the superior tolerability of probiotics compared with antibiotics, further, larger, controlled studies are warranted to better define the therapeutic role of probiotic products in pouchitis.

Notes on the Quoted Products

The VSL#3 product employed in the studies on pouchitis is available in 3-g packets. Each packet contains 900 billion bacteria. It includes 4 strains of *Lactobacillus* (*L. casei, L. plantarum, L. acidophilus, and L. bulgaricus*), 3 strains of *Bifidobacterium* (*B. longum, B. breve*, and *B. infantis*), and *Streptococcus salivarius* spp. *thermophilus*.

Cultura is a fermented milk product containing lactobacilli (La-5) and bifidobacteria (Bb-12).

REFERENCES

1. Johnson E, Carlsen E, Nazir M, Nygaard K. Morbidity and functional outcome after restorative proctocolectomy for ulcerative colitis. *Eur J Surg.* 2001;167:40-45.
2. Fazio VW, Ziv Y, Church JM, et al. Ileal pouch-anal anastomoses complications and function in 1005 patients. *Ann Surg.* 1995;222:120-127.
3. Meagher AP, Farouk R, Dozois RR, Kelly KA, Pemberton JH. J ileal pouch-anal anastomosis for chronic ulcerative colitis: complications and long-term outcome in 1310 patients. *Br J Surg.* 1998;85:800-803.
4. Sandborn WJ. Pouchitis following ileal pouch-anal anastomosis: definition, pathogenesis and treatment. *Gastroenterology.* 1994;107:1856-1860.
5. Pardi DS, Sandborn WJ. Management of pouchitis. *Aliment Pharmacol Ther.* 2006;23:1087-1096.
6. Simchuck E, Thirlby R. Risk factors and true incidence of pouchitis in patients after ileal pouc-anal anastomosis. *World J Surg.* 2000;24:851-856.
7. Mowschenson PM, Critchlow JF, Peppercorn MA. Ileo-anal pouch operation: long-term outcome with or without diverting ileostomy. *Arch Surg.* 2000;135:463-466.
8. Madden MV, Farthing MJ, Nicholls RJ. Inflammation in ileal reservoirs: "pouchitis." *Gut.* 1990;31:247-249.
9. Sandborn WJ, Tremaine WJ, Batts KP, Pemberton JH, Phillips SF. Pouchitis after ileal pouch-anal anastomosis: a Pouchitis Disease Activity Index. *Mayo Clin Proc.* 1994;69:409-415.
10. Ruseler-van Embden JG, Schouten WR, van Lieshout LM. Pouchitis: result of microbial imbalance? *Gut.* 1994;35:658-664.
11. Iwaya A, Iiai T, Okamoto H, et al. Change in the bacterial flora of pouchitis. *Hepato-Gastroenterology.* 2006;53:55-59.
12. Kmiot WA, Youngs D, Tudor R, et al. Mucosal morphology, cell proliferation and faecal bacteriology in acute pouchitis. *Br J Surg.* 1993;80:1445-1449.
13. Kuchbacher T, Ott SJ, Helwig U, et al. Bacterial and fungal microbiota in relation to probiotic therapy (VSL#3) in pouchitis. *Gut.* 2006;55:833-841.
14. Madden M, McIntyre A, Nicholls RJ. Double-blind cross-over trial of metronidazole versus placebo in chronic unremitting pouchitis. *Dig Dis Sci.* 1994;39:1193-1196.
15. Nygaard K, Bergan T, Bjorneklett A, et al. Topical metronidazole treatment in pouchitis. *Scand J Gastroenterol.* 1994;29:462-467.
16. Shen B, Achkar JP, Lashner BA, et al. A randomized clinical trial of ciprofloxacin and metronidazole to treat acute pouchitis. *Inflamm Bowel Dis.* 2001;7:301-305.
17. Gionchetti P, Rizzello F, Venturi A, et al. Antibiotic combination therapy in patients with chronic, treatment-resistant pouchitis. *Aliment Pharmacol Ther.* 1999;13:713-718.
18. Mimura T, Rizzello F, Helwig U, et al. Four week open-label trial of metronidazole and ciprofloxacin for the treatment of recurrent or refractory pouchitis. *Aliment Pharmacol Ther.* 2002;16:909-917.
19. Shen B, Remzi FH, Lopez AR, Queener E. Rifaximin for maintenance therapy in antibiotic-dependent pouchitis. *BMC Gastroenterol.* 2008;8:26-32.
20. Sambuelli A, Boerr L, Negreira S, et al. Budesonide enema in pouchitis: a double-blind, double-dummy, controlled trial. *Aliment Pharmacol Ther.* 2002;16:27-34.

21. Gionchetti P, Rizzello F, Poggioli G, et al. Oral budesonide in the treatment of chronic refractory pouchitis. *Aliment Pharmacol Ther.* 2007;25:1231-1236.
22. Winter TA, Dalton HR, Merrett MN, et al. Cyclosporine A retention enemas in refractory distal ulcerative colitis and pouchitis. *Scand J Gastroenterol.* 1993;28:701-704.
23. Wyschmeyer P, Pemberton JH, Phillips SF. Chronic pouchitis after ileal pouch-anal anastomosis: responses to butyrate and glutamine suppositories in a pilot study. *Mayo Clin Proc.* 1993;68:978-981.
24. Gionchetti P, Rizzello F, Venturi A, et al. Long-term efficacy of bismuth carbomer enemas in patients with treatment-resistant chrounic pouchitis. *Aliment Pharmacol Ther.* 1997;11:673-678.
25. Tremaine WJ, Sandborn WJ, Kenan ML. Bismuth subsalicylate tablets for chronic antibiotic-resistant pouchitis. *Gastroenterology.* 1998;114:A1101.
26. Jones JL, Foxx-Orenstein AE. The role of probiotics in inflammatory bowel disease. *Dig Dis Sci.* 2007;52:607-611.
27. Schultz M, Veltkamp C, Dieleman LA, et al. *Lactobacillus plantarum* 299Vs in the treatment and prevention if spontaneous colitis in interleukin-10-deficient mice. *Inflamm Bowel Dis.* 2002;8:71-80.
28. Madsen KL, Doyle JS, Jewell LD, et al *Lactobacillus* species prevents colitis in interleukin 10-gene deficient mice. *Gastroenterology.* 1999;116:1107-1114.
29. Fabia R, Ar'Rajab A, Johansson ML, et al. The effect of exogenous administration of *Lactobacillus reuteri* R2LC and oat fiber on acetic acid-induced colitis in the rat. *Scand J Gastroenterol.* 1993;28:155-162.
30. Mao Y, Nobaek S, Kasravi B, et al. The effects *of Lactobacillus* strains and oat fiber on methotrexate-induced enterocolitis in rats. *Gastroenterology.* 1996;111:334-344.
31. Lammers KM, Vergopoulos A, Babel N, et al. Probiotic therapy in the prevention of pouchitis onset: decreased interleukin-1beta, interleukin-8 and interferon-gamma gene expression. *Inflamm Bowel Dis.* 2005;11:447-454.
32. Kujisma J, Mentula S, Jarvinen H, et al. Effect of *Lactobacillus rhamnosus* GG on ileal pouch inflammation and microbial flora. *Aliment Pharmacol Ther.* 2003;17:509-515.
33. Laake KO, Bjrneklett A, Aamodt G, et al. Outcome of four weeks' intervention with probiotics on symptoms and endoscopic appearance after surgical reconstruction with a J-configurated ileal-pouch-anal anastomosis in ulcerative colitis. *Scand J Gastroenterol.* 2005;40:43-51.
34. Kuzela L, Kascak M, Vavrecka A. Induction and maintenance of remission with nonpathogenic *Escherichia coli* in patients with pouchitis. *Am J Gastroenterol.* 2001;96:3218-3219.
35. Gionchetti P, Rizzello F, Morselli C, et al. High-dose probiotics for the treatment of active pouchitis. *Dis Colon Rectum.* 2007;50:2075-2084.
36. Gionchetti P, Rizzello F, Venturi A, et al. Oral bacteriotherapy as maintenance treatment in patients with chronic pouchitis: a double-blind, placebo-controlled trial. *Gastroenterology.* 2000;119:305-309.
37. Mimura T, Rizzello F, Helwig U, et al. Once daily high dose probiotic therapy (VSL#3) for maintaining remission in recurrent or refractory pouchitis. *Gut.* 2004;53:108-114.
38. Shen B, Brezinski A, Fazio VW, et al. Maintenance therapy with a probiotic in antibiotic-dependent pouchitis: experience in clinical practice. *Aliment Pharmacol Ther.* 2005;22:721-728.
39. Gosselink MP, Schouten WP, van Lieshout LMC, et al. Delay of the first onset of pouchitis by oral intake of the probiotic strain *Lactobacillus rhamnosus* GG. *Dis Colon Rectum.* 2004;47:876-884.
40. Gionchetti P, Rizzello F, Helwig U, et al. Prophylaxis of pouchitis onset with probiotic therapy: a double-blind, placebo-controlled trial. *Gastroenterology.* 2003;124:1202-1209.
41. Elahi B, Nikfar S, Derakhshani S, et al. On the benefit of probiotics in the management of pouchitis in patients underwent ileal pouch anal anastomosis: a meta-analysis of controlled clinical trials. *Dig Dis Sci.* 2008;53:1278-1284.

20

Irritable Bowel Syndrome

Eamonn M. M. Quigley, MD, FRCP, FACP, FACG, FRCPI

IBS is one of the most common disorders encountered in modern medicine; community surveys in Western Europe and North America suggest a prevalence of around 10% in the adult population.[1] It should be stressed, in addition, that IBS appears to be common worldwide, regardless of geography or socioeconomic status. There is no single specific diagnostic test for IBS; its definition relies, therefore, either on the exclusion of diseases that may share its symptomatology in whole or in part, or on the application of symptom-based criteria whose integrity has been validated in cross-sectional and longitudinal studies. The cardinal symptoms of IBS are abdominal pain/discomfort and bowel dysfunction. Typically, these are interrelated such that, for example, affected patients may report that their symptoms worsen when constipated, only to be relieved once a bowel movement has been achieved. In clinical research, most studies apply the definitions enshrined in the Rome criteria, whose third iteration (Rome III) was released in early 2006, which defined IBS as follows:

Recurrent abdominal pain or discomfort (an uncomfortable sensation not described as pain) at least 3 days per month in the last 3 months associated with 2 or more of the following:
1. improvement with defecation,
2. onset associated with a change in frequency of stool,
3. onset associated with a change in form (appearance) of stool.

These criteria should have been fulfilled for the last 3 months with symptom onset at least 6 months prior to diagnosis.[2]

Currently, therefore, IBS lacks an objective test or biomarker to confirm or refute the diagnosis, monitor progress, or evaluate response to treatment; this remains a major obstacle to progress. As individual IBS symptoms are very nonspecific and may occur in a host of other clinical conditions, the potential for diagnostic confusion is considerable. Even when taken collectively, as in the Rome criteria, the potential for diagnostic overlap persists unless the criteria become overly restrictive. Furthermore, a condition such as IBS, whose definition rests exclusively on the interpretation of symptoms, is

Floch MH, Kim AS, eds.
Probiotics: A Clinical Guide (pp 273-282)
© 2010 Taylor & Francis Group

certain to encompass a heterogeneous population whose constituents may ultimately be found to have different causes. Not surprisingly, the search for a unifying hypothesis to explain all IBS has proven unfruitful. Several phenomena undoubtedly contribute to symptom genesis, including disordered bowel motility ("spasm"), increased bowel sensitivity (visceral hypersensitivity or hyperalgesia), altered cerebral processing of gut events, environmental stressors, and intrinsic psychopathology. The interplay between such gut and central nervous system factors has led to the concept of gut-brain axis dysfunction as fundamental to the induction of symptoms in IBS. According to this concept, the interaction or interplay between gut dysfunction and a central factor, such as stress or anxiety, leads to the development of symptoms. More recently, the emphasis in IBS research has changed and, somewhat surprisingly, has been focused on interactions between the intestinal flora (or microbiota) and the immune system of the host, in both the mucosal and systemic compartments. This is the scientific context in which the application of probiotics to the therapy of IBS should be viewed. Simultaneously, the IBS sufferer has been exploring this same avenue. Reflecting, perhaps, the paucity of truly disease-modifying therapies that are available to relieve the disorder, irritable bowel sufferers commonly have recourse to the use of complimentary and alternative medical remedies and practices.[3] Foremost among such approaches have been various dietary manipulations, including exclusion diets,[4,5] and a variety of dietary supplements. In Europe, in particular, where several such products are advertised widely for their general "immune-boosting" and "health-enhancing" properties, probiotics have been widely used as dietary supplements by IBS patients. Recently, based on data from the experimental laboratory as well as some evidence from clinical trials, the concept of probiotic use in IBS has begun to wend its way into the realm of conventional medicine,[6] and an assessment of the potential role of these agents in IBS is now timely.

Is There a Rational Basis for the Use of Probiotics in Irritable Bowel Syndrome?

While the precise cause of IBS remains obscure and theories of symptom pathogenesis abound, most hypotheses center on 1 or more of the following areas: an altered intraluminal milieu, immune activation, enteric neuromuscular dysfunction, and brain-gut axis dysregulation. Of these, alterations in the intraluminal milieu and immune activation provide the most obvious basis for the use of probiotics in IBS; as we will see later, evidence for the effects of probiotics on other putative factors in IBS pathogenesis also exists.

For some time, various studies, using a variety of methodologies, have suggested the presence of qualitative changes in the colonic flora in IBS patients, a relative decrease in the population of bifidobacteria being one reasonably consistent finding.[7-15] It should be noted, however, that these findings have not always been reproduced and the methods employed have been subject to question. Given the fact that the majority of the fecal microbiota is unculturable by conventional means and that the molecular analysis of the fecal flora is in its infancy, it is reasonable to state that the accurate delineation of the fecal microbiota in IBS is yet to be accomplished; initial results, however, consistently describe qualitative differences.[9,15] Such qualitative changes in the colonic flora, be they primary or secondary, could lead to the proliferation of species that produce more gas[16] and SCFA, and are more avid in the deconjugation of bile acids. The latter could, in turn, lead to clinically significant changes in water and electrolyte transport in the colon and affect colonic motility and/or sensitivity. More recently, the role of the gut flora in IBS has been taken a stage further with the suggestion that some IBS patients may harbor quantitative changes in the indigenous flora, in the small intestine: that is, they have developed small intestinal bacterial overgrowth (SIBO).[17-21] The occurrence of SIBO has been associated with abnormalities in small intestinal motor function[22] and its eradication with symptomatic relief.[17,18] Further evidence for a role for an altered indigenous flora in IBS is provided by one study that described improvements in IBS symptomatology, in the short term, following the administration of the nonabsorbable antibiotic rifaximin to a group of patients who did not have SIBO at baseline.[23] Furthermore, a recent RCT[24] has suggested more sustained effects for rifaximin therapy in IBS. Limitations to the sensitivity and specificity of the hydrogen breath test, the methodology most commonly employed for the diagnosis of SIBO in the aforementioned studies, as well as negative aspiration studies,[25] have led some to question the role of SIBO in IBS and to suggest that the effect of antibiotics is on the colonic rather than on the small intestinal flora.[26,27] Nevertheless, and pending the resolution of this controversial issue, one can readily visualize opportunities for probiotic administration in this context.

There is now a considerable body of evidence to support the concept of post-infectious IBS (PI-IBS).[28,29] Certain probiotics possess potent antibacterial and antiviral properties. Probiotic antibacterial activity may derive from the direct secretion of bacteriocins,[30] the elaboration of proteases directed against bacterial toxins,[31] or through their ability to adhere to epithelial cells and thus exclude pathogens. An effective antibacterial probiotic could well play a role in preventing the 5% to 10% incidence of IBS that may follow an episode of confirmed bacterial gastroenteritis, especially among high-risk individuals.[32,33]

Evidence now accumulates to suggest an association between IBS, in general, and immune activation. Colonic biopsies have demonstrated, in some cases, frank inflammation and, in others, more subtle evidence of immune activation.[34] More recently, studies on cytokine levels in peripheral blood mononuclear cells[35,36] and even in serum[37] have revealed a proinflammatory state. It is interesting to note that constipation has also been associated with a partially reversible inflammatory activation of the colonic mucosa.[38] These studies have, to date, been performed in relatively small patient numbers and require confirmation. Furthermore, the origin of these immune signals is unknown, and relationships between the mucosal and the systemic compartments remain to be defined. Even if, ultimately, only a subset of IBS is found to be associated with mucosal inflammation, it still provides yet another rationale for the use of probiotics. Thus, in experimental animal models of inflammatory bowel disease, various probiotics and probiotic cocktails have demonstrated potent anti-inflammatory properties, suppressing mucosal inflammation and restoring cytokine balance toward an anti-inflammatory state.[39] The suggestion that bifidobacteria may be especially potent as immunomodulatory agents is consistent with our own observation that a symptomatic response to *B. infantis* 35624, in IBS, was associated with a normalization of a baseline abnormality in the ratio of IL-10 to IL-12 in peripheral blood mononuclear cells, which was tilted toward a proinflammatory state.[35]

For decades, dysmotility and visceral hypersensitivity have reigned supreme as the dominant factors in the pathophysiology of IBS.[40] Of late, visceral hypersensitivity has been in the ascendancy. This is not to deny a role for dysmotility in symptom pathogenesis but, rather, to indicate that disturbed motor function may not be the primary abnormality in IBS. Both dysmotility and visceral hypersensitivity may, indeed, be secondary to other primary etiological factors. There is, for example, abundant literature, largely derived from animal models, to indicate that immune activation can lead to disturbed motor function and increased activity in sensory pathways from the gut. Recent studies have extended this concept in humans. Relevant findings have included the following:

an increased density of mast cells in the colonic mucosa, evidence of increased levels of mast cell degranulation, the demonstration of a close correlation between the proximity of mast cells to neural elements and pain severity and reports, not only of increased concentrations of mast cell products, such as proteases, in the lumen, but also of the ability of such proteases to induce visceral hypersensitivity in appropriate animal models.[41-43]

Probiotics have the potential to influence both motility and visceral sensation. In an animal model of PI-IBS, Collins' group has demonstrated the ability of a probiotic to prevent and reverse dysmotility consequent upon an intestinal infestation.[44] Probiotics could, in theory, reverse many of the processes involved in the initiation or perpetuation of immune-mediated hypersensitivity through antipathogenic, barrier-enhancing, and immunomodulating effects.[6] Experimental data, indeed, now support an effect of probiotics on visceral hypersensitivity[45-47] and have linked these benefits to anti-inflammatory,[45] barrier-enhancing,[46] and neuromodulatory[45,46] actions. Most recently, Rousseaux and colleagues found that oral administration of specific *Lactobacillus* strains induced the expression of mu-opioid and cannabinoid receptors in intestinal epithelial cells and mediated analgesic functions in the gut, similar to the effects of morphine.[48]

The advent of functional brain imaging, as well as tests of autonomic function and the hypothalamic-pituitary-adrenal (HPA) axis, has permitted an exploration of the various components of the gut-brain axis in IBS. Such studies have revealed aberrant cerebral activation, exaggerated HPA responses, and autonomic nervous dysfunction among some IBS subjects.[49-53] There is ample evidence from experimental animal studies for the ability of proinflammatory cytokines, and TNFα in particular, to influence the HPA axis,[54] and evidence is also beginning to accrue to suggest a role for inflammation in cerebral processes, such as depression.[55] Dinan and colleagues have been able to detect elevated levels of the proinflammatory cytokine IL-6 in plasma, among IBS patients, and have documented a direct correlation between IL-6 and exaggerated ACTH and cortisol responses to corticotrophin-releasing factor.[37] This intriguing finding suggests a direct link, in IBS, between inflammation, presumably of intestinal origin, and brain-gut axis dysregulation. Alternatively, central dysfunction could be driving the cytokine response; indeed, IBS subjects also demonstrate an exaggerated release of IL-6 in response to the systemic administration of cholinergic agents.[56] Given the aforementioned demonstration of a normalization of systemic cytokine balance by a probiotic in IBS,[35] it is appropriate to speculate that at least some of the efficacy of probiotics in IBS may be related to this effect. That orally administered probiotics could modulate central pathways is supported by the recent demonstration of effects of a *Bifidobacterium* in an animal model of depression.[57] Probiotics, therefore, have the potential to influence IBS pathophysiology at a variety of levels.

WHAT IS THE EVIDENCE FOR PROBIOTIC EFFICACY IN IBS?

A growing number of studies have evaluated the response of IBS to probiotic preparations, and while results between studies are difficult to compare because of differences in study design, probiotic dose, and strain, there has been some, but by no means consistent, evidence of symptom improvement.[6,35,39,58-88] Hamilton-Miller, reviewing the evidence relating to the efficacy of probiotics in IBS in 2001, drew attention to the shortcomings of trials performed prior to then in terms of study design but concluded that there was, overall, sufficient evidence of efficacy to warrant further evaluation.[89] Most studies reviewed were small in size and almost certainly underpowered to demonstrate anything other than a very striking benefit. Several did not verify bacterial transit and survival by confirmatory stool studies. Many different organisms and strains were employed, and dosage varied from as little as 10^5 to as much as 10^{13}. Furthermore, some studies employed probiotic "cocktails" rather than single isolates, rendering it impossible to induce what, if any, were the active moieties. Nevertheless, even in these earlier studies, some positive results were noted. Studies since 2000, though generally better in terms of quality of study design and execution, have yielded conflicting results; however, some trends have begun to emerge. A number of recent systematic reviews and meta-analyses have critically summarized the current status of the role of probiotics in IBS.[90-94] There does appear to be evidence for a benefit for probiotics, in general, in IBS. More detailed analyses suggest that such effects may apply to specific species or, even, strains. Thus, Moayyedi and colleagues concluded that while lactobacilli were not effective, bifidobacteria, either alone or in combination (or "cocktail") preparations, were,[92] a finding confirmed by the only head-to-head comparison of a *Lactobacillus* and a *Bifidobacterium*.[35] Brenner and colleagues went further to assert that only one strain, *B. infantis* 35624, had good evidence from clinical trials to support overall efficacy in IBS.[94] Dose may also be important; in a large, 4-week duration, dose-ranging study of *B. infantis* 35624 in more than 360 community-based subjects with IBS, a dose of 10^8 CFU/day, but not 10^6, significantly improved all of the primary symptoms of IBS and provided substantial global relief.[71]

A number of these recent studies have provided hints for mechanisms of action of various probiotics in IBS; some accelerate transit[88] and appear especially suited for those with constipation-predominant IBS,[77] while others may affect fermentation,[64,79] thus explaining why a number of trials, while failing to demonstrate global relief, have reduced bloating and/or flatulence.[61,65,67,77,88] Indeed, when formally tested, one strain, *B lactis* DN-173-010, was shown to produce objective effects on abdominal distension in IBS. Other organisms have demonstrated beneficial effects on the intestinal barrier[85] and immune responses.[35]

THE FUTURE

Further large, RCTs of probiotics and of bifidobacteria, in particular, are warranted in IBS and detailed explorations of their mechanism(s) of action are indicated. Several other issues remain to be resolved. What is the optimal strain and dose? There are very few comparative studies and only one known dose-ranging study in this area.[71] The ideal duration of probiotic therapy is also unknown; most studies have been short term, and those that have demonstrated benefit have witnessed a relapse soon after cessation of active therapy. This is consistent with the observation that while probiotic therapy can modulate the fecal flora during its administration, the microbiota reverts to normal soon after the end of feeding.[84] Given what we know of the natural history of IBS, lifelong therapy with a probiotic may, therefore, prove necessary for those who respond. This concept is also supported by 6- and 5-month studies with one particular "cocktail," which demonstrated continuing, and even increasing, benefit over these time periods.[68,84] More long-term studies are indicated. Finally, we currently can only speculate on the actual mechanism (or mechanisms) of action of probiotics in IBS. Are these agents only effective in a select subgroup or are they of value in all? Do we need to administer live organisms in order to obtain benefit? In the future, will a component or a derivative of a probiotic be the ideal therapy? The possible roles of co-therapy or sequential therapy with antibiotics, probiotics, prokinetics, or other agents also deserve further study.

REFERENCES

1. Hungin AP, Whorwell PJ, Tack J, Mearin F. The prevalence, patterns and impact of irritable bowel syndrome: an international survey of 40,000 subjects. *Aliment Pharmacol Ther.* 2003;17:643-650.
2. Longstreth GF, Thompson WG, Chey WD, Houghton LA, Mearin F, Spiller RC. Functional bowel disorders. *Gastroenterology.* 2006;130:1480-1491.
3. Hussein Z, Quigley EM. Complementary and alternative medicine in irritable bowel syndrome. *Aliment Pharmacol Ther.* 2006;15:465-471.
4. Atkinson W, Sheldon TA, Shaath N, Whorwell PJ. Food elimination based on IgG antibodies in IBS: a randomised controlled trial. *Gut.* 2004;53:1459-1464.
5. Zar S, Mincher L, Benson MJ, Kumar D. Food specific IgG4 antibodies guided exclusion diet improves symptoms and rectal compliance in IBS. *Scand J Gastroenterol.* 2005;40:800-807.
6. Quigley EM. The use of probiotics in functional bowel disease. *Gastroenterol Clin North Am.* 2005;34:533-545.
7. Madden JA, Hunter JO. A review of the role of the gut microflora in irritable bowel syndrome and the effects of probiotics. *Br J Nutr.* 2002;(Suppl 1)88:S67-S72.
8. Si JM, Yu YC, Fan YJ, Chen SJ. Intestinal microecology and quality of life in irritable bowel syndrome patients. *World J Gastroenterol.* 2004;10:1802-1805.
9. Malinen E, Rinttila T, Kajander K, et al. Analysis of the fecal microbiota of irritable bowel patients and healthy controls with real-time PCR. *Am J Gastroenterol.* 2005;100:373-382.
10. Sun X, Cai G, Wang WJ. Observation on intestinal flora in patients of IBS after treatment of Chinese integrative medicine. *Zhong Xi Yi Jie He Xue Bao.* 2004;2:340-342.
11. Balsari A, Ceccarelli A, Dubini F, et al. The fecal microbial population in the irritable bowel syndrome. *Microbiologica.* 1982;5:185-194.
12. Bradley HK, Wyatt GM, Bayliss CE, et al. Instability in the faecal flora of a patient suffering from food-related irritable bowel syndrome. *J Med Microbiol.* 1987;23:29-32.
13. Matto J, Maunuksela L, Kajander K, et al. Composition and temporal stability of gastrointestinal microbiota in irritable bowel syndrome: a longitudinal study in IBS and control subjects. *FEMS Immunol Med Microbiol.* 2005;43:213-222.
14. Maukonen J, Satokari R, Mättö J, Söderlund H, Mattila-Sandholm T, Saarela M. Prevalence and temporal stability of selected clostridial groups in irritable bowel syndrome in relation to predominant faecal bacteria. *J Med Microbiol.* 2006;55:625-633.
15. Kassinen A, Krogius-Kurikka L, Makivuokko H, et al. The fecal microbiota of irritable bowel syndrome patients differs significantly from that of healthy subjects. *Gastroenterology.* 2007;133:24-33.
16. King TS, Elia M, Hunter JO. Abnormal colonic fermentation in the irritable bowel syndrome. *Lancet.* 1998;352:1187-1189.
17. Pimentel M, Chow EJ, Lin HC. Eradication of small bowel bacterial overgrowth reduces symptoms of irritable bowel syndrome. *Am J Gastroenterol.* 2000;95:3503-3506.
18. Pimentel M, Chow E, Lin H. Normalization of lactulose breath testing correlates with symptom improvement in irritable bowel syndrome: a double-blind, randomized, placebo-controlled study. *Am J Gastroenterol.* 2003;98:412-419.
19. Pimentel M, Wallace D, Hallegua D, et al. A link between irritable bowel syndrome and fibromyalgia may be related to findings on lactulose breath testing. *Ann Rheum Dis.* 2004;63:450-452.
20. Pimentel M, Lin HC, Enayati P, et al. Methane, a gas produced by enteric bacteria, slows intestinal transit and augments small intestinal contractile activity. *Am J Physiol (Gastrointest Liver Physiol).* 2006;29:G1089-G1095.
21. Lin HC. Small intestinal bacterial overgrowth: a framework for understanding irritable bowel syndrome. *JAMA.* 2004;292:852-858.
22. Pimentel M, Soffer EE, Chow EJ, Kong Y, Lin HC. Lower frequency of MMC is found in IBS subjects with abnormal lactulose breath test suggesting bacterial overgrowth. *Dig Dis Sci.* 2002;47:2639-2642.
23. Sharara AI, Aoun E, Abdul-Baki H, Mounzer R, Sidani S, Elhajj I. A randomized double-blind placebo-controlled trial of rifaximin in patients with abdominal bloating and flatulence. *Am J Gastroenterol.* 2006;101:326-333.
24. Pimentel M, Park S, Mirocha J, Kane SV, Kong Y. The effect of a nonabsorbed antibiotic (rifaximin) on the symptoms of the irritable bowel syndrome: a randomized trial. *Ann Intern Med.* 2006;145:557-563.
25. Posserud I, Stotzer PO, Bjornsson E, et al. Small intestinal bacterial overgrowth in patients with irritable bowel syndrome. *Gut.* 2006;56:802-808.
26. Quigley EM. Germs, gas and the gut; the evolving role of the enteric flora in IBS. *Am J Gastroenterol.* 2006;101:334-335.

27. Quigley EM. A 51-year old with with irritable bowel syndrome: test or treat for bacterial overgrowth? *Clin Gastroenterol Hepatol.* 2007;5:1140-1143.
28. Spiller RC. Postinfectious irritable bowel syndrome. *Gastroenterology.* 2003;124:1662-1671.
29. Mearin F, Perez-Oliveras M, Perello A, et al. Dyspepsia and irritable bowel syndrome after a Salmonella outbreak: a one year follow-up cohort study. *Gastroenterology.* 2005;129:98-104.
30. Cotter PD, Hill C, Ross RP. Bacteriocins: developing innate immunity for food. *Nat Rev Microbiol.* 2005;3:777-788.
31. Castigliuolo I, Riegler MF, Valenick L, et al. *Saccharomyces boulardii* protease inhibits the effects of *Clostridium difficile* toxins A and B in human colonic mucosa. *Infect Immun.* 1999;67:302-307.
32. Quigley EM. Bacterial flora in irritable bowel syndrome: role in pathophysiology, implications for management. *Chin J Dig Dis.* 2007;8:2-7.
33. Spiller RC. Estimating the importance of infection in IBS. *Am J Gastroenterol.* 2003;98:238-241.
34. Chadwick V, Chen W, Shu D, et al. Activation of the mucosal immune system in irritable bowel syndrome. *Gastroenterology.* 2002;122:1778-1783.
35. O'Mahony L, McCarthy J, Kelly P, et al. A randomized, placebo-controlled, double-blind comparison of the probiotic bacteria lactobacillus and *Bifidobacterium* in irritable bowel syndrome (IBS): symptom responses and relationship to cytokine profiles. *Gastroenterology.* 2005;128:541-551.
36. Liebregts T, Adam B, Bredack C, et al. Immune activation in patients with irritable bowel syndrome. *Gastroenterology.* 2007;132:913-920.
37. Dinan TG, Quigley EM, Ahmed SM, et al. Hypothalamic-pituitary-gut axis dysregulation in irritable bowel syndrome: plasma cytokines as a potential biomarker? *Gastroenterology.* 2006;130:304-311.
38. Khalif IL, Quigley EM, Konovitch EA, Maximova ID. Alterations in the colonic flora and intestinal permeability and evidence of immune activation in chronic constipation. *Dig Liver Dis.* 2005;37:838-849.
39. Quigley EM, Flourie B. Probiotics and irritable bowel syndrome: a rationale for their use and an assessment of the evidence to date. *Neurogastroenterol Motil.* 2007;19:166-172.
40. Quigley EM. Disturbances of motility and visceral hypersensitivity in irritable bowel syndrome: biological markers or epiphenomenon. *Gastroenterol Clin North Am.* 2005;34:221-233.
41. Barbara G, Stanghellini V, De Giorgio R, et al. Activated mast cells in proximity to colonic nerves correlate with abdominal pain in irritable bowel syndrome. *Gastroenterology.* 2004;126:693-702.
42. Barbara G, Wang B, Stanghellini V, et al. Mast cell-dependent excitation of visceral-nociceptive sensory neurons in irritable bowel syndrome. *Gastroenterology.* 2007;132:26-37.
43. Cenac N, Andrews CN, Holzhausen M, et al. Role for protease activity in visceral pain in irritable bowel syndrome. *J Clin Invest.* 2007;117:636-647.
44. Verdu EF, Bercik P, Bergonzelli GE, et al. *Lactobacillus paracasei* normalizes muscle hypercontractiltiy in a murine model of postinfective gut dysfunction. *Gastroenterology.* 2004;127:826-837.
45. Verdu EF, Bercik P, Verma-Gandhu M, et al. Specific probiotic therapy attenuates antibiotic induced visceral hypersensitivity in mice. *Gut.* 2006;55:182-190.
46. Ait-Belgnaoui A, Han W, Lamine F, et al. *Lactobacillus farciminis* treatment suppresses stress-induced visceral hypersensitivity: a possible action through interaction with epithelial cells cytoskeleton contraction. *Gut.* 2006;55:1090-1094.
47. Kamiya T, Wang L, Forsythe P, et al. Inhibitory effects of *Lactobacillus reuteri* on visceral pain induced by colorectal distension in Sprague-Dawley rats. *Gut.* 2006;55:191-196.
48. Rousseaux C, Thuru X, Gelot A, et al. *Lactobacillus acidophilus* modulates intestinal pain and induces opioid and cannabinoid receptors. *Nat Med.* 2007;13:35-37.
49. Hobday D, Thompson DG. Role of functional brain imaging in gastroenterology in health and disease. *Dig Liver Dis.* 2000;32:101-103.
50. Aziz Q, Thompson DG. Clinical relevance of the gut brain axis. *Gastroenterology.* 1997;114:559-578.
51. Mertz H, Morgan V, Tanner G, et al. Regional cerebral activation in irritable bowel syndrome with painful and nonpainful stimuli. *Gastroenterology.* 2000;118:842-848.
52. Patacchioli FR, Angelucci L, Delleba G, et al. Actual stress, psychopathology and salivary cortisol levels in the irritable bowel syndrome (IBS). *J Endocrinol Invest.* 2001;24:173-177.
53. Ellenbruch S, Orr WC. Diarrhea- and constipation-predominant IBS patients differ in postprandial autonomic and cortisol responses. *Am J Gastroenterol.* 2001;96:460-466.
54. Beishuizen A, Thijs LG. Endotoxin and the hypothalamic-pituitary-adrenal (HPA) axis. *J Endotoxin Res.* 2003;9:3-24.
55. O'Brien SM, Scully P, Scott LV, Dinan TG. Cytokine profiles in bipolar affective disorders: focus on acutely ill patients. *Affect Disord.* 2006;90:263-267.
56. Dinan TG, Clarke G, Quigley EM, et al. Enhanced cholinergic-mediated increase in the pro-inflammatory cytokine IL-6 in irritable bowel syndrome: role of muscarinic receptors. *Am J Gastroenterol.* 2008;103:2570-2576.

57. Desbonnet L, Garrett L, Clarke G, Bienenstock J, Dinan TG. The probiotic *Bifidobacteria infantis*: an assessment of potential antidepressant properties in the rat. *J Psychiatr Res*. 2008;43:164-174.
58. Halpern GM, Prindiville T, Blankenburg M, Hsia T, Gershwin ME. Treatment of irritable bowel syndrome with lacteol fort: a randomized, double-blind, cross-over trial. *Am J Gastroenterol*. 1996;91:1579-1585.
59. Bittner AC, Croffut RM, Stranahan MC. Prescript-assist probiotic-prebiotic treatment for irritable bowel syndrome: a methodologically oriented, 2-week, randomized, placebo-controlled, double-blind clinical study. *Clin Ther*. 2005;27:755-761.
60. O'Sullivan MA, O'Morain CA. Bacterial supplementation in the irritable bowel syndrome. A randomised double-blind placebo-controlled crossover study. *Dig Liver Dis*. 2000;32:302-304.
61. Nobaek S, Johansson ML, Molin G, Ahrné S, Jeppsson B. Alteration of intestinal microflora is associated with reduction in abdominal bloating and pain in patients with irritable bowel syndrome. *Am J Gastroenterol*. 2000;95:1231-1238.
62. Brigidi P, Vitali B, Swennen E, et al. Effects of probiotic administration upon the composition and enzymatic activity of human fecal microbiota in patients with irritable bowel syndrome or functional diarrhea. *Res Microbiol*. 2001;152:735-741.
63. Niedzielin K, Kordecki H, Birkenfeld B. A controlled, double-blind, randomized study on the efficacy of *Lactobacillus plantarum* 299V in patients with irritable bowel syndrome. *Eur J Gastroenterol Hepatol*. 2001;13:1143-1147.
64. Sen S, Mulan MM, Parker TJ, et al. Effect of *Lactobacillus plantarum* 299V on colonic fermentation and symptoms of irritable bowel syndrome. *Dig Dis Sci*. 2002;47:2615-2620.
65. Kim HJ, Camilleri M, McKenzie S, et al. A randomized controlled trail of a probiotic, VSL#3 on gut transit and symptoms in diarrhoea-predominant IBS. *Aliment Pharmacol Ther*. 2003;17:895-904.
66. Tsuchiya J, Barreto R, Okura R, Kawakita S, Fesce E, Marotta F. Single-blind follow-up study on the effectiveness of a symbiotic preparation in irritable bowel syndrome. *Chin J Dig Dis*. 2004;5:169-174.
67. Kim HJ, Vazquez Roque MI, Camilleri M, et al. A randomised controlled trial of probiotic combination VSL#3 and placebo in IBS with bloating. *Neurogastroenterol Motil*. 2005;17:687-696.
68. Kajander K, Hatakka K, Poussa T, et al. A probiotic mixture alleviates symptoms in irritable bowel syndrome patients: a controlled 6-month intervention. *Aliment Pharmacol Ther*. 2005;22:387-394.
69. Niv E, Naftali T, Hallak R, Vaisman N. The efficacy of *Lactobacillus reuteri* ATCC 55730 in the treatment of patients with irritable bowel syndrome—a double blind, placebo-controlled, randomized study. *Clin Nutr*. 2005;24;925-931.
70. Bausserman M, Michail S. The use of *Lactobacillus* GG in irritable bowel syndrome in children: a double-blind randomized control trial. *J Pediatr*. 2005;147:197-201.
71. Whorwell PJ, Altringer L, Morel J, et al. Efficacy of an encapsulated probiotic *Bifidobacterium infantis* 35624 in women with irritable bowel syndrome. *Am J Gastroenterol*. 2006;101:1581-1590.
72. Drisko J, Bischoff B, Hall M, McCallum R. Treating irritable bowel syndrome with a food elimination diet followed by food challenge and probiotics. *J Am Coll Nutr*. 2006;25:514-522.
73. Fanigliulo L, Comparato G, Aragona G, et al. Role of gut microflora and probiotic effects in the irritable bowel syndrome. *Acta Biomed*. 2006;77:85-89.
74. Gawronska A, Dziechciarz P, Horvath A, Szajewska H. A randomized double-blind trial of *Lactobacillus* GG for abdominal pain disorders in children. *Aliment Pharmacol Ther*. 2007;25:177-184.
75. Dughera L, Elia C, Navino M, Cisarò F; ARMONIA Study Group. Effects of symbiotic preparations on constipated irritable bowel syndrome symptoms. *Acta Biomed*. 2007;78:111-116.
76. Bittner AC, Croffut RM, Stranahan MC, Yokelson TN. Prescript-assist probiotic-prebiotic treatment for irritable bowel syndrome: an open-label, partially controlled, 1-year extension of a previously published controlled clinical trial. *Clin Ther*. 2007;29:1153-1160.
77. Guyonnet D, Chassany O, Ducrotte P, et al. Effect of a fermented milk containing *Bifidobacterium animalis* DN-173 010 on the health-related quality of life and symptoms in irritable bowel syndrome in adults in primary care: a multicentre, randomized, double-blind, controlled trial. *Aliment Pharmacol Ther*. 2007;26:475-486.
78. Kajander K, Krogius-Kurikka L, Rinttilä T, Karjalainen H, Palva A, Korpela R. Effects of multispecies probiotic supplementation on intestinal microbiota in irritable bowel syndrome. *Aliment Pharmacol Ther*. 2007;26:463-473.
79. Barrett JS, Canale KE, Gearry RB, Irving PM, Gibson PR. Probiotic effects on intestinal fermentation patterns in patients with irritable bowel syndrome. *World J Gastroenterol*. 2008;14:5020-5024.
80. Andriulli A, Neri M, Loguercio C, et al. Clinical trial on the efficacy of a new symbiotic formulation, Flortec, in patients with irritable bowel syndrome: a multicenter, randomized study. *J Clin Gastroenterol*. 2008;42(suppl 3, pt 2):S218-S223.

81. Enck P, Zimmermann K, Menke G, Müller-Lissner S, Martens U, Klosterhalfen S. A mixture of *Escherichia coli* (DSM 17252) and *Enterococcus faecalis* (DSM 16440) for treatment of the irritable bowel syndrome: a randomized controlled trial with primary care physicians. *Neurogastroenterol Motil.* 2008;20:1103-1109.
82. Drouault-Holowacz S, Bieuvelet S, Burckel A, Cazaubiel M, Dray X, Marteau P. A double blind randomized controlled trial of a probiotic combination in 100 patients with irritable bowel syndrome. *Gastroenterol Clin Biol.* 2008;32:147-152.
83. Sinn DH, Song JH, Kim HJ, et al. Therapeutic effect of *Lactobacillus acidophilus*-SDC 2012, 2013 in patients with irritable bowel syndrome. *Dig Dis Sci.* 2008;53:2714-2718.
84. Kajander K, Myllyluoma E, Rajilić-Stojanović M, et al. Clinical trial: multispecies probiotic supplementation alleviates the symptoms of irritable bowel syndrome and stabilizes intestinal microbiota. *Aliment Pharmacol Ther.* 2008;27:48-57.
85. Zeng J, Li YQ, Zuo XL, Zhen YB, Yang J, Liu CH. Clinical trial: effect of active lactic acid bacteria on mucosal barrier function in patients with diarrhoea-predominant irritable bowel syndrome. *Aliment Pharmacol Ther.* 2008;28:994-1002.
86. Guyonnet D, Woodcock A, Stefani B, Trevisan C, Hall C. Fermented milk containing *Bifidobacterium lactis* DN-173 010 improved self-reported digestive comfort amongst a general population of adults. A randomized, open-label, controlled, pilot study. *J Dig Dis.* 2009;10:61-70.
87. Williams E, Stimpson J, Wang D, et al. Clinical trial: a multistrain probiotic preparation significantly reduces symptoms of irritable bowel syndrome in a double-blind placebo-controlled study. *Aliment Pharmacol Ther.* Sep 10, 2008. (epublication ahead of print.)
88. Agrawal A, Houghton LA, Morris J, et al. Clinical trial: the effects of a fermented milk product containing *Bifidobacterium lactis* DN-173-010 on abdominal distension and gastrointestinal transit in irritable bowel syndrome with constipation. *Aliment Pharmacol Ther.* Sep 17, 2008. (epublication ahead of print.)
89. Hamilton-Miller JMT. Probiotics in the management of irritable bowel syndrome: a review of clinical trials. *Microb Ecol Health Dis.* 2001;13:212-216.
90. Nikfar S, Rahimi R, Rahimi F, Derakhshani S, Abdollahi M. Efficacy of probiotics in irritable bowel syndrome: a meta-analysis of randomized, controlled trials. *Dis Colon Rectum.* 2008;51:1775-1780.
91. McFarland LV, Dublin S. Meta-analysis of probiotics for the treatment of irritable bowel syndrome. *World J Gastroenterol.* 2008;14:2650-2661.
92. Moayyedi P, Ford AC, Talley NJ, et al. The efficacy of probiotics in the therapy of irritable bowel syndrome: a systematic review. *Gut.* Dec 17, 2008. (epublication ahead of print.)
93. Hoveyda N, Heneghan C, Mahtani KR, Perera R, Roberts N, Glasziou P. A systematic review and meta-analysis: probiotics in the treatment of irritable bowel syndrome. *BMC Gastroenterol.* 2009;9:15.
94. Brenner DM, Moeller MJ, Chey WD, Schoenfeld PS. The utility of probiotics in the treatment of irritable bowel syndrome: a systematic review. *Am J Gastroenterol.* 2009;104(4):1033-1049.

21

Use of Probiotics in the Prevention and Treatment of Radiation Enteritis

Giuseppe Famularo, MD, PhD; Vito Trinchieri, MD;
Luciana Mosca, PhD; and Giovanni Minisola, MD

THE CLINICAL PROBLEM

Radiotherapy plays an important role in the treatment of abdominal and pelvic malignancies and has significantly contributed during the past decades to improved outcomes and prognoses of those patients. The potential of radiation to also cause injury to normal tissue is well understood, and this still represents an important and unresolved issue. Walsh's first description of enteritis following abdominal exposure to radiation dates back to 1897—ie, just 2 years after the landmark discovery of X-rays.[1] Technical improvements have helped reduce the frequency and severity of radiotherapy-related complications in recent years.[2] However, despite these encouraging improvements in care of patients treated with radiotherapy, radiation enteritis still accounts for a substantial early and late morbidity in at least 1 of 5 patients treated with radiotherapy because of abdominal or pelvic cancers.[3] Besides worsening quality of life of patients treated with radiotherapy, radiation enteritis is an important cause of interruptions of treatment, and may also account for a huge increase in the economic burden in the management of cancer patients through utilization of supportive and adjuvant measures.

The incidence of radiation enteritis among patients with abdominal or pelvic neoplasms ranges from 5% to 40%. In a series of 386 patients undergoing radiotherapy for rectal carcinoma, about 20% of patients have been reported to develop clinically apparent radiation enteritis or proctitis,[4] and in another series an 8% incidence of moderate proctitis was recognized among patients undergoing radiotherapy for prostate cancer within 10 years of the end of treatment.[5] In a review that focused on late-development radiation proctitis, the incidence rates were between 5% and 20% among patients treated with radiotherapy for pelvic cancers.[6]

Mortality directly or indirectly linked with radiation enteritis caused by pelvic or abdominal radiotherapy has not been accurately estimated in the clinical setting; nonetheless, most studies have reported mortality rates as high as 11% of treated patients.[7-9]

Floch MH, Kim AS, eds.
Probiotics: A Clinical Guide (pp 283-294)
© 2010 Taylor & Francis Group

Clinical and experimental evidence has clearly demonstrated that gut is the most important dose-limiting organ in patients treated with abdominal or pelvic radiotherapy, at least in terms of safety treatment and risk of serious adverse effects. Mild or moderate symptoms consistent with acute radiation enteritis are observed in most treated patients though those symptoms are normally transient and in most cases resolve after completion of radiotherapy.[10]

There are also radiotherapy-related complications that occur late after the treatment is completed, and these complications need to be distinguished from those occurring during or immediately after the end of therapy, which are usually self-limiting and respond well to conservative medical and noninvasive management. Late complications of abdominal or pelvic radiotherapy are less frequent than acute radiation enteritis and comprise a number of specific entities, including radiation chronic fibrosing enteritis and proctitis, and the formation of both strictures and fistulae. These complications that typically arise after 3 to 6 months up to 6 years after radiotherapy may be sometimes progressive, especially in severe cases, and may also persist indefinitely.[11] Researchers have estimated that up to 40% of patients receiving abdominal or pelvic radiotherapy may be involved with delayed-onset radiation enteritis.[8,10] Clinical features include dysmotility and malabsorption, fibrosis, and, in some cases, overt bowel obstruction that may develop years or even decades after radiation exposure.

A latency period was previously thought to exist between the time of radiation exposure and the onset of radiation-induced damage, including enteritis, but many studies now show that this is not the case. Experimental evidence indicates that the onset of delayed radiation effects is a continuous process that starts immediately at irradiation.[12]

Evidence is now available that the incidence and severity of radiation enteritis is closely dependent on several factors that are both patient- and treatment-specific, such as the dose of radiotherapy, the volume treated, fractionation schedule, and the length of follow-up. Additional risk factors have also been proposed, which include age, the presence of comorbidities, tobacco abuse, prior operation, and concurrent chemotherapy.[10]

Typical symptoms reported by patients exposed to radiotherapy for abdominal or pelvic malignancies include diarrhea, tenesmus, rectal blood and/or mucus, and abdominal pain, and can be graded according to the Radiation Therapy Oncology Group from 0 to 5 (Table 21-1). These symptoms usually arise from radiation enteritis or proctitis and generally are well managed with conservative medical management. Chronic or more extensive and severe injuries typical of delayed-onset radiation enteritis, such as fistulae, abscesses, or strictures, require surgical intervention in a percentage of patients ranging from 2% to 17%.[13,14]

One important point is that a significant proportion of patients with radiation enteritis may have 2 or more radiation-induced injuries, especially those who have refractory injuries that are not effectively managed with medical treatment alone, or progress despite optimal medical management, and this appears to be the critical factor responsible for their refractory course. For example, Turina and colleagues have reported that two-thirds of their patients developed 2 or more complications from radiotherapy,[15] and Kimose and colleagues found a combination of more than 2 radiotherapy injuries affecting the colon, rectum, small bowel, or the urinary tract in 62% of their 182 patients.[16]

Whether preoperative radiotherapy may be more safe than postoperative radiotherapy in terms of maintaining a normal long-term bowel function is not firmly established as of today. Nathanson and colleagues suggested that postoperative radiotherapy may be associated with more postoperative bowel movements and more episodes of clustered bowel movements as compared to preoperative radiotherapy.[17] However, this finding remains to be confirmed in further large-scale trials.

TABLE 21-1

ACUTE AND CHRONIC RADIATION MORBIDITY SCORING CRITERIA FROM THE RADIATION THERAPY ONCOLOGY GROUP

GRADE	ACUTE RADIATION	CHRONIC RADIATION
0	No change	No change
1	Increased frequency/ change in bowel habits not requiring medication, rectal discomfort not requiring analgesics	Mild diarrhea, mild cramping bowel movement 5 times/day, slight rectal discharge or bleeding
2	Diarrhea requiring parasympatholytic drugs, mucus discharge not necessitating sanitary pads, rectal or abdominal pain requiring analgesics	Moderate diarrhea and colic, bowel movement >5 times/day, excessive rectal mucus or intermittent bleeding
3	Diarrhea requiring parenteral support, severe mucus or blood discharge necessitating sanitary pads, abdominal distension	Obstruction or bleeding requiring operation
4	Obstruction, fistula, or perforation, gastrointestinal bleeding requiring transfusion, abdominal pain or tenesmus requiring decompression or bowel diversion	Necrosis, perforation, fistula
5		Death directly related to late radiation effect

An additional problem is represented by the potential risk of developing a secondary new cancer among patients with radiation enteritis. A recently published, large retrospective cohort study has found an independent association, with an adjusted odds ratio 1.7, and the future development of rectal cancer in more than 30,000 patients receiving radiotherapy because of prostate cancer.[18] Other studies, however, have produced conflicting results about the potential risk of the development of a new cancer in patients treated with radiotherapy for prostate cancer. Brenner and colleagues have reported a 34% increase in solid tumors of the pelvis in patients surviving longer than 10 years after radiotherapy of prostate cancer,[19] whereas Neugut and colleagues have found only a slightly increased risk of bladder cancer following prostatic radiotherapy but no increased risk of rectal cancer.[20]

Finally, the most important issue is that as yet we do not know why some patients develop radiation enteritis or proctitis when exposed to radiotherapy while other patients do not, and this remains a long-standing and unresolved question. As with many other disorders of the gastrointestinal tract, radiation enteritis is a challenging issue for basic researchers and clinicians for at least 2 crucial points: we need a better understanding of the underlying mechanisms of disease pathobiology, and more effective and safe therapeutic strategies are also urgently required.

A MICROBIAL HYPOTHESIS FOR RADIATION ENTERITIS

Several etiologies have been postulated for radiation enteritis, and there is now agreement that its causes and mechanisms of pathobiology are probably multifactorial. Nonetheless, those mechanisms remain incompletely understood as of today, and many problems are still obscure. Changes in intestinal motility, malabsorption, and mucosal inflammation triggered by direct exposure to radiation have been advocated as critical key points in the pathogenesis of radiation enteritis.[10] However, available experimental and clinical data suggest that almost all regimens of radiation therapy should be expected to disturb the colonization resistance of the indigenous gut flora, and recent studies have pointed out that investigation of gut microbial ecology may hold great promise in the identification of mechanisms involved in pathobiology of radiation-induced diarrhea and also of new therapeutic targets. In fact, since the early 1900s, radiation enteritis has been thought to be exacerbated by the gut microbiota, that is, the gut microbial ecosystem.[21] Furthermore, on the basis of the background of the claimed hypothesis of a microbial cause of radiation enteritis, antibiotics have been used in human clinical trials with the aim to manipulate gut radiosensitivity and enhance gut resistance to radiotoxicity, but, unfortunately, no definitive results and no clearly effective antibiotic protocol have emerged to date.[22,23] The impact of ionizing radiation on germ-free animals was first studied in the late 1950s, and one important point that has emerged is that responses of germ-free animals strongly differ in a number of ways from those of conventionally raised animals—that is, those that either acquire a microbiota from birth or are initially germ free and then experimentally colonized at various stages of postnatal life or adulthood with a gut microbiota. The first important point is that the minimum dose required to induce a 50% mortality is higher in germ-free mice and, in addition, germ-free animals appear to survive longer than their conventionally raised counterparts after receiving lethal doses of total body irradiation.[24] Furthermore, the minimum radiation dose that causes the appearance of the histological hallmarks of radiation enteritis—ie, mucosal atrophy, mesenchymal inflammation, and fibrosis—is significantly higher in germ-free mice as compared to animals carrying a microbiota.[24] One additional important point is that the overgrowth of Gram-negative bacilli in the gut lumen seems to be an essential requisite for triggering radiation enteritis in experimental animals.[25] On the basis of these observations, researchers have suggested that the enhanced lethality of radiation in conventionally raised mice could be related to systemic infection and/or to a greater susceptibility to irreversible gut damage. However, the precise nature of the cellular damage at the gut level, its relationship to survival, and the molecular pathways through which the microbiota operates to influence gut radiosensitivity and radiotoxicity remain poorly defined.

More recent investigations have confirmed that animals harboring a normal microbiota exhibit enhanced gut sensitivity to radiation as compared to germ-free animals and also that indigenous microbes alter the radiosensitive or radioresistant gut phenotype independently of whether bacterial translocation and systemic infection do occur.[26] There is also increasing evidence that progression from mild diarrhea to more severe or chronic symptoms of radiation enteritis correlates with the extent of radiation-induced endothelial apoptosis,[27,28] and this may be related to the ability of microbiota to modulate the susceptibility of mesenchymal endothelial cells to radiation-induced apoptosis.

The hypothesis that qualitative and quantitative changes in gut microbial ecology could be caused by radiation exposure is also lent support by studies performed in humans. We know that fecal microbial diversity and its bacterial composition, which are thought to closely mirror the qualitative and quantitative composition of gut microbial ecology, are features specific to each individual, and different individuals have no more than 40% similarity with respect to the bacterial species and strains present in their indigenous digestive flora.[29] One additional crucial point is that the microbial profile of the more dominant bacterial species and strains is generally maintained in each individual subject over time with about a 60% reported similarity over a period of about 2 years.[30] This finding suggests that the stability of the microbiota is also important for the maintenance of a healthy gut functional equilibrium in each individual subject, including the gut sensitivity to toxic effects of radiation. It is therefore reasonable to suppose that if each single individual subject harbors a unique, specific gut microbial ecosystem, harboring specific sets of bacteria rather than others could also act as a specific risk, or otherwise protective factor for different intestinal disorders and radiation enteritis could well be included among them. For example, a reduction in diversity of the firmicutes has been associated with the risk of developing inflammatory bowel disorders,[31,32] and a decrease in the proportion of bacteroidetes has been linked with obesity.[33] There is some evidence also in the field of radiation enteritis. A recent study performed with amplification of the bacterial 16S rRNA, DNA fingerprinting, and cloning-sequencing techniques has indeed demonstrated an association between individual fecal microbial profiles and the appearance of radiation enteritis.[30] This finding implicates that susceptibility or resistance against the onset of radiation enteritis may be linked with the specific gut microbial colonization at baseline, that is, before the course of radiotherapy is started, which is different among different individuals and, in particular, the distribution and proportion of dominant bacterial species and strains. In other words, the qualitative and quantitative composition of the indigenous digestive flora, which is specific to each single individual subject, seems to represent a key and, so far, underestimated determinant of the risk of developing enteritis when each individual subject is exposed to radiation, including radiotherapy. Whether the characteristics of the quantitative and qualitative composition of the indigenous digestive flora could represent a potentially helpful tool in the clinical setting to estimate and predict the risk of developing radiation enteritis remains to be established and requires further investigation.

Another interesting observation provided by Manichanh and colleagues is that the microbial profile is markedly changed over time in the group of patients with radiation enteritis.[30] These changes do not appear to be restricted to some bacterial species or strains rather than to others, which points to a general imbalance of the gut microbial ecology and underlines the important concept that bacterial instability in the gastrointestinal tract should be regarded as the central mechanism responsible for the pathobiology of radiation enteritis.

AN IMMUNE HYPOTHESIS FOR RADIATION ENTERITIS

The view that changes in the quantitative and qualitative composition of gut microbial ecology are implicated in the pathobiology of radiation enteritis is closely linked with the recognition that radiation may affect a wide spectrum of cellular functions, which could ultimately lead to disruption of the epithelial barrier and mucosal inflammation. One important mechanism in the pathobiology of radiation enteritis includes the dysregulated production of cytokines and reactive oxygen species. Recent studies have demonstrated that radiation induces the synthesis of a wide range of cytokines in several tissues, including gut[34] and lungs.[35] These cytokines lead to cell infiltration and fibroblast stimulation, thus enhancing collagen synthesis.[36] One interesting observation is that disorders that share several clinical features with radiation enteritis, such as IBD, are associated with imbalances between Th1 (T helper cell type 1) and Th2 (T helper cell type 2) cytokines.[37] Th1 cytokines can activate macrophages, regulate cell-mediated immune responses, and promote tumoricidal activity whereas Th2 cells promote humoral immunity, resistance to parasites, and allergic inflammation.

Because these cell subpopulations tend to function antagonistically toward each other, the profile of susceptibility or resistance to IBD, and perhaps radiation enteritis as well, could depend at least to a certain degree on the profiles of the cytokines that each type secretes. There is evidence that ionizing radiation induces the preferential differentiation of Th cells into Th2 cells in the spleen[38,39] and also in the gut,[40] where this Th2 dominance is functionally characterized by suppressed interferon (IFN)-γ synthesis and release. Furthermore, Th2 cells have been shown to play a critical role in the pathobiology of radiation-induced pneumonitis and lung fibrosis.[41]

A recent study by Grémy and colleagues has confirmed this view by showing in a rat model that alterations of immune mechanisms, in particular T helper cell polarization with suppressed IFN-γ in the colon, may assume crucial importance during the early stages of radiation enteritis.[42] This shift occurred through transcriptional regulation of the level of cytokine mediators, through modification of specific signal transducers of IFN signaling, and through the secretion of a feedback inhibitor of Th1 polarization, with overall final result potentiating the Th2 profile.[42] This shift toward a Th2 profile was also associated in the early phase of exposure to ionizing radiation with increased expression of TNF-α and induction of inducible nitric oxide synthase (iNOS) and thus nitric oxide (NO) synthesis.[42] Of interest, iNOS is capable of inducing TNF-α synthesis,[43] and previous studies have also suggested the involvement of iNOS-derived NO in acute ionizing radiation syndrome. The immunomodulatory activity of iNOS is reported to influence Th cell development and to downregulate the induction of Th1 responses, thereby promoting a Th2 response.[44] These results are in line with the results of other investigations reporting on the initiation of a Th2 response in the early phase of abdominal radiation.[40]

One further important advance provided by Grémy and colleagues is that those immunity alterations appear to persist over time in the long term after the end of the radiotherapy protocol.[42] These data could be in agreement with the hypothesis that the postirradiation Th2 polarization in the gut, irrespective of whether acute or delayed, may represent the ultimate result of changes in the dynamics of lymphocyte recirculation. This hypothesis remains to be confirmed.

The radiation-induced immune damage has not yet been studied in great detail; however, the understanding of these immunity alterations and their relationship with the acute and late clinical effects from exposure to ionizing radiation could represent a huge forward step in the search for decreasing tissue toxicity in patients exposed to abdominal or pelvic radiotherapy.

PROBIOTICS FOR PREVENTION AND THERAPY FOR RADIATION ENTERITIS

Radiation enteritis is in most cases a self-limiting disorder, although it may evolve to a more severe and complicated form in a subset of patients. Thus, the usual goal of treatment is to control the disease while keeping potential toxic effects of treatment to a minimum. Good progress has been made in recent years with a wide spectrum of nonoperative treatment modalities for radiation injuries including hyperbaric oxygen, endoscopic formalin therapy, argon plasma coagulation, and laser therapy.[15] In contrast, attempts to treat radiation-induced diarrhea with antibiotics, sucralfate, anti-inflammatory drugs such as mesalazine and balsalazide, glutamine, octreotide, and proteolytic enzymes have so far provided inconclusive clinical results with failure of treatment occurring in a substantial proportion of patients.[10] Furthermore, prophylactic use of sucralfate has been shown not to reduce the burden of radiation-induced bowel toxicity; rather, it is associated with more severe gastrointestinal symptoms such as bleeding and long-term severe and disabling sequelae, ie, fecal incontinence.[10] On the basis of this background, it is clear that priority needs to be given in the field of radiotherapy to assess simple methods of preventing bowel toxicity, without compromising the control of the tumor and the efficacy of radiotherapy. It is clear as well, in light of the contradictory findings of therapeutic trials for radiation enteritis, that we urgently need innovative approaches that target the crucial steps in the pathobiology of radiation enteritis.

The term probiotic refers to a product or preparation containing viable and defined microorganisms in a number thought to be sufficient to alter by implantation or colonization the host's microflora and thereby exert beneficial effects.[45,46] Experimental studies in animal models and clinical trials of patients with IBD have consistently shown that use of probiotic organisms may effectively down-modulate the severity of intestinal inflammation through altering the composition and the metabolic and functional properties of gut indigenous flora.[45,46]

There is some suggestion provided by pivotal experimental and clinical studies that probiotics might represent a potentially effective strategy for both treatment and prevention of radiation enteritis. Experimental models with particular interest in endotoxinemia and bacterial translocation have confirmed that the manipulation of gut ecosystem by biologically effective probiotic preparations might be a worthwhile therapeutic and preventive tool in the field of radiation enteritis.[47,48] Furthermore, at least in experimental models, probiotics added as substrates can be given by an oral or enteral route to prevent radiation enteritis and related malnutrition. Experience with probiotic organisms for the prevention of radiation enteritis in cancer patients receiving radiotherapy is nonetheless limited, except for the double-blind and randomized trial by Urbancsek and colleagues who reported favorable results with LGG treatment.[49] However, this was a small-size, exploratory, and pilot study, and its encouraging results remain to be confirmed.

We have focused our interest on VSL#3, a new high-potency preparation of probiotic lactobacilli, that is known to effectively modulate intestinal inflammation through altering the composition and the metabolic and functional properties of enteric flora.[45,46] We hypothesized that preemptive treatment with VSL#3 may decrease the rate and severity of radiation enteritis during adjuvant radiotherapy after surgery for abdominal and pelvic cancer. In our 2 trials,[50,51] 490 consecutive patients attending the outpatient clinics of the Cancer X-Ray Unit of the University of Messina, Italy, who had adjuvant postoperative radiotherapy after surgery for sigmoid, rectal, or cervical cancer, were randomly assigned treatment with VSL#3 (VSL Pharmaceuticals, Gaithersburg, Maryland), 1 sachet tid, or placebo starting from the first day of radiation therapy. The design of the study was approved by the Ethics Committee at our hospital, and all patients gave written and informed consent to participate. The study was performed in accordance with the Declaration of Helsinki and with standards of good clinical practice.

Each sachet of VSL#3 contained 450 billions/g of viable lyophilized bacteria, including 4 strains of lactobacilli (*L. casei*, *L. plantarum*, *L. acidophilus*, and *L. delbruekii* ssp.

bulgaricus), 3 strains of bifidobacteria (*B. longum*, *B. breve*, and *B. infantis*), and 1 strain of *Streptococcus salivarius* ssp. *thermophilus*.

Patients were eligible for inclusion if they had no contraindication to probiotic or antibiotic therapy or radiation therapy. We excluded from randomization patients with a Karnofsky performance score ≤70, a life expectancy ≤1 year, persistent vomiting or diarrhea, fistulizing disease, known CD or UC, intra-abdominal abscesses or fever (more than 37.5°C) at the time of enrollment, or clinical, microbiological, or imaging evidence of sepsis syndrome, and requirement for continuous antibiotic treatment or use of antibiotics in the last 2 week before initiation of VSL#3 therapy. At baseline, patients provided a medical history and had a physical examination (consisting of vital signs, 12-lead electrocardiogram, neurological examination, and laboratory testing). Study subjects were followed up weekly during the scheduled cycle of radiation therapy and then 1 month after completion of radiation therapy. At each visit, clinical disease symptoms, concomitant medications, and any adverse events were reviewed, and a physical examination and laboratory studies were performed. Efficacy endpoints were incidence and severity of radiation-induced diarrhea, number of patients who discontinued radiotherapy because of diarrhea, daily number of bowel movements, and the time from the start of the study to the use of loperamide as rescue medication for diarrhea. The randomization was balanced between treatment groups in terms of gender, age, nodal involvement, tumor grade and size, local invasion at operation, invasion of contiguous structures at histology, and postoperative complications. The total X-ray dose the patients were given was between 60 and 70 Gy. We measured the severity of gastrointestinal toxicity according to World Health Organization grading, with grade 0 indicating no toxicity, grade 1 indicating self-limited toxicity lasting less than 2 days, grade 2 indicating self-limited symptoms lasting more than 2 days, grade 3 referring to symptoms requiring treatment, and grade 4 indicating severe toxicity with dehydration and/or hemorrhage.

Of the 245 patients in the placebo group, 239 (97.5%) completed the study as 6 patients were withdrawn after a few sessions of radiation therapy due to the occurrence of severe diarrhea resistant to loperamide and the usual standard of care; these patients were excluded from the analysis of results. Of the 245 patients in the VSL#3 group, 243 (99.1%) completed the study, 1 patient withdrew his consent after the first session of radiation therapy, and 1 patient died of myocardial infarction after 3 sessions of radiation therapy; both patients were excluded from analysis of the results.

More patients in the placebo group had radiation enteritis compared with the VSL#3 group (124 of 239, 51.8%, vs 77 of 243 patients, 31.6%; $P < .001$). Furthermore, patients given the placebo suffered more severe toxicity compared with VSL#3 recipients as grade 3 or 4 diarrhea was documented in 69 of 124 (55.4%) placebo-treated patients and 8 of 77 (1.4%) VSL#3-treated patients ($P < .001$), whereas 50 of 124 placebo-treated patients had grade 1 or 2 diarrhea compared with 34 of 77 VSL#3 recipients. Even though the difference did not reach statistical significance, there was clearly a trend in favor of the treatment with VSL#3 compared to the placebo.

The mean daily number of bowel movements for patients with radiation enteritis was 14.7 ± 6 and 5.1 ± 3 among placebo and VSL#3 recipients, respectively ($P < .05$), and the mean time to the use of loperamide as rescue medication for diarrhea was 86 ± 6 hours for patients receiving placebo versus 122 ± 8 hours for patients receiving VSL#3 ($P < .001$).

No tumor- or treatment-related deaths or deaths from other causes were recorded in either group during the period of radiation therapy, and no case of bacteremia, sepsis, or septic shock due to the probiotic lactobacilli was reported among the VSL#3 recipients during the treatment period with the probiotic preparation or during the 6 months beyond active treatment. Likewise, no case of bacteremia, sepsis, or septic shock due to organisms other than the probiotic lactobacilli was recognized during the period of active treatment. We did not recognize any other toxicity reasonably attributable to VSL#3.

The results of these 2 pilot clinical trials indicate that bacteriotherapy with the use of probiotic lactobacilli may protect patients against the risk of radiation enteritis. This could have an additional clinical fallout as fewer patients treated with probiotic lacto-bacilli should be expected to discontinue radiotherapy or require a reduction in the radiation dose because of severe gastrointestinal toxicity. This might ultimately allow patients treated with probiotic lactobacilli to receive a greater cumulative radiation tumor dose with a potentially important benefit in terms of efficacy of radiotherapy. We have not specifically addressed this issue in our studies; however, no subject in the VSL#3 group discontinued radiotherapy because of gastrointestinal toxicity as compared with 2 patients in the placebo group. This finding appears to be in line with the above hypothesis.

Although a recent study has reported favorable results with LGG bacteriotherapy for radiation-induced colitis,[49] we designed to use VSL#3 rather than LGG or other traditional preparations of probiotic lactobacilli for several reasons. The clinical potential of VSL#3 in the treatment of IBD has been validated by several studies,[45,46] whereas reports of LGG have been somewhat conflicting.[52,53] VSL#3 is a high-potency preparation with innovative characteristics compared to traditional probiotics, in particular the enormously high bacterial concentration and the presence of a consortium of different bacterial species with potential synergistic relations between different strains enhancing suppression of potential pathogens.[45,46] The composite mixture of this preparation with a large number of probiotic strains possessing very different and specialized metabolic and immunoregulatory activities is a unique feature of VSL#3, which might explain its wide spectrum of biological activities.[45,46] This is most impor-tant as the different species of probiotic lactobacilli may exert very different biological and immunomodulatory effects,[8] and the health benefits ultimately resulting from pro-biotic bacteriotherapy strictly depend on the metabolic and biologic diversity of the ingested lactobacilli.[45,46] In this view, the widely different biological, immunoregulatory, and metabolic characteristics contained within the probiotic lactobacilli and bifido-bacteria of VSL#3 greatly enhance its therapeutic potential, compared to traditional probiotic preparations. We have not analyzed the bacterial content of stool samples from patients treated with VSL#3. However, previous experience with this probiotic preparation has shown that colonization of intestinal niches with protective lactobacil-li and bifidobacteria and reconditioning of the endogenous digestive microflora occurs in almost all the subjects treated with VSL#3.[45,46] In vitro experiments with VSL#3 have demonstrated the ability of the bacterial strains contained in this probiotic prepara-tion to regulate the process of apoptosis.[45,46] This property of VSL#3 may be crucial for explaining the protective effect against radiation-induced colitis in patients treated with radiotherapy. Recent studies in experimental models have indeed demonstrated that an unregulated process of apoptosis is the primary mechanism of radiation-induced intestinal damage.[45,46] Furthermore, VSL#3 lowers the production of proinflam-matory cytokines and several other effectors of inflammation and tissue injury, such as nitric oxide and metalloproteinases.[45,46] Taken together, these mechanisms ultimately account for the significant protection exerted by VSL#3 upon the integrity of the gas-trointestinal intestinal epithelial barrier.[45,46] Although we do not have direct proof, it is conceivable that VSL#3 is operating through these same mechanisms in patients at risk for radiation-induced colitis. In our study, none among the patients given VSL#3 experienced treatment-related toxicity. Previous clinical experience with this probiotic preparation has indeed demonstrated the remarkable safety of VSL#3 bacteriotherapy even with dosages significantly greater than those we used in this trial. Therefore, it is our opinion that VSL#3 is a safe treatment even for cancer patients receiving radiotherapy. Our preliminary observation, of course, needs to be independently confirmed in a larger number of patients. However, our data suggest that treatment with probiotic bacteriotherapy has the potential to protect the gastrointestinal tract against radiation injury. Furthermore, this study indirectly lends support to the view that the severe and potentially lethal gastrointestinal syndrome caused by abdominal radiotherapy is related to a quantitative and/or qualitative alteration in the microecology of resident intestinal bacteria. If confirmed, the results of this study could pave the way to preemptive treatment with probiotic preparations for subjects at risk for radiation-induced diarrhea to reduce both the incidence and severity of this complication.

REFERENCES

1.   Walsh DW. Deep tissue traumatism from Roentgen ray exposure. *Br Med J.* 1897;11:272-273.
2.   Abbasakoor F, Vaizey CJ, Boulos PB. Improving the morbidity of anorectal injury from pelvic radiotherapy. *Colorectal Dis.* 2006;8(1):2-10.
3.   Hayne D, Vaizey CJ, Boulos PB. Anorectal injury following pelvic radiotherapy. *Br J Surg.* 2001;88(8):1037-1048.
4.   Miller AR, Martenson JA, Nelson H, et al. The incidence and clinical consequences of treatment-related bowel injury. *Int J Radiat Oncol Biol Phys.* 1999;43(4):817-825.
5.   Perez CA, Lee HK, Georgiou A, Lockett MA. Technical factors affecting morbidity in definitive irradiation for localized carcinoma of the prostate. *Int J Radiat Oncol Biol Phys.* 1994;28(4):811-819.
6.   Babb RR. Radiation proctitis: a review. *Am J Gastroenterol.* 1996;91(7):1309-1311.
7.   Lucarotti ME, Mountford RA, Bartolo DC. Surgical management of intestinal radiation injury. *Dis Colon Rectum.* 1991;34(10):865-869.
8.   Miller AR, Martenson JA, Nelson H, et al. The incidence and clinical consequences of treatment-related bowel injury. *Int J Radiat Oncol Biol Phys.* 1999;43(4):817-825.
9.   Muttillo IA, Elias D, Bolognese A, et al. Surgical treatment of severe late radiation injury to the bowel: a retrospective analysis of 83 cases. *Hepatogastroenterology.* 2002;49(46):1023-1026.
10. Zimmerer T, Wenz F, Singer MV. Medical prevention and treatment of acute and chronic radiation induced enteritis: is there any proven therapy? A short review. *Z Gastroenterol.* 2008;46(5):441-448.
11. Gilinsky NH, Burns DG, Barbezat GO, et al. The natural history of radiation-induced proctosigmoiditis: an analysis of 88 patients. *Q J Med.* 1983;52(205):40-53.
12. McBride WH, Chiang CS, Olson JL, et al. A sense of danger from radiation. *Radiat Res.* 2004;162(1):1-19.
13. Allen-Mersh TG, Wilson EJ, Hope-Stone HF, Mann CV. Has the incidence of radiation-induced bowel damage following treatment of uterine carcinoma changed in the last 20 years? *J R Soc Med.* 1986;79(7):387-390.
14. Hatcher PA, Thomson HJ, Ludgate SN, Small WP, Smith AN. Surgical aspects of intestinal injury due to pelvic radiotherapy. *Ann Surg.* 1985;201(4):470-475.
15. Turina M, Mulhall AM, Mahid SS, Yashar C, Galandiuk S. Frequency and surgical management of chronic complications related to pelvic radiation. *Arch Surg.* 2008;143(1):46-52.
16. Kimose HH, Fischer L, Spjeldnaes N, Wara P. Late radiation injury of the colon and rectum: surgical management and outcome. *Dis Colon Rectum.* 1989;32(8):684-689.
17. Nathanson DR, Espat NJ, Nash GM, et al. Evaluation of preoperative and postoperative radiotherapy on long-term functional results of straight coloanal anastomosis. *Dis Colon Rectum.* 2003;46(7):888-894.
18. Baxter NN, Tepper JE, Durham SB, Rothenberger DA, Virnig BA. Increased risk of rectal cancer after prostate radiation: a population-based study. *Gastroenterology.* 2005;128(4):819-824.
19. Brenner DJ, Curtis RE, Hall EJ, Ron E. Second malignancies in prostate carcinoma patients after radiotherapy compared with surgery. *Cancer.* 2000;88(2):398-406.
20. Neugut AI, Ahsan H, Robinson E, Ennis RD. Bladder carcinoma and other second malignancies after radiotherapy for prostate carcinoma. *Cancer.* 1997;79(8):1600-1604.
21. Somosy Z, Horvath G, Telbisz A, Rez G, Palfia Z. Morphological aspects of ionizing radiation response of small intestine. *Micron.* 2002;33(2):167-178.
22. Brook I, Walker RI, MacVittie TJ. Effect of antimicrobial therapy on bowel flora and bacterial infection in irradiated mice. *Int J Radiat Biol Relat Stud Phys Chem Med.* 1988;53(5):709-716.

23. Brook I, Ledney GD. Short and long courses of ofloxacin therapy of *Klebsiella pneumoniae* sepsis following irradiation. *Radiat Res.* 1992;130(1):61-64.
24. Onoue M, Uchida K, Yokokura T, Takahashi T, Mutai M. Effect of intestinal microflora on the survival time of mice exposed to lethal whole-body gamma irradiation. *Radiat Res.* 1981;88(3):533-541.
25. Husebye E, Skar V, Høverstad T, et al. Abnormal intestinal motor patterns explain enteric colonization with gram-negative bacilli in late radiation enteropathy. *Gastroenterology.* 1995;109(4):1078-1089.
26. Crawford PA, Gordon JI. Microbial regulation of intestinal radiosensitivity. *Proc Natl Acad Sci USA.* 2005;102(37):13254-13259.
27. Paris F, Fuks Z, Kang A, et al. Endothelial apoptosis as the primary lesion initiating intestinal radiation damage in mice. *Science.* 2001;293(5528):293-297.
28. Cho CH, Kammerer RA, Lee HJ, et al. Designed angiopoietin-1 variant, COMP-Ang1, protects against radiation-induced endothelial cell apoptosis. *Proc Natl Acad Sci U S A.* 2004;101(15):5553-5558.
29. Zoetendal EG, Akkermans AD, De Vos WM. Temperature gradient gel electrophoresis analysis of 16S rRNA from human fecal samples reveals stable and host-specific communities of active bacteria. *Appl Environ Microbiol.* 1998;64(10):3854-3859.
30. Manichanh C, Varela E, Martinez C, et al. The gut microbiota predispose to the pathophysiology of acute postradiotherapy diarrhea. *Am J Gastroenterol.* 2008;103(7):1754-1761.
31. Manichanh C, Rigottier-Gois L, Bonnaud E, et al. Reduced diversity of faecal microbiota in Crohn's disease revealed by a metagenomic approach. *Gut.* 2006;55(2):205-211.
32. Frank DN, St Amand AL, Feldman RA, et al. Molecular phylogenetic characterization of microbial community imbalances in human inflammatory bowel diseases. *Proc Natl Acad Sci U S A.* 2007;104(34):13780-13785.
33. Ley RE, Turnbaugh PJ, Klein S, et al. Microbial ecology: human gut microbes associated with obesity. *Nature.* 2006;444(7122):1022-1023.
34. Linard C, Marquette C, Mathieu J, Pennequin A, Clarencon D, Mathe D. Acute induction of inflammatory cytokine expression after gamma-irradiation in the rat: effect of an NF-kappaB inhibitor. *Int J Radiat Oncol Biol Phys.* 2004;58(2):427-434.
35. Hong JH, Chiang CS, Tsao CY, Lin PY, McBride WH, Wu CJ. Rapid induction of cytokine gene expression in the lung after single and fractionated doses of radiation. *Int J Radiat Biol.* 1999;75(11):1421-1427.
36. Strup-Perrot C, Mathe D, Linard C, et al. Global gene expression profiles reveal an increase in mRNA levels of collagens, MMPs, and TIMPs in late radiation enteritis. *Am J Physiol Gastrointest Liver Physiol.* 2004;287(4):G875-G885.
37. MacDonald TT, Monteleone G, Pender SL. Recent developments in the immunology of inflammatory bowel disease. *Scand J Immunol.* 2000;51(1):2-9.
38. Park HR, Jo SK, Paik SG. Factors effecting the Th2-like immune response after gamma-irradiation: low production of IL-12 heterodimer in antigen-presenting cells and small expression of the IL-12 receptor in T cells. *Int J Radiat Biol.* 2005;81(3):221-231.
39. Han SK, Song JY, Yun YS, Yi SY. Effect of gamma radiation on cytokine expression and cytokine-receptor mediated STAT activation. *Int J Radiat Biol.* 2006;82(9):686-697.
40. Grémy O, Benderitter M, Linard C. Caffeic acid phenethyl ester modifies the Th1/Th2 balance in ileal mucosa after gamma-irradiation in the rat by modulating the cytokine pattern. *World J Gastroenterol.* 2006;12(31):4996-5004.
41. Westermann W, Schobl R, Rieber EP, Frank KH. Th2 cells as effectors in postirradiation pulmonary damage preceding fibrosis in the rat. *Int J Radiat Biol.* 1999;75(5):629-638.
42. Grémy O, Benderitter M, Linard C. Acute and persisting Th2-like immune response after fractionated colorectal γ-irradiation. *World J Gastroenterol.* 2008;14(46):7075-7085.
43. Huang FP, Niedbala W, Wei XQ, et al. Nitric oxide regulates Th1 cell development through the inhibition of IL-12 synthesis by macrophages. *Eur J Immunol.* 1998;28(12):4062-4070.
44. Lawrence CE, Paterson JC, Wei XQ, Liew FY, Garside P, Kennedy MW. Nitric oxide mediates intestinal pathology but not immune expulsion during *Trichinella spiralis* infection in mice. *J Immunol.* 2000;164(8):4229-4234.
45. Famularo G, De Simone C, Matteuzzi D, Pirovano F. Traditional and high-potency probiotic preparations: advances, perspectives and safety of oral bacteriotherapy. *Biodrugs.* 1999;12(6):455-470.
46. Famularo G, Mosca L, Minisola G, Trinchieri V, De Simone C. Probiotic lactobacilli: a new perspective for the treatment of inflammatory bowel disease. *Curr Pharm Des.* 2003;9(24):1973-1980.
47. Seal M, Naito Y, Barreto R, Lorenzatti A, Safran P, Marotta F. Experimental radiotherapy-induced enteritis: a probiotic interventional study. *J Dig Dis.* 2007;8(3):143-147.
48. Demirer S, Aydintug S, Aslim B, et al. Effects of probiotics on radiation-induced intestinal injury in rats. *Nutrition.* 2006;22(2):179-186.
49. Urbancsek H, Kazar T, Mezes I, Neumann K. Results of a double-blind, randomized study to evaluate the efficacy and safety of Antibiophilus in patients with radiation-induced diarrhoea. *Eur J Gastroenterol Hepatol.* 2001;13(4):391-396.

50. Delia P, Sansotta G, Donato V, et al. Prevention of radiation-induced diarrhea with the use of VSL#3, a new high-potency probiotic preparation. *Am J Gastroenterol.* 2002;97(8):2150-2152.

51. Delia P, Sansotta G, Donato V, et al. Use of probiotics for prevention of radiation-induced diarrhea. *World J Gastroenterol.* 2007;13(6):912-915.

52. Malin M, Suomalainen H, Saxelin M, et al. Promotion of IgA immune response in patients with Crohn's disease by oral bacteriotherapy with *Lactobacillus* GG. *Ann Nutr Metab.* 1996;40(3):137-145.

53. Prantera C, Scribano ML, Falasco G, et al. Inefficacy of probiotic in preventing recurrence after curative resection for Crohn's disease: a randomised controlled trial with *Lactobacillus* GG. *Gut.* 2002;51(3): 405-409.

22

Probiotics and
Helicobacter pylori

Adam S. Kim, MD

Helicobacter pylori is one of the most common pathogens in the world. It has infected humans for at least 3000 years, and traces of it have been found in the feces of mummified human remains from the South American Andes.[1] It was first recognized in the late nineteenth century by Italian pathologists who found spiral bacteria in the stomach of dogs.[2] In the early twentieth century, spiral bacteria were found in the stomach of humans.[3] These bacteria did not grow in culture, were thought to be an oral contaminant, and were mostly forgotten until the 1980s. Barry Marshall and J. Robin Warren studied these spiral or curved bacteria and later received the 2005 Nobel Prize in Medicine for their early descriptions of *H. pylori* and its association with human diseases. They first published their discoveries on curved bacilli in the stomach in *The Lancet* in 1984.[4] In this early case series, they reported on 100 consecutive patients undergoing gastroscopy in Perth, Australia. Spiral or curved bacilli were found in 58% of patients and in 87% of patients with an ulcer. They were only able to culture bacilli in 11 subjects, and they described a Gram-negative microaerophilic species related to *Campylobacter*. They also found that the bacilli was related to the histologic finding of gastritis, and bacilli were found in 30 out of 40 (75%) patients with gastritis, but only 1 out of 29 (3%) patients without gastritis. At the time, colonization with *C. pyloridis* was not associated with any clinical symptoms, and it was not clear if the bacteria were the cause of peptic ulcer or gastritis.

In a much publicized incident, Dr Marshall deliberately inoculated himself with *H. pylori* and then developed new gastritis and severe symptoms that resolved after eradication therapy. This experiment helped to solidify the causative role that *H. pylori* plays in gastritis and peptic ulcer disease. It has since been confirmed that *H. pylori* is a causative agent in chronic gastritis and peptic ulcer disease[5,6] and is present in 60% to 80% of gastric and 90% to 95% of duodenal ulcers.[7] Eradication of *H. pylori* has been proven effective at decreasing recurrence of peptic ulcers in many instances.[8,9] *H. pylori* is also known to be a causative agent in the development of gastric cancer, as shown in epidemiologic studies,[10-12] and was first named as a carcinogen by a panel of international cancer experts in 1994.[13] Primary prevention trials aimed at decreasing rates of gastric cancer in *H. pylori*-infected individuals at high risk have been mixed.[14,15]

Floch MH, Kim AS, eds.
Probiotics: A Clinical Guide (pp 295-306)
© 2010 Taylor & Francis Group

CURRENT THERAPY

H. pylori is difficult to eradicate, and current treatments feature the use of combination antibiotics. None of the current treatments have 100% efficacy, in part because of antibiotic resistance to commonly used antimicrobials such as metronidazole and clarithromycin. In fact, antimicrobial resistance of *H. pylori* has been increasing over time,[16,17] and antimicrobial resistance is one of the major factors in treatment failure.[18-21] The recommended antimicrobial therapy has been reported by the Maastricht III Consensus Report.[22] First choice for eradication treatment is a proton pump inhibitor (PPI), clarithromycin, and either amoxicillin or metronidazole (often referred to as "triple therapy"). Second choice therapies are either PPI-based triple therapy with different antibiotics than were previously used (metronidazole, and either amoxicillin or tetracycline), or quadruple therapy with bismuth (bismuth, metronidazole, tetracycline, and PPI/or histamine receptor 2 antagonist [H2 blocker]). If treatment still fails after 2 rounds of therapy, the recommendation is to check antibiotic susceptibility and to consider using levofloxacin- or rifabutin-based therapies.

Recently, there is expanding evidence for the use of "sequential therapy," and in some instances, it may even be preferred vs triple therapy. In 10-day sequential therapy regimens, patients are treated for 5 days with a PPI and a single antibiotic (often amoxicillin), followed by 5 days with 2 other antibiotics (often clarithromycin and tinidazole). A recent meta-analysis, largely consisting of trials from Europe, showed improved eradication rates using sequential therapy vs standard triple therapy.[23]

RATIONALE LEADING TO THE CLINICAL USE OF PROBIOTICS IN *H. PYLORI* INFECTION

Probiotics are useful because of their ability to maintain the integrity of the mucosal barrier and to maintain or restore intestinal ecoflora. Probiotics have been useful and efficacious in several human diseases, and many have speculated about their usefulness in *H. pylori* infection. The rationale for using probiotics to treat or prevent *H. pylori* infection is varied and multifaceted. In rat models of induced gastric ulcers, altering the gut flora with antibiotics decreases the size of the ulcers,[24] suggesting the benefit of altering the gut flora in patients with gastritis and peptic ulcers. The probiotics *B. breve* YIT4014 and 4043 and *B. bifidum* YIT4007 prevent ethanol-induced gastric ulcers in rats,[25] suggesting that certain probiotics can prevent peptic ulcers. A group from Texas led by Dr Oh showed that lactobacilli and yeast isolated from fermented milk products limited *H. pylori* growth and/or killed *H. pylori* in vitro,[26] but did not explain how this occurred. The mechanism of action against *H. pylori* is likely multifactorial and may be from lowering pH, secreting antimicrobial substances, blocking adhesion, restoring mucus production, or through immunologic mediators.[27] Each of these mechanisms will be explored.

Many probiotics are crucial to the production of SCFA such as acetic, butyric, and lactic acids that lower intraluminal pH. Common LAB that are considered probiotics are *Lactobacillus*, *Leuconostoc*, *Pediococcus*, and *Streptococcus*. In vitro, certain types of LAB can produce large amounts of lactic acid and inhibit *H. pylori* growth (eg, *L. salivarius*), whereas other LAB (*L. casei* and *L. acidophilus*) fail to inhibit *H. pylori* growth in culture.[28] Yet other studies have shown that several probiotics, such as *L. casei* Shirota[29] and *L. acidophilus* LA1,[30] can inhibit *H. pylori* growth independent of lactic acid.

If not by the production of acid and by lowering pH, how do probiotics inhibit growth of *H. pylori*? Several authors have shown that proteinaceous compounds secreted by probiotics have an inhibitory effect on *H. pylori*. Coconnier et al in 1998 showed that supernatant from growing *L. acidophilus* contains an antibacterial substance that dramatically decreases the viability of *H. pylori* in vitro, as well as decreases adhesion of *H. pylori* to cultured epithelial cells.[31] *L. johnsonii* Lal also has bactericidal activity against *H. pylori*, owing to release of bacteriocin-like compounds that were found in the supernatant of spent cultures.[32] Bacteriocins are proteinaceous compounds produced by bacteria that inhibit the growth of other bacteria. Kim et al also showed in vitro inhibition of *H. pylori* growth by a number of different bacteriocins produced by *Lactococcus lactis*.[33] Of note, the amount of bacteriocins produced by the probiotic differed between individual strains, again indicating the importance of not only organism choice of probiotics but also strain choice.

One of the main factors in *H. pylori*-related disease is the organisms' ability to adhere to epithelial cells.[34] Several in vitro studies have shown that probiotics can inhibit the adherence of *H. pylori* to intestinal epithelial cells.[31,32,35] The exact mechanism of this blockage is not entirely clear. In certain probiotics, such as *L. reuteri*, inhibition is via the glycolipid receptors gangliotetraosylceramide and sulfatide.[36] Of note, only 2 of 9 strains of *L. reuteri* studied were able to block binding of *H. pylori*. Although a few specific mechanisms of *H. pylori* binding inhibition are known, it is most likely that nonspecific mechanisms are largely responsible because probiotics can inhibit the adhesion of large varieties of pathogenic bacteria.[27]

A common finding in *H. pylori*-associated gastritis is a reduction in mucus secretion, another area in which probiotics may be beneficial. *H. pylori* can decrease gene expression of mucin genes MUC5AC and MUC1,[37] whereas *L. plantarum* and *L. rhamnosus* can increase expression of MUC2 and MUC3,[38] with a corresponding increase in mucin secretion.[39] This mechanism is partially responsible for the ability of probiotics to block adherence of pathogenic bacteria.

Finally, probiotics may work through blocking inflammatory mediators triggered by *H. pylori*. *H. pylori* infection can provoke the release of interleukin-8 (IL-8), a powerful chemoattractant of other inflammatory cells.[40] Other mediators of *H. pylori*-induced inflammation are TNF-α, IL-1, and IL-6.[41] Kabir et al have demonstrated that *L. salivarius* can inhibit the *H. pylori*-mediated release of IL-8 by intestinal epithelial cells.[42] *L. paracasei* NCC2461 can block the proliferative activity of CD4(+) T cells in a dose-dependent fashion, accompanied by a marked decrease in both T helper (Th)1 and Th2 effector cytokines, including gamma interferon, IL-4, and IL-5.[43] Overall, our understanding of the mechanisms of immunologic signaling by probiotics is poor. Bacterial signaling at the mucosal surface is dependent on a network of cellular interactions, which will take some time to be fully understood.[44]

ANIMAL STUDIES

Many animal studies have been performed that demonstrate the efficacy of probiotics to limit *H. pylori*-mediated disease or to decrease numbers of *H. pylori* in vivo. A few prominent examples have been selected for review here. Two studies using *L. salivarius* demonstrated prevention of *H. pylori* colonization and gastritis in mice.[28,42] In another study, Coconnier and colleagues used spent supernatant of *L. acidophilus* in a mouse model of *Helicobacter* infection and were able to decrease colonization and inflammation as well as urease activity in vivo.[31] Finally, Sgouras et al showed that *L. casei* Shirota could decrease *H. pylori* colonization and gastric mucosal inflammation in a mouse model of *H. pylori* infection.[45]

EARLY CLINICAL STUDIES

Successful animal trials have led to an abundance of early clinical trials or pilot studies aimed at determining the effect of probiotics on *H. pylori* in human subjects. Imase and colleagues published a trial in 2007 in which *L. reuteri* SD2112 tablets could suppress urease activity and *H. pylori* density in asymptomatic volunteers.[46] An epidemiologic study out of Poland noted that those who were re-infected with *H. pylori* after successful eradication were less likely to have consumed fermented dairy products, presumed to contain probiotic organisms such as *Lactobacillus* species.[47] Felley et al showed that acidified milk containing *L. johnsonii* La1 could decrease *H. pylori* density and inflammation in healthy volunteers with *H. pylori* colonization.[48] Also from the same center in Switzerland, they studied the effects of fermented milk containing *L. johnsonii* Lj1 on endoscopic and histologic gastritis in healthy *H. pylori*-positive volunteers.[49] They found that treatment with *L. johnsonii*, but not placebo, decreased *H. pylori* density in the antrum and decreased severity and activity of antral gastritis. In addition, mucus layer thickness in the stomach was significantly increased in the probiotic-treated group. Finally, Shimbo et al demonstrated that *Clostridium butyricum* MIYAIRI 588 can halt the decrease in fecal counts of obligate anaerobes associated with PPI-based eradication therapy.[50] All of these epidemiologic and early clinical studies have led to the study of probiotics as an adjunct to eradication therapy for *H. pylori* infection.

PROBIOTICS AS ADJUNCT TO
H. PYLORI ERADICATION THERAPY

Numerous studies have attempted to show increased rates of *H. pylori* eradication by adding probiotics to conventional antibiotic combination therapy. Several studies reported results as change in urease breath test, although this technique seems problematic as evidenced by other studies that have failed to correlate changes in urease breath test to eradication status.[51] Most of the studies referenced herein will not report results as change in urease breath test (or delta urease), but on eradication rate as confirmed by stool antigen, gastric biopsy samples (via histology or urease activity), and absolute urease breath test activity.

The first *H. pylori* eradication trial using probiotics as an adjunct was performed by Canducci et al.[52] They used a lyophilized and inactivated culture of *L. acidophilus* to increase *H. pylori* eradication rates when combined with standard triple therapy for 7 days. In their intention-to-treat analysis, the group with the inactivated *L. acidophilus* had a significant increase in eradication compared to the standard therapy group (87% vs 70%, respectively, *P* = .02).

Sheu and colleagues randomized 160 patients to 7 days of triple therapy with or without yogurt containing *Lactobacillus* and *Bifidobacterium* (AB-Yogurt, President Corp, Taiwan).[53] In the intention-to-treat analysis, eradication was improved in the yogurt group compared to standard triple-therapy alone group (91% vs 78%, respectively, *P* < .05). Interestingly, the probiotic yogurt may not improve eradication rates on its own, but may decrease side effects and allow more people to complete eradication therapy. In the per-protocol analysis, there was no statistically significant difference in eradication rates (94% vs 89%), suggesting that probiotics did not increase eradication in those who completed the 7 days of triple therapy. However, the rates of treatment completion were significantly improved in the group with yogurt (68% vs 44%, $P < .05$), and there were significantly fewer side effects in the yogurt group (19% vs 65%, $P < .05$).

An Italian group (de Bortoli and colleagues) published a RCT in 2007 comparing standard 7-day triple therapy with triple therapy plus a combination of bovine lactoferrin and probiotics in 206 patients.[54] The probiotic used was a combination of 9 lactic acid-producing organisms, sold as Probinul by Cadigroup. In both intention-to-treat and per-protocol analyses, the group that received bovine lactoferrin and probiotics had significantly higher rates of eradication ($P < .01$) at 8 weeks. There were also significantly fewer side effects in the group treated with bovine lactoferrin and probiotics ($P < .005$). In this trial, it is impossible to determine whether it was the probiotics, the lactoferrin, or a combination of both that caused the improved eradication of *H. pylori*. Probinul includes *L. plantarum*, *L. reuteri*, *L. casei* subsp. *rhamnosus*, *B. infantis*, *B. longum*, *L. salivarius*, *L. acidophilus*, *S. thermophilus*, and *L. sporogenes*. Bovine lactoferrin is a glycoprotein of the transferrin family that transports iron. It is found in milk, as well as tears, saliva, bile, and other mucosal secretions.[55] Bovine lactoferrin has in vitro antimicrobial activity against numerous microbes,[56,57] including *H. pylori*.[58]

Kim and colleagues in Korea conducted a randomized controlled trial of 347 patients comparing PPI-based triple therapy with PPI-based triple therapy plus a Korean yogurt.[59] The yogurt was called Will and contained *L. acidophilus* HY2177, *L. casei* HY2743, *B. longum* HY8001, and *S. thermophilus* B-1. There was no difference in eradication in the intention-to-treat analysis, but there was a statistically significant increase in eradication in the per-protocol analysis for the group that received the yogurt (78.7% vs 87.5%, $P < .05$). Interestingly, there was also an increase in frequency of adverse effects in the yogurt group (26.3% vs 41.1%, $P < .01$), although the adverse events were mostly very mild symptoms.

In the only clinical trial using probiotics as an adjunct to second-line eradication therapy after an initial treatment failure, Sheu et al[60] in 2006 enrolled 138 patients in a RCT. Subjects were randomized to receive quadruple therapy with or without 4 weeks of pretreatment with probiotic yogurt containing *Lactobacillus* and *Bifidobacterium* (AB-Yogurt, President Corporation, Taiwan). Those treated with the yogurt had increased eradication compared to standard therapy alone (intention-to-treat analysis: 85% vs 71%, $P < .05$).[60]

Not all clinical trials that have used probiotics as an adjunct to PPI- and antibiotic-based eradication treatment have been effective. There are several studies of probiotics being added to triple therapy with no improvement in eradication rates of *H. pylori*. Cindoruk et al[61] conducted a randomized placebo-controlled trial of 124 subjects with dyspepsia and *H. pylori*. The addition of *S. boulardii* to standard therapy had no effect on eradication rates, but did decrease the frequency of diarrhea and epigastric pain associated with triple-therapy treatment.[61] Francavilla and colleagues reported negative results on *L. reuteri's* effect on *H. pylori* eradication as monotherapy in a randomized, placebo-controlled trial of 40 subjects with dyspepsia.[62] In this study similar to the pediatric trial by Gotteland et al,[63] there was no antibiotic or PPI therapy given, in an attempt to see if probiotics alone can eradicate *H. pylori* in some subjects. Although the probiotic did not alter eradication rates, there was a significant improvement in gastrointestinal symptoms of the probiotic-treated group at the end of treatment, which was not seen in the placebo group. Goldman et al in 2006 reported on the negative results of a probiotic yogurt on increasing *H. pylori* eradication when the yogurt was added to PPI-based triple therapy, in a RCT of 65 subjects.[64]

There have been pediatric clinical trials investigating the use of probiotics as an adjunct aimed at improving eradication rates when given along with triple therapy.

A group from the Czech Republic (Sykora and colleagues) showed increased rates of *H. pylori* eradication when a fermented milk product containing *L. casei* DN-114 was administered along with standard triple therapy to 86 symptomatic children with *H. pylori* (P < .01).[65] There has also been one pediatric clinical trial that failed to show an increase in eradication rates with probiotics. In this trial by Lionetti et al, *L. reuteri* SD2112 (marketed as Reuterin by Nóos in Sweden) and triple-therapy failed to improve eradication rates over triple-therapy plus placebo in 40 pediatric patients (ages 3 to 18 years) with gastrointestinal symptoms.[66]

PROBIOTIC IN ASYMPTOMATIC CHILDREN WITH *H. PYLORI* INFECTION

An interesting trial was reported by Gotteland et al[63] in 2008 involving 271 asymptomatic children who were colonized with *H. pylori*. Children were randomized to placebo or a combination of *L. johnsonii* (La1) and/or cranberry juice, and eradication was measured at 3 weeks. The placebo-treated children had a spontaneous rate of eradication of only 1.5%, whereas the groups treated with probiotic and/or cranberry juice had eradication rates between 14.9% and 22.9%, which were significantly higher than placebo. However, there was no significant difference between the cranberry juice and probiotic group. This indicates that cranberry juice alone, or probiotic alone or in combination with cranberry juice, has a modest effect on the eradication of *H. pylori* in asymptomatic children. This raises the possibility of community-wide treatment strategies in areas of high prevalence.

MANAGEMENT OF SIDE EFFECTS ASSOCIATED WITH ERADICATION THERAPY

The primary outcome of most *H. pylori* trials is eradication rates, an outcome in which probiotics have had varied success. Another useful outcome is the frequency or severity of side effects associated with standard triple-therapy regimens, especially if a decreased amount of side effects may increase the number of patients who complete the regimen. If more patients complete their regimen, this may have a small effect on eradication rates and/or decrease antibiotic resistance. Many studies have shown beneficial effects at limiting side effects when taking traditional combination therapy antibiotics. De Bortoli's study demonstrated fewer side effects overall, as well as less nausea, diarrhea, metallic taste, and abdominal pain, when patients were treated with a combination probiotic plus bovine lactoferrin.[54] Francavilla and colleagues showed that dyspepsia symptoms in the setting of *H. pylori* infection could be improved with probiotic monotherapy with *L. reuteri*, a change that was not seen in placebo-treated patients.[62] Cindoruk et al showed decreased diarrhea and epigastric pain when *S. boulardii* was added to standard triple therapy in dyspeptic adults.[61] Interestingly, Kim et al showed an increase in side effects in the group that received a probiotic yogurt.[59] The yogurt contained *L. acidophilus* HY2177, *L. casei* HY2743, *B. longum* HY8001, and *S. thermophilus* B-1, implying that these particular organisms or strains may not be beneficial for minimizing the side effects associated with *H. pylori* eradication therapy.

In the pediatric population, Lionetti and colleagues showed a significant improvement in gastrointestinal symptoms after triple therapy when *L. reuteri* SD2112 was

TABLE 22-1

ADULT: RECOMMENDATIONS FOR PROBIOTIC USE IN HELICOBACTER PYLORI INFECTION

INDICATION	LEVEL OF RECOMMENDATION	ORGANISM	DOSE	REFERENCES
Augmentation of eradication therapy	C	Lyophilized L. acidophilus (Lactéol Fort)	tid	51
	B	AB-Yogurt	200 mL bid	52
	C	Will Korean Yogurt	150 mL qd	58
	C	Probinul + Bovine Lactoferrin (Lf100)	5 g Probinul bid + 100 mg Lf100 bid	53
Augmentation of second-line therapy	B	AB-Yogurt	200 mL bid	59
Prevention of eradication therapy side effects	C	L. reuteri ATCC 55730 (Reuterin)	1 tablet qd	61
	C	S. boulardii (Reflor)	500 mg bid	60
	C	Probinul + Bovine Lactoferrin (Lf100)	5 g Probinul bid + 100 mg Lf100 bid	61

AB-Yogurt contains L. acidophilus La5, B. lactis Bb12, L. bulgaricus, and S. thermophilus and is produced by the President Corp, Taiwan.

Will Yogurt contains L. acidophilus HY2177, L. casei HY2743, B. longum HY8001, and S. thermophilus B-1 and is produced by Korea Yakult Company Limited, South Korea.

Probinul contains L. plantarum, L. reuteri, L. casei ssp. rhamnosus, B. infantis, B. longum, L. salivarius, L. acidophilus, S. thermophilus, and L. sporogenes and is produced by Cadigroup.

Bovine Lactoferrin is sold as Lf100 and is produced by Dicofarm.

Lactéol Fort contains L. acidophilus strain LB (heat-killed organism) spent culture supernatant 80 mg, lactose monohydrate 50 mg, calcium carbonate 5 mg, silicic acid 20 mg, talc 7 mg, magnesium stearate 3 mg, anhydrous lactose 35 mg, and is produced by Bruschettini s.r.l., Italy.

Reuterin is L. reuteri ATCC 55730, produced by Nóos in Sweden.

Reflor is made by Sanofi-Synthelabo Ilac A.S. in Turkey

TABLE 22-2

PEDIATRIC: RECOMMENDATIONS FOR PROBIOTIC USE IN *HELICOBACTER PYLORI* INFECTION

INDICATION	LEVEL OF RECOMMENDATION	ORGANISM	DOSE	REFERENCES
Augmentation of eradication therapy	Insufficient data to recommend	*L. casei* DN114 in fermented milk	100 mL	63
Prevention of eradication therapy side effects	Insufficient data to recommend	*L. reuteri* SD2112	1 pill (10^8 CFU) qd	64
Probiotic monotherapy in asymptomatic kids	Insufficient data to recommend	*L. johnsonii* (La1)	80 mL (>10^7 CFU/mL) qd	65

Levels of recommendation based on The UK National Health Service categories.
- Level A: Consistent randomized controlled clinical trial, cohort study, clinical decision rule validated in different populations.
- Level B: Consistent retrospective cohort, exploratory cohort, ecological study, outcomes research, case-control study; or extrapolations from level A studies.
- Level C: Case-series study or extrapolations from level B studies.
- Level D: Expert opinion without explicit critical appraisal, or based on physiology, bench research or first principles.

added to the regimen.[66] This is the same trial cited above that failed to show an effect on eradication rates.

CONCLUSION

The rationale for the use of probiotics in the treatment of *H. pylori* infections is solid. Several animal and early clinical studies have shown promise using various probiotic organisms to decrease *H. pylori* colonization or increase eradication of *H. pylori*. Despite very promising results in single studies showing efficacy of probiotics for *H. pylori* infection, there are no replication trials in the literature that confirm these findings. As such, it is hard to make any definitive recommendations for the use of probiotics in the treatment or prevention of *H. pylori* infection or for its use to decrease the side effects associated with standard eradication therapy. For example, 2 different probiotic yogurts were effective in increasing eradication rates of *H. pylori* in combination with triple therapy,[53,59] while a third probiotic yogurt trial showed no change in eradication rates.[63] The only probiotic product that has shown success in more than one RCT involving *H. pylori* is the Taiwanese AB-Yogurt.[53,60] Yet the interventions in the trials were performed for different indications and cannot necessarily be interpreted as effective replication. For now, tentative recommendations have been given for the use of specific probiotic products that show promise (Tables 22-1 and 22-2).

REFERENCES

1. Allison MJ, Bergman T, Gerszten E. Further studies on fecal parasites in antiquity. *Am J Clin Pathol.* 1999;112(5):605-609.
2. Bizzozero G. Sulle ghiandole tubulari del tubo gastroenterico e sui rapporti del loro coll'epitelio di givestimento della mucosa. *Arch Mikr Anat.* 1893;42(1):82-152.
3. Egan BJ, O'Morain CA. A historical perspective of *Helicobacter gastroduodenitis* and its complications. *Best Pract Res Clin Gastroenterol.* 2007;21(2):335-346.
4. Marshall BJ, Warren JR. Unidentified curved bacilli in the stomach of patients with gastritis and peptic ulceration. *Lancet.* 1984;1(8390):1311-1315.
5. Dooley CP, Cohen H, Fitzgibbons PL, et al. Prevalence of *Helicobacter pylori* infection and histologic gastritis in asymptomatic persons. *N Engl J Med.* 1989;321(23):1562-1566.
6. Peterson WL. *Helicobacter pylori* and peptic ulcer disease. *N Engl J Med.* 1991;324(15):1043-1048.
7. Hunt RH. The role of *Helicobacter pylori* in pathogenesis: the spectrum of clinical outcomes. *Scand J Gastroenterol Suppl.* 1996;220:3-9.
8. Forbes GM, Glaser ME, Cullen DJ, et al. Duodenal ulcer treated with *Helicobacter pylori* eradication: seven-year follow-up. *Lancet.* 1994;343(8892):258-260.
9. Graham DY, Lew GM, Klein PD, et al. Effect of treatment of *Helicobacter pylori* infection on the long-term recurrence of gastric or duodenal ulcer. A randomized, controlled study. *Ann Intern Med.* 1992;116(9):705-708.
10. An international association between *Helicobacter pylori* infection and gastric cancer. The EUROGAST Study Group. *Lancet.* 1993;341(8857):1359-1362.
11. Graham DY. *Helicobacter pylori* infection is the primary cause of gastric cancer. *J Gastroenterol.* 2000;35(suppl 12):90-97.
12. Uemura N, Okamoto S, Yamamoto S, et al. *Helicobacter pylori* infection and the development of gastric cancer. *N Engl J Med.* 2001;345(11):784-789.
13. Schistosomes, liver flukes and *Helicobacter pylori*. IARC Working Group on the Evaluation of Carcinogenic Risks to Humans. Lyon, 7-14 June 1994. *IARC Monogr Eval Carcinog Risks Hum.* 1994;61:1-241.
14. Wong BC, Lam SK, Wong WM, et al. *Helicobacter pylori* eradication to prevent gastric cancer in a high-risk region of China: a randomized controlled trial. *JAMA.* 2004;291(2):187-194.
15. Mera R, Fontham ET, Bravo LE, et al. Long term follow up of patients treated for *Helicobacter pylori* infection. *Gut.* 2005;54(11):1536-1540.
16. Glupczynski Y. Antimicrobial resistance in *Helicobacter pylori*: a global overview. *Acta Gastroenterol Belg.* 1998;61(3):357-366.
17. Megraud F, Doermann HP. Clinical relevance of resistant strains of *Helicobacter pylori*: a review of current data. *Gut.* 1998;43(suppl 1):S61-S65.
18. Adamek RJ, Suerbaum S, Pfaffenbach B, Opferkuch W. Primary and acquired *Helicobacter pylori* resistance to clarithromycin, metronidazole, and amoxicillin—influence on treatment outcome. *Am J Gastroenterol.* 1998;93(3):386-389.
19. Murakami K, Kimoto M. Antibiotic-resistant *H. pylori* strains in the last ten years in Japan. *Nippon Rinsho.* 1999;57(1):81-86.
20. Fraser AG, Moore L, Hackett M, Hollis B. *Helicobacter pylori* treatment and antibiotic susceptibility: results of a five-year audit. *Aust N Z J Med.* 1999;29(4):512-516.
21. McMahon BJ, Hennessy TW, Bensler JM, et al. The relationship among previous antimicrobial use, antimicrobial resistance, and treatment outcomes for *Helicobacter pylori* infections. *Ann Intern Med.* 2003;139(6):463-469.
22. Malfertheiner P, Megraud F, O'Morain C, et al. Current concepts in the management of *Helicobacter pylori* infection: the Maastricht III Consensus Report. *Gut.* 2007;56(6):772-781.
23. Jafri NS, Hornung CA, Howden CW. Meta-analysis: sequential therapy appears superior to standard therapy for *Helicobacter pylori* infection in patients naive to treatment. *Ann Intern Med.* 2008;148(12):923-931.
24. Elliott SN, Buret A, McKnight W, Miller MJ, Wallace JL. Bacteria rapidly colonize and modulate healing of gastric ulcers in rats. *Am J Physiol.* 1998;275(3, pt 1):G425-G432.
25. Nagaoka M, Hashimoto S, Watanabe T, Yokokura T, Mori Y. Anti-ulcer effects of lactic acid bacteria and their cell wall polysaccharides. *Biol Pharm Bull.* 1994;17(8):1012-1017.
26. Oh Y, Osato MS, Han X, Bennett G, Hong WK. Folk yoghurt kills *Helicobacter pylori*. *J Appl Microbiol.* 2002;93(6):1083-1088.
27. Lesbros-Pantoflickova D, Corthesy-Theulaz I, Blum AL. *Helicobacter pylori* and probiotics. *J Nutr.* 2007;137(3, suppl 2):812S-818S.

28. Aiba Y, Suzuki N, Kabir AM, Takagi A, Koga Y. Lactic acid-mediated suppression of *Helicobacter pylori* by the oral administration of *Lactobacillus salivarius* as a probiotic in a gnotobiotic murine model. *Am J Gastroenterol.* 1998;93(11):2097-2101.

29. Cats A, Kuipers EJ, Bosschaert MA, Pot RG, Vandenbroucke-Grauls CM, Kusters JG. Effect of frequent consumption of a *Lactobacillus casei*-containing milk drink in *Helicobacter pylori*-colonized subjects. *Aliment Pharmacol Ther.* 2003;17(3):429-435.

30. Bernet-Camard MF, Lievin V, Brassart D, Neeser JR, Servin AL, Hudault S. The human *Lactobacillus acidophilus* strain LA1 secretes a nonbacteriocin antibacterial substance(s) active in vitro and in vivo. *Appl Environ Microbiol.* 1997;63(7):2747-2753.

31. Coconnier MH, Lievin V, Hemery E, Servin AL. Antagonistic activity against *Helicobacter* infection in vitro and in vivo by the human *Lactobacillus acidophilus* strain LB. *Appl Environ Microbiol.* 1998;64(11):4573-4580.

32. Michetti P, Dorta G, Wiesel PH, et al. Effect of whey-based culture supernatant of *Lactobacillus acidophilus* (*johnsonii*) La1 on *Helicobacter pylori* infection in humans. *Digestion.* 1999;60(3):203-209.

33. Kim TS, Hur JW, Yu MA, et al. Antagonism of *Helicobacter pylori* by bacteriocins of lactic acid bacteria. *J Food Prot.* 2003;66(1):3-12.

34. Guruge JL, Falk PG, Lorenz RG, et al. Epithelial attachment alters the outcome of *Helicobacter pylori* infection. *Proc Natl Acad Sci U S A.* 1998;95(7):3925-3930.

35. Nam H, Ha M, Bae O, Lee Y. Effect of Weissella confusa strain PL9001 on the adherence and growth of *Helicobacter pylori. Appl Environ Microbiol.* 2002;68(9):4642-4645.

36. Mukai T, Asasaka T, Sato E, Mori K, Matsumoto M, Ohori H. Inhibition of binding of *Helicobacter pylori* to the glycolipid receptors by probiotic *Lactobacillus reuteri. FEMS Immunol Med Microbiol.* 2002;32(2):105-110.

37. Byrd JC, Yunker CK, Xu QS, Sternberg LR, Bresalier RS. Inhibition of gastric mucin synthesis by *Helicobacter pylori. Gastroenterology.* 2000;118(6):1072-1079.

38. Mack DR, Michail S, Wei S, McDougall L, Hollingsworth MA. Probiotics inhibit enteropathogenic *E. coli* adherence in vitro by inducing intestinal mucin gene expression. *Am J Physiol.* 1999;276(4, pt 1):G941-G950.

39. Mack DR, Ahrne S, Hyde L, Wei S, Hollingsworth MA. Extracellular MUC3 mucin secretion follows adherence of *Lactobacillus* strains to intestinal epithelial cells in vitro. *Gut.* 2003;52(6):827-833.

40. Ernst PB, Michetti P, Smith PD. *The Immunobiology of H. pylori: From Pathogenesis to Prevention.* Philadelphia, PA: Lippincott-Raven; 1997.

41. Noach LA, Bosma NB, Jansen J, Hoek FJ, van Deventer SJ, Tytgat GN. Mucosal tumor necrosis factor-alpha, interleukin-1 beta, and interleukin-8 production in patients with *Helicobacter pylori* infection. *Scand J Gastroenterol.* 1994;29(5):425-429.

42. Kabir AM, Aiba Y, Takagi A, Kamiya S, Miwa T, Koga Y. Prevention of *Helicobacter pylori* infection by lactobacilli in a gnotobiotic murine model. *Gut.* 1997;41(1):49-55.

43. von der Weid T, Bulliard C, Schiffrin EJ. Induction by a lactic acid bacterium of a population of CD4(+) T cells with low proliferative capacity that produce transforming growth factor beta and interleukin-10. *Clin Diagn Lab Immunol.* 2001;8(4):695-701.

44. Haller D, Bode C, Hammes WP, Pfeifer AM, Schiffrin EJ, Blum S. Non-pathogenic bacteria elicit a differential cytokine response by intestinal epithelial cell/leucocyte co-cultures. *Gut.* 2000;47(1):79-87.

45. Sgouras D, Maragkoudakis P, Petraki K, et al. In vitro and in vivo inhibition of *Helicobacter pylori* by *Lactobacillus casei* strain Shirota. *Appl Environ Microbiol.* 2004;70(1):518-526.

46. Imase K, Tanaka A, Tokunaga K, Sugano H, Ishida H, Takahashi S. *Lactobacillus reuteri* tablets suppress *Helicobacter pylori* infection—a double-blind randomised placebo-controlled cross-over clinical study. *Kansenshogaku Zasshi.* 2007;81(4):387-393.

47. Jarosz M, Rychlik E, Siuba M, et al. Dietary and socio-economic factors in relation to *Helicobacter pylori* re-infection. *World J Gastroenterol.* 2009;15(9):1119-1125.

48. Felley CP, Corthesy-Theulaz I, Rivero JL, et al. Favourable effect of an acidified milk (LC-1) on *Helicobacter pylori* gastritis in man. *Eur J Gastroenterol Hepatol.* 2001;13(1):25-29.

49. Pantoflickova D, Corthesy-Theulaz I, Dorta G, et al. Favourable effect of regular intake of fermented milk containing *Lactobacillus johnsonii* on *Helicobacter pylori* associated gastritis. *Aliment Pharmacol Ther.* 2003;18(8):805-813.

50. Shimbo I, Yamaguchi T, Odaka T, et al. Effect of *Clostridium butyricum* on fecal flora in *Helicobacter pylori* eradication therapy. *World J Gastroenterol.* 2005;11(47):7520-7524.

51. Zullo A, Perna F, Ricci C, et al. 13C-urea breath test values and *Helicobacter pylori* eradication. *Dig Dis Sci.* 2008;53(2):370-374.

52. Canducci F, Armuzzi A, Cremonini F, et al. A lyophilized and inactivated culture of *Lactobacillus acidophilus* increases *Helicobacter pylori* eradication rates. *Aliment Pharmacol Ther.* 2000;14(12):1625-1629.

53. Sheu BS, Wu JJ, Lo CY, et al. Impact of supplement with *Lactobacillus-* and *Bifidobacterium*-containing yogurt on triple therapy for *Helicobacter pylori* eradication. *Aliment Pharmacol Ther.* 2002;16(9): 1669-1675.

54. de Bortoli N, Leonardi G, Ciancia E, et al. *Helicobacter pylori* eradication: a randomized prospective study of triple therapy versus triple therapy plus lactoferrin and probiotics. *Am J Gastroenterol.* 2007;102(5):951-956.

55. Britigan BE, Serody JS, Cohen MS. The role of lactoferrin as an anti-inflammatory molecule. *Adv Exp Med Biol.* 1994;357:143-156.

56. Ellison RT III. The effects of lactoferrin on gram-negative bacteria. *Adv Exp Med Biol.* 1994;357:71-90.

57. Lonnerdal B, Iyer S. Lactoferrin: molecular structure and biological function. *Annu Rev Nutr.* 1995;15: 93-110.

58. Dial EJ, Hall LR, Serna H, Romero JJ, Fox JG, Lichtenberger LM. Antibiotic properties of bovine lactoferrin on *Helicobacter pylori. Dig Dis Sci.* 1998;43(12):2750-2756.

59. Kim MN, Kim N, Lee SH, et al. The effects of probiotics on PPI-triple therapy for *Helicobacter pylori* eradication. *Helicobacter.* 2008;13(4):261-268.

60. Sheu BS, Cheng HC, Kao AW, et al. Pretreatment with *Lactobacillus-* and *Bifidobacterium*-containing yogurt can improve the efficacy of quadruple therapy in eradicating residual *Helicobacter pylori* infection after failed triple therapy. *Am J Clin Nutr.* 2006;83(4):864-869.

61. Cindoruk M, Erkan G, Karakan T, Dursun A, Unal S. Efficacy and safety of *Saccharomyces boulardii* in the 14-day triple anti-*Helicobacter pylori* therapy: a prospective randomized placebo-controlled double-blind study. *Helicobacter.* 2007;12(4):309-316.

62. Francavilla R, Lionetti E, Castellaneta SP, et al. Inhibition of *Helicobacter pylori* infection in humans by *Lactobacillus reuteri* ATCC 55730 and effect on eradication therapy: a pilot study. *Helicobacter.* 2008;13(2):127-134.

63. Gotteland M, Poliak L, Cruchet S, Brunser O. Effect of regular ingestion of *Saccharomyces boulardii* plus inulin or *Lactobacillus acidophilus* LB in children colonized by *Helicobacter pylori. Acta Paediatr.* 2005;94(12):1747-1751.

64. Goldman CG, Barrado DA, Balcarce N, et al. Effect of a probiotic food as an adjuvant to triple therapy for eradication of *Helicobacter pylori* infection in children. *Nutrition.* 2006;22(10):984-988.

65. Sykora J, Valeckova K, Amlerova J, et al. Effects of a specially designed fermented milk product containing probiotic *Lactobacillus casei* DN-114 001 and the eradication of *H. pylori* in children: a prospective randomized double-blind study. *J Clin Gastroenterol.* 2005;39(8):692-698.

66. Lionetti E, Miniello VL, Castellaneta SP, et al. *Lactobacillus reuteri* therapy to reduce side-effects during anti-*Helicobacter pylori* treatment in children: a randomized placebo controlled trial. *Aliment Pharmacol Ther.* 2006;24(10):1461-1468.

Probiotics in Liver Disease

Adam S. Kim, MD and Anish Sheth, MD

Liver disease is a broad term that implies liver dysfunction or damage, and covers anything from slight abnormalities in biochemical tests to cirrhosis and fulminant liver failure. The liver performs many functions including the formation and excretion of bile, regulation of carbohydrate homeostasis, lipid synthesis, control of cholesterol metabolism, formation of numerous proteins (such as albumin and clotting factors), and metabolism or detoxification of drugs and other substances.[1] Abnormalities in any of these functions can be considered "liver disease." Common symptoms associated with liver disease are mostly nonspecific and include pruritus, jaundice, GI bleeding, right upper quadrant abdominal pain, fatigue, weakness, and nausea. When liver disease becomes advanced, common complications include variceal hemorrhage, ascites, edema, encephalopathy, and bacterial infections. Those with advanced liver disease are especially prone to infections by Gram-negative bacteria, and this is likely attributable to increased bacterial translocation of gut flora as well as increased small intestinal bacterial overgrowth.[2]

The use of probiotics in the treatment of liver diseases may not be entirely obvious, but their use is based on logical assumptions. Several mainstays of treatment for complications of end-stage liver disease, such as lactulose and poorly absorbable antibiotics, are targeted at intestinal bacteria. Lactulose, a poorly absorbable sugar used for treating hepatic encephalopathy, breaks down to SCFA that acidify the gut and thereby limit the systemic absorption of ammonia[3,4] (ammonia being a key neurotoxin implicated in the pathogenesis of hepatic encephalopathy[5]). Lactulose also increases fecal bifidobacterial counts and decreases the counts of urease-producing bacteria that are capable of producing ammonia.[6] Poorly absorbable antibiotics, such as rifaximin, are also successful in treating hepatic encephalopathy,[7] by decreasing counts of urease-producing bacteria that produce ammonia.[8] Another antibiotic commonly used in end-stage liver disease is the quinolone norfloxacin. Norfloxacin can decrease spontaneous infections in cirrhotic patients[9,10] and is commonly used as a prophylactic medication to prevent infections or reinfections.

The observed benefits of lactulose and poorly absorbable antibiotics may work by limiting bacterial translocation of intestinal bacteria (or their surrogate marker,

Floch MH, Kim AS, eds.
Probiotics: A Clinical Guide (pp 307-320)
© 2010 Taylor & Francis Group

endotoxins) to mesenteric lymph nodes and to the systemic circulation. Bacterial translocation is known to occur not only in situations such as sepsis or trauma,[11] but also in cirrhosis.[12] In cirrhosis, bacterial translocation is thought to play a major role in spontaneous infections and in the hyperdynamic circulatory state of cirrhosis[13] that is defined by portal hypertension, ascites, and the hepatorenal syndrome. Bacterial translocation in cirrhosis models has specifically been shown to coincide with pronounced endotoxin-driven proinflammatory cytokine release.[14,15] Because probiotics have been shown to decrease bacterial translocation in burn models,[16] colitis models,[17] and animal models of pancreatitis,[18] it was assumed that they could decrease bacterial translocation in liver diseases. On the basis of this background knowledge, probiotics were tested in animal models of liver disease and later in clinical trials.

This chapter will focus on areas with the most data regarding the use of probiotics in liver disease: fatty liver disease, infection prevention, hepatic encephalopathy, and modulation of liver function (Table 23-1).

FATTY LIVER DISEASE

Hepatic steatosis is a reversible condition of fat vacuole accumulation inside of the liver, whereas steatohepatitis refers to fat accumulation together with inflammation. In the past, steatohepatitis was commonly found with alcoholic liver disease and hepatitis C infection, but, of late, it has become increasingly identified in patients without significant alcohol use or hepatitis C infection. Many of these newly recognized patients with steatohepatitis have the metabolic syndrome, characterized by abdominal obesity, elevated fasting glucose, hypertension, and dyslipidemia. When steatohepatitis is not associated with excessive alcohol use, it is termed nonalcoholic steatohepatitis (NASH) or the more widely accepted term, nonalcoholic fatty liver disease (NAFLD). NAFLD is a broad term that can refer to steatosis, steatohepatitis, steatohepatitis with progression to fibrosis, or even to cirrhosis. It is now recognized as the most common cause of abnormal liver tests in the United States.[19] NAFLD should also be differentiated from other secondary causes of steatosis and steatohepatitis, such as from malnutrition, drugs or other toxins, acute fatty liver of pregnancy, HIV, and IBD.[20] NAFLD affects 10% to 24% of the general population in industrialized countries, and the prevalence is as high as 57% to 75% in obese persons. There are also alarming rates of NAFLD in children, with a prevalence of 2.6% in children and 22% to 53% in obese children. On the basis of recent estimates, there may be 30 million Americans with steatosis and 9 million with steatohepatitis.[20]

Many patients with NAFLD experience no symptoms, although some report malaise or right upper quadrant pain. There are few physical examination findings with NAFLD, but some patients may have an enlarged liver. Laboratory tests often reveal isolated elevations of aspartate aminotransferase (AST) and/or alanine aminotransferase (ALT), while findings of elevated International Normalized Ratio (INR), low albumin, low platelets, and elevated bilirubin may indicate progression to cirrhosis. The evaluation may include liver ultrasound or abdominal CT scan to help make the diagnosis: both modalities have very good sensitivity and specificity for steatosis.[21,22] While liver biopsy commonly reveals steatosis, a mixed-inflammatory cell infiltrate, hepatocyte ballooning, Mallory's hyaline, and fibrosis, these are nonspecific for NAFLD. Liver biopsy is also helpful in establishing the stage of liver disease (or the degree of fibrosis). The diagnosis is largely one of exclusion, and one of the utilities of liver biopsy is to exclude other causes of abnormal liver aminotransferases. Although most patients with NAFLD have a very benign course, it is known that this disease can progress to significant

TABLE 23-1

RECOMMENDATIONS FOR PROBIOTIC USE IN LIVER DISEASE

DISEASE	LEVEL OF RECOMMENDATION	ORGANISM	DOSE	REFERENCES
NAFLD	Insufficient data to recommend			
Prevention of infection: peri-liver transplantation	B	Synbiotic 2000	1 sachet twice daily	61
	B	L. plantarum 299	1×10^9 twice daily	60
Minimal hepatic encephalopathy	B	Cocktail 2000	10^{10} CFU daily	53
	B	Combination Therapy (yogurt with live active cultures; Medilac; Bifco)	Varied	69,70
	B	B. longum	Not reported	71
Improving liver function	Insufficient data to recommend			

Our levels of recommendation will be based on The UK National Health Service categories:
- Level A: consistent randomized controlled clinical trial, cohort study, clinical decision rule validated in different populations.
- Level B: consistent retrospective cohort, exploratory cohort, ecological study, outcomes research, case-control study; or extrapolations from level A studies.
- Level C: Case-series study or extrapolations from level B studies.
- Level D: Expert opinion without explicit critical appraisal, or based on physiology, bench research or first principles.

fibrosis and even to cirrhosis and hepatocellular carcinoma (HCC).[20] As many as 13% of all cases of HCC in the United States can be attributed to NAFLD.[23] The mainstays of NAFLD treatment focus on gradual weight loss and increased physical activity, along with improved control of blood glucose and lipids. Other therapies have been studied but are not clearly proven, and were recently reviewed by Vuppalanchi et al.[24] For the morbidly obese with NAFLD and significant liver fibrosis, bariatric surgery has been recommended as a last resort before patients develop frank cirrhosis.

The rationale for the use of probiotics for fatty liver diseases stems from the ability of probiotics to prevent bacterial translocation and to reduce proinflammatory cytokines such as TNF-α.[25] It is thought that by decreasing bacterial translocation in liver diseases, probiotics can lessen the stimulatory effects that bacterial translocation and endotoxemia have on the production of TNF-α by hepatic macrophages (also known as Kupffer cells). Endotoxin is a structural component of bacteria, such as lipopolysaccharide (LPS) in Gram-negative bacteria, and is a major factor in the ability of certain bacteria to cause disease. In many studies, endotoxin levels are used as a surrogate for bacterial translocation of Gram-negative bacteria. Because Gram-negative bacteria are known to trigger numerous complications of liver disease, it is hypothesized that decreasing bacterial translocation (or endotoxin levels) could reduce the negative effects of fatty liver disease. TNF-α has been shown to both stimulate hepatic fibrosis and to contribute to the development of fatty liver disease,[26] and anti-TNF therapy has even been shown to be effective in improving liver function in NAFLD.[27,28]

There are numerous animal studies that have opened the door for the use of probiotics in humans with fatty liver disease. One mouse model with a combination probiotic, VSL#3, used the methionine choline-deficient diet-induced mouse model of NASH. VSL#3 is a patented probiotic product containing 8 different LAB: *B. breve, B. longum, B. infantis, L. acidophilus, L. plantarum, L. casei, L. bulgaricus,* and *S. thermophilus.* In this trial, probiotics had no effect on histologic steatosis, histologic inflammation, or liver TNF-α, but did ameliorate the increase in liver collagen and α-smooth muscle actin, and may have had an effect on preventing liver fibrosis.[29]

A study by Li et al used ob/ob mice, which have a mutation in the gene for leptin causing them to eat excessively and become extremely obese. These mice were fed a high-fat diet for 4 weeks and had significant improvements in histologic steatosis, liver fatty acid content, and serum ALT and NF-κB after VSL#3 treatment.[30] Interestingly, the same effects were also found by treating the mice with the anti-TNF antibody Infliximab.

Another mouse study showed amelioration of fatty liver caused by ethanol intake after the intake of heat-killed *L. brevis* SBC8803.[31] They postulated that the killed LAB inhibited gut-derived endotoxin migration to the liver by showing that cytoprotective heat-shock proteins were upregulated in the small intestine. In addition, this study showed that they could suppress the overexpression of TNF-α and sterol regulatory element-binding proteins in the liver by using a heat-killed organism. This suggests that cellular components of probiotics could be effective in humans, even if the probiotics are not alive when consumed. They were expanding upon work from the 1990s that showed that LGG could ameliorate serum endotoxin levels and pathologic liver damage during ethanol-induced liver injury in rats.[25] In a final mouse study, VSL#3 treatment ameliorated weight gain, histologic steatosis, and elevated serum glucose levels in C57BL6 mice fed a high-fat diet for 12 weeks.[32]

Currently, there are only 3 human trials that have investigated the use of probiotics for the treatment of NAFLD. The first trial was a very small open-label trial using VSL#3. Four human subjects with NAFLD were given 1 sachet of VSL#3 daily for 4 months, and liver fat was measured by proton magnetic resonance spectroscopy.[33] Unfortunately, all 4 subjects had an increase in liver fat at the end of 4 months, and 3 of the 4 subjects experienced the predefined "meaningful" increase (greater than 3% change). The second human trial was also a very small open-label study comprising 10 patients with biopsy-proven steatohepatitis with elevated ALT and/or gamma glutamyl transpeptidase (GGT) at baseline. After 2 months of treatment with a combination of LAB, FOS, vitamins, and minerals, the patients had a significant decrease in ALT (by 65%) and GGT (by 55%) at the end of treatment ($P < .01$).[34] Unfortunately, this effect was not maintained, and both ALT and GGT levels increased above baseline (+136% and +15%, $P < .01$ and $P < .05$) after 1 month washout. The probiotic used in this second trial, by Loguercio et al, contained *L. acidophilus, Bifidus, Rhamnosus, Plantarum, Salivarius, Bulgaricus, Lactis, Casei, Breve,* + FOS as prebiotic + vitamins B6, B2, B12, D3, and C + folic acid, zinc oxide, iron gluconate, and potassium iodide (Bio-Flora, Dermo Duemila, Italy).

The final clinical trial was also from Loguercio et al in Italy. They gave VSL#3 to 22 patients with biopsy-proven NAFLD for 3 months in an open-label fashion without controls. They showed a significant decrease in AST and ALT, and this effect was maintained after 1 month washout.[35] Given the lack of any randomized clinical trials using probiotics in NAFLD, no conclusions can be made about their use in human patients.[36]

PREVENTING INFECTIONS IN PATIENTS WITH LIVER DISEASE

It has long been known that patients with liver disease, and specifically those with cirrhosis, have high rates of bacterial infection.[37-39] Two large prospective series of cirrhotic patients showed that bacterial infections were documented in 32%[40] and 34%[41] of all hospitalizations. A population-based study in Denmark revealed that the incidence of bacteremia in more than 1300 cirrhotic patients was 10.5 times higher than the expected incidence in Danish adults living in the same geographic area.[42] The cirrhotic patients at the highest risk of developing bacterial infections are those with decompensated cirrhosis and those with GI bleeding. In a retrospective analysis of 1140 cirrhotic patients[43] and in a prospective analysis of 170 cirrhotic patients,[44] the highest rates of bacterial infection were in those with the most decompensated liver disease (based on Child-Pugh classification, a marker of severity of cirrhosis, taking into account 5 clinical variables). These infections come with significant morbidity, and higher mortality rates are observed in those cirrhotic patients who develop infections.[41] Variceal hemorrhage is a major risk factor for bacterial infection,[45,46] and the presence of bacterial infection after variceal bleed increases rates of variceal rebleeding.[47]

When cirrhotic patients become infected, the most common infection is spontaneous bacterial peritonitis, followed by urinary tract infections and pneumonia.[48] These infections are most commonly caused by Gram-negative bacilli such as *Escherichia coli*, indicating that the main source of bacteria is derived from the gut. More recent studies have shown a significantly higher rate of Gram-positive cocci infections,[40] thought to be related to increasing numbers of invasive procedures and the use of chronic antibiotic prophylaxis against Gram-negative bacteria. Increased intestinal permeability and increased bacterial translocation have been observed in cirrhotic patients in a number of different scenarios,[2] hinting at the possible mechanisms of increased infections. Cirrhotic patients, in particular, are thought to have a defective innate immune response with decreased neutrophil phagocytosis and intracellular killing of organisms.[49]

As stated earlier in this chapter, bacterial translocation is thought to be a major cause of bacterial infections in cirrhosis and of the hyperdynamic circulatory state of cirrhosis.[13] Because probiotics are known to decrease rates of bacterial translocation in a number of clinical scenarios, it is plausible that they would have a beneficial effect on limiting bacterial translocation in cirrhosis. Antibiotics targeting the enteric flora, such as fluoroquinolones, have long been used to prevent infections in cirrhosis.[10] In addition, infections can be catastrophic in cirrhotic patients, and often trigger events such as variceal rebleeding.[47] Therefore, there were supportive data to begin animal studies in order to test the hypothesis that probiotics could prevent infections in liver diseases.

There are many animal models of liver disease that have shown the effectiveness of probiotics to reduce rates of bacterial translocation. Ewaschuk et al used IL-10 gene-deficient mice and induced a sepsis-like state with LPS and D-galactosamine.[50] After pretreating the mice with VSL#3 for 7 days, they were able to prevent the breakdown of colonic barrier function, prevent bacterial translocation to the liver, as well as attenuate acute liver injury.

Two studies using probiotics to decrease bacterial translocation in cirrhotic rats had differing results, depending on which probiotic was used. The first used *L. johnsonii* La1 and antioxidants and showed a decrease in bacterial translocation and endotoxemia after 10 days of treatment.[51] The second used *L. rhamnosus* GG for 10 days in cirrhotic rats, but failed to show a decrease in bacterial translocation despite cecal colonization of LGG in 90% of treated subjects.[52]

Liu et al showed that cirrhotic patients with even minimal hepatic encephalopathy (MHE) had significantly higher levels of fecal *E. coli* and *Staphylococcus* species when compared to healthy controls.[53] After 30 days of treatment with a synbiotic preparation (containing *Pediacoccus pentosaceus* 5-33:3, *Leuconostoc mesenteroides* 32-77:1, *L. paracasei* subspecies *paracasei* 19, and *L. plantarum* 2592, and bioactive, fermentable fibers [Cocktail 2000; Medipharm, Kagerod, Sweden]), patients had significant reductions in *E. coli* and *Staphylococcus* species and increases in nonurease-producing *Lactobacillus* species. Lata et al also showed that in 39 cirrhotic patients randomized to 42 days of *E. coli* Nissle or placebo, the treated individuals had increased fecal *Lactobacillus* species and *Bifidobacterium* species with decreased pathogenic bacteria *Proteus hauseri*, *Citrobacter* species, and *Morganella* species, as well as decreased endotoxemia.[54]

Major liver resection is known to be a risk factor for bacterial infection, with infection rates reported in 11%[55] to 34% of patients.[56] One study of surgical mortality followed 165 patients and showed significantly increased mortality in combination liver resection and colonic resection when compared to liver resection alone (17 vs 1%).[57] In an animal study, rats subjected to liver resection and synchronous colonic anastamosis had lower rates of bacterial translocation to mesenteric lymph nodes when given oral probiotics and fiber pre- and postoperative, compared to those without probiotics.[58] The probiotic combination used contained *P. pentoseceus* 5-33:3, *Lactococcus raffinolactis* 32-77:1, *L. paracasei* subspecies *paracasei* 19, and *L. plantarum* 2362, as well as 0.2 g beta-glukan, inulin, pectin, and resistant starch.

Despite promising mechanistic and animal studies, there have not been many clinical trials that have used probiotics to treat or prevent infections in cirrhotic patients. There is 1 open-label clinical trial validating a proposed mechanism for the use of probiotics for preventing infection. In this trial, there was a return to baseline in neutrophil phagocytic capacity in 12 cirrhotic patients after 4 weeks of the probiotic *L. casei* Shirota.[59]

There are 2 single-center, prospective, randomized, placebo-controlled trials investigating the use of probiotics for limiting infections surrounding liver transplantation. The first of the 2 involved 105 liver transplantation patients who received early enteral nutrition beginning on the second postoperative day and continuing to postoperative day 12.[60] Patients were excluded if they had preoperative severe renal insufficiency, intestinal obstruction, cerebral disorders, or had anything other than a side-to-side biliary anastamosis. Ten patients did not complete the study because of early postoperative complications that precluded them from receiving early enteral nutrition such as laparotomy, ileus, or acute renal failure. The remaining 95 patients completed the intervention and were analyzed. The patients were randomized into 3 different groups that received (1) tube feeds plus selective bowel decontamination with antibiotics and antifungals, (2) tube feeds supplemented with fiber and *L. plantarum* 299, or (3) tube feeds supplemented with fiber and heat-killed *L. plantarum* 299 (placebo). The overall rate of bacterial infections was lower in the group that received *L. plantarum* 299 compared to those that received selective bowel decontamination (13% vs 48%, $P = .017$), but was not decreased in those that received heat-killed *L. plantarum* 299. There were no significant differences in number of days in the ICU or in the hospital, cumulative days of antibiotic therapy, or in any of the measured side effects.

The second study included 66 adult liver transplantation recipients who received early enteral nutrition.[61] Patients were randomized to receive supplements that contained 4 bioactive fibers, or 4 bioactive fibers plus a combination of 4 LAB (Synbiotic 2000: *P. pentosaceous* 5-33:3, *Leuc mesenteroides* 77:1, *L. paracasei* ssp. *paracasei* F19, *L. plantarum* 2362, betaglucan, inulin, pectin, and resistant starch). The primary endpoint was bacterial infections in the first 30 days postoperative. The group that received fibers plus LAB had lower rates of infection compared to those that did not receive the LAB (3% vs 48%, $P < .05$), without any differences in side effects. The group that received LAB also had a shorter duration of antibiotic therapy (0.1 vs 3.8 days, $P < .05$) but no change in length of hospital stay. In addition, no serious adverse events were found in either of these liver transplantation studies.

These 2 well-controlled studies should open the door for the use of probiotics surrounding liver transplantation. A recent Cochrane Review regarding preventing infections at the time of liver transplantation concluded that, "The use of prebiotics and probiotics offers promise."[62] It remains to be determined which exact probiotic, combination of probiotics, or combination of prebiotics and probiotics will be the most beneficial in this realm. RCTs should also be designed to investigate the use of probiotics in preventing bacterial infections in cirrhotic patients at high risk for infection, such as those with decompensation or GI bleeding, or those who are hospitalized. Although probiotics appear very safe for use in liver diseases, careful monitoring of adverse events should be maintained when probiotics are used in these transplant or cirrhotic patients with abnormal immune systems, especially after the unexpected deaths reported with the use of probiotics in severe acute pancreatitis.[63]

HEPATIC ENCEPHALOPATHY

Hepatic encephalopathy is a common complication of liver cirrhosis. It is defined as:

a syndrome of neuropsychiatric dysfunction caused by portosystemic venous shunting, with or without intrinsic liver disease. Patients with hepatic encephalopathy often present with the onset of mental status changes ranging from subtle psychological abnormalities to profound coma.[64]

It is often seen in conjunction with ascites, jaundice, and GI variceal bleeding. Hepatic encephalopathy is often disabling, and can prevent patients from working, driving, and caring for themselves. Patients with diabetes mellitus or malnutrition are more likely to develop encephalopathy.[65] Subclinical hepatic encephalopathy is also called MHE and presents a risk for developing overt hepatic encephalopathy.[66] Current treatments for hepatic encephalopathy center around the cathartic agent lactulose and poorly absorbable antibiotics. They work by decreasing stool transit time, which limits the absorption of toxic bacterial metabolites (eg, ammonia), and by inhibiting the growth of intestinal bacteria capable of producing ammonia (eg, urease-producing bacteria). As stated earlier, probiotics could have effects similar to these widely used treatments for hepatic encephalopathy, paving the way for animal studies to test this theory.

Animal studies have laid the groundwork for the use of probiotics in hepatic encephalopathy. In a study from Belgium, probiotics were used in 3 different rodent models of hyperammonemia.[67] The models were constitutive hyperammonemia in ornithine transcarbamoylase-deficient sparse-fur mice, thioacetamide-induced acute liver injury in C57BL/6 mice, and chronic liver insufficiency using phenobarbital and carbon tetrachloride in Lewis rats. In each of the models, oral treatment with *L. plantarum* NCIMB8826 significantly reduced serum levels of ammonia after treatment.

Another study, by Jia and Zhang, showed that probiotics or lactulose were equally good at preventing and treating MHE in rats.[68] Both the probiotic mixture and lactulose groups had significantly decreased serum ammonia and endotoxin levels when compared to the no-treatment arm, but did not have altered serum AST, ALT, or bilirubin levels. The probiotic mixture used was a combination of bifidobacteria, lactobacilli, and *S. thermophilus* strains (Golden Bifid, Shuangqi Pharmaceutical Co, Inner Mongolia, China).

Most of the clinical work on probiotics for hepatic encephalopathy is targeted at treating or preventing MHE. Liu et al studied the use of probiotics and fermentable fibers in the treatment of MHE.[53] In a randomized, placebo-controlled trial, they showed that patients receiving probiotics and/or fermentable fibers had decreased serum ammonia levels, decreased serum endotoxin levels, and significant improvements in MHE when compared to patients receiving placebo for 30 days. Their probiotic combination was called Cocktail 2000, which contains *P. pentoseceus* 5-33:3, *Leuc mesenteroides* 32-77:1, *L. paracasei* subspecies *paracasei* 19, and *L. plantarum* 2592, and bioactive, fermentable fibers.

Yogurts containing live cultures are a good vehicle for probiotic supplementation and have been studied in MHE. Yogurt is produced by the fermentation of lactic acid in milk, and the end product contains live *Lactobacillus* species. A clinical trial at the Medical College of Wisconsin used an over-the-counter yogurt (CC Jersey Crème, no longer produced) in the treatment of MHE.[69] This particular yogurt contains live active cultures of *L. bulgaricus*, *L. acidophilus*, *L. casei*, and *Bifidobacteria*, and *S. thermophilus* with good bacterial stability over 4 weeks time. In this small (n = 25), randomized, placebo-controlled trial, 71% of treated patients had resolution of their MHE after 60 days of use of yogurt, compared to 0% in the untreated group (P = .003). No patients in the yogurt group developed overt hepatic encephalopathy compared to 2 of 8 in the no-treatment group, but this was not statistically significant (P = 0.1).

A trial by a Chinese group used 2 commercially available probiotic combinations in 25 cirrhotic patients each.[70] After 14 days of treatment with Bifico (Shanhai Sine Pharmaceutical, containing *Bifidobacterium*, *L. acidophilus*, and *Enterococcus*) or Medilac-s (Beijing Hanmi Pharmaceutical, containing *B. subtilis* and *E. faecium*), subjects had a significant decrease (P < .05) in blood ammonia, fecal ammonia, and fecal pH, as well as increase in fecal *Bifidobacterium*. In addition, treatment with probiotics containing *B. subtilis* and *E. faecium* reduced the level of endotoxin in cirrhotic patients with endotoxemia.

A trial from Italy enrolled 60 cirrhotic patients with MHE into a randomized, placebo-controlled trial of *B. longum* W11 plus prebiotics in the form of FOS.[71] After 30, 60, and 90 days of treatment, the prebiotic plus probiotic group had significant improvements, when compared to placebo, in serum ammonia levels and in multiple neuropsychiatric tests such as trail-making tests A and B, the block design test, and the Mini Mental State Examination. These improvements were maintained up to 30 days posttreatment.

MODULATING LIVER FUNCTION

Probiotic use is associated with improved liver function in a number of animal and human studies. As stated earlier, probiotics have been shown to decrease bacterial translocation and, therefore, decrease proinflammatory cytokines. If proinflammatory cytokines, such as TNF-α, can be decreased by probiotics, then probiotics may be able to limit liver injury and improve liver function.

Animal studies have shown that acute liver injury can be improved by probiotics. After acute liver injury in rats with LPS and D-galactosamine, 8 days of supplementation with probiotics resulted in decreased levels of ALT (*B. infantis* DSM 15159), decreased total bilirubin (*B. infantis* and *L. plantarum* DSM 15313), and decreased rates of bacterial translocation (*L. plantarum*).[72] This study expanded upon an earlier study by some of the same authors with similar results, published in 2001.[73] Segawa et al showed that heat-inactivated *L. brevis* can ameliorate alcohol-induced liver injury in mice, with inhibition of increases in serum AST, ALT, liver TNF-α, and liver steatosis.[31] Nicaise et al showed that treatment with *L. plantarum* NCIMB8826 significantly improved survival when compared to placebo (80% vs 47.5% survival, respectively, $P < .05$) in a mouse model of acute liver injury using thioacetamide.[67] Ewaschuk et al showed decreased hepatic damage in a mouse model of sepsis by using VSL#3.[50] Finally, Marotta et al used probiotics (combination of *L. acidophilus*, *L. helveticus*, and *Bifidobacterium* in an enriched medium) to ameliorate cerulein- and alcohol-mediated pancreatitis and liver injury in rats.[74]

There are a handful of trials in humans with liver disease that looked at liver function or markers of acute liver injury after administration of probiotics, with somewhat mixed results. An open-label trial using a combination of probiotics (VSL#3) showed that chronic liver disease patients had significant improvement in their liver function tests (total protein, albumin, and total bilirubin) after treatment with the probiotics.[35] This included 22 patients with NAFLD, 20 with alcoholic cirrhosis, 20 with Hepatitis C hepatitis, and 16 with Hepatitis C cirrhosis. In addition, proinflammatory cytokines (IL-6, IL-10, and TNF-α) were improved in alcoholic cirrhosis patients, and markers of lipid peroxidation (malondialdehyde and 4-hydroxynonenal) were improved in NAFLD patients after use of probiotics.

A trial by Liu et al primarily investigating the treatment of MHE showed improvements in liver function after treatment with a combination of probiotics and fibers (Cocktail 2000).[53] In this trial, 55 cirrhotic patients (most with Hepatitis B cirrhosis) with MHE were randomized to receive probiotics plus fibers, fermentable fibers alone, or placebo with nonfermentable fiber for 30 days. After treatment, there was a significant improvement in not only Child-Pugh score in the probiotics and fibers group ($P = .04$), but also in total bilirubin ($P < .01$, $P = .03$), albumin ($P < .01$, $P < .01$), and ALT levels ($P < .01$, $P < .01$) in both the combination group and the fermentable-fibers-alone group (respectively).

A third human trial that was double-blind and randomized with 39 cirrhotic patients showed a nonsignificant trend toward improvement in Child-Pugh score after treatment with *E. coli* Nissle for 42 days ($P = .06$).[54] A more recent human trial showed improvements in liver enzymes with probiotics after alcohol injury.[75] In this study, 66 Russian patients with mild alcoholic hepatitis and psychiatric illness were randomized to 5 days of *B. bifidum* and *L. plantarum* 8PA3 vs standard therapy, which was abstinence and vitamins. And the end of treatment, the probiotic arm had significantly lower AST and ALT levels compared to standard therapy. In a post-hoc subgroup, analysis of patients with AST and ALT above 30 U/L and an AST-to-ALT ratio greater than 1, there were also significant decreases in lactate dehydrogenase and total bilirubin in the probiotic treatment arm.

MISCELLANEOUS

There are 2 important clinical trials that evaluated the use of probiotics in primary sclerosing cholangitis (PSC) and in decreasing hepatic carcinogens. One human trial investigated the use of probiotics in patients with PSC.[76] The authors theorized that by decreasing bacterial translocation and proinflammatory cytokines, probiotics may be able to improve the liver injury and bacterial infections common to PSC. Fourteen PSC patients with concurrent IBD were randomized to 3 months with probiotics or placebo, followed by 1-month washout, and then a crossover to the opposite treatment for 3 months. No significant changes were noted between the groups when looking at pruritus, fatigue, stool frequency, bilirubin, alkaline phosphatase, GGT, AST, ALT, prothrombin, albumin, or bile salts. In this trial, the probiotic combination was 6 bacteria (*L. acidophilus*, *L. casei*, *L. salivarius*, *Lact lactis*, *B. bifidum*, and *B. lactis*) along with starch, sugar, minerals, and amylases, which is sold as Ecologic 641 (Winclove Bio Industries, Amsterdam, The Netherlands).

One early mechanistic clinical trial examined the effects of probiotics on decreasing levels of a class of carcinogens known to cause HCC, the aflatoxins.[77] The study authors hypothesized that probiotics could decrease serum levels of the hepatocarcinogen aflatoxin B_1, which is found in food products and is thought to increase rates of HCC, particularly in chronic hepatitis B patients. After showing that *L. rhamnosus* could bind aflatoxins in vitro[78] and in vivo (in chickens),[79] the authors planned this clinical trial. Ninety healthy male Chinese students with elevated baseline levels of serum aflatoxins were randomized to receive 5 weeks of placebo or *L. rhamnosus* LC705 and *Propionibacterium freudenreichii* ssp. *shermanii*. Treatment with probiotics significantly decreased urinary excretion of a surrogate marker for serum aflatoxin B_1 called aflatoxin B_1-N^7-guanine (AFB-N^7-guanine). This may be clinically relevant as increased urinary AFB-N^7-guanine levels have been associated with increased risk of liver cancer in a case-control study,[80] and decreased AFB-N^7-guanine levels in animal models has been associated with decreased rates of HCC.[81]

SAFETY

Probiotics appear extremely safe for use in patients with liver disease. Although side effects such as bloating, nausea, and headache have been reported, there are no reports of serious adverse events (bacteremia, sepsis, multiorgan failure, death) in any of these studies or in a search for other related case reports. However, not all of the clinical trials referenced in this chapter reported on side effects or adverse events, which makes it difficult to generalize about safety. In light of the above-mentioned deaths in a randomized, placebo-controlled trial using probiotics in severe acute pancreatitis, all future clinical trials using probiotics in liver disease should monitor for and report on adverse events, signs of infection, and death.

FUTURE DIRECTIONS

The use of probiotics in liver disease remains in its infancy. Although there is plausible mechanistic theories for their effectiveness and numerous animal studies that may lead to promising treatments in humans, much of this realm remains unstudied. In NAFLD, there are only open-label studies of probiotics, and randomized controlled trials are needed, potentially with VSL#3 or another combination product. In the prevention of infections, open-label and small, randomized trials are first needed to investigate the use of probiotics in at-risk cirrhotic patients, such as those with GI bleeding, spontaneous bacterial infection, or significant liver decompensation. With regard to liver transplantation, the positive findings need to be replicated in an independent cohort of patients. The use of yogurts or probiotics for the treatment of MHE looks especially promising and should also be replicated. For improving liver function in cirrhotics, replication studies with VSL#3 or Cocktail 2000 are needed. Currently, there is an ongoing study using combination probiotics, aimed at reducing the hyperdynamic circulatory state of cirrhosis. In acute liver injury from alcohol, replication of the positive findings with *B. bifidum* and *L. plantarum* 8PA3 also require replication. Finally, the use of probiotics to decrease risk of HCC in at-risk (Hepatitis B) patients needs further clarification.

REFERENCES

1. Simon JB. Approach to the patient with liver disease. The Merck Manual Online Web site. http://www.merck.com/mmpe/sec03/ch022/ch022a.html. Published 2005. Updated 2009. Accessed 04/02/2009.
2. Almeida J, Galhenage S, Yu J, Kurtovic J, Riordan SM. Gut flora and bacterial translocation in chronic liver disease. *World J Gastroenterol*. 2006;12(10):1493-1502.
3. Patil DH, Westaby D, Mahida YR, et al. Comparative modes of action of lactitol and lactulose in the treatment of hepatic encephalopathy. *Gut*. 1987;28(3):255-259.
4. De Preter V, Vanhoutte T, Huys G, Swings J, Rutgeerts P, Verbeke K. Effect of lactulose and *Saccharomyces boulardii* administration on the colonic urea-nitrogen metabolism and the bifidobacteria concentration in healthy human subjects. *Aliment Pharmacol Ther*. 2006;23(7):963-974.
5. Butterworth RF. The neurobiology of hepatic encephalopathy. *Semin Liver Dis*. 1996;16(3):235-244.
6. Bouhnik Y, Attar A, Joly FA, Riottot M, Dyard F, Flourie B. Lactulose ingestion increases faecal bifidobacterial counts: a randomised double-blind study in healthy humans. *Eur J Clin Nutr*. 2004;58(3):462-466.
7. Williams R, James OF, Warnes TW, Morgan MY. Evaluation of the efficacy and safety of rifaximin in the treatment of hepatic encephalopathy: a double-blind, randomized, dose-finding multi-centre study. *Eur J Gastroenterol Hepatol*. 2000;12(2):203-208.
8. Hoover WW, Gerlach EH, Hoban DJ, Eliopoulos GM, Pfaller MA, Jones RN. Antimicrobial activity and spectrum of rifaximin, a new topical rifamycin derivative. *Diagn Microbiol Infect Dis*. 1993;16(2):111-118.
9. Maclayton DO, Eaton-Maxwell A. Rifaximin for treatment of hepatic encephalopathy. *Ann Pharmacother*. 2009;43(1):77-84.
10. Gines P, Rimola A, Planas R, et al. Norfloxacin prevents spontaneous bacterial peritonitis recurrence in cirrhosis: results of a double-blind, placebo-controlled trial. *Hepatology*. 1990;12(4, pt 1):716-724.
11. Woodruff PW, O'Carroll DI, Koizumi S, Fine J. Role of the intestinal flora in major trauma. *J Infect Dis*. 1973;128(suppl):290-294.
12. Garcia-Tsao G, Lee FY, Barden GE, Cartun R, West AB. Bacterial translocation to mesenteric lymph nodes is increased in cirrhotic rats with ascites. *Gastroenterology*. 1995;108(6):1835-1841.
13. Garcia-Tsao G, Wiest R. Gut microflora in the pathogenesis of the complications of cirrhosis. *Best Pract Res Clin Gastroenterol*. 2004;18(2):353-372.
14. Perez-Paramo M, Munoz J, Albillos A, et al. Effect of propranolol on the factors promoting bacterial translocation in cirrhotic rats with ascites. *Hepatology*. 2000;31(1):43-48.
15. Wiest R, Das S, Cadelina G, Garcia-Tsao G, Milstien S, Groszmann RJ. Bacterial translocation in cirrhotic rats stimulates eNOS-derived NO production and impairs mesenteric vascular contractility. *J Clin Invest*. 1999;104(9):1223-1233.
16. Gun F, Salman T, Gurler N, Olgac V. Effect of probiotic supplementation on bacterial translocation in thermal injury. *Surg Today*. 2005;35(9):760-764.
17. Pavan S, Desreumaux P, Mercenier A. Use of mouse models to evaluate the persistence, safety, and immune modulation capacities of lactic acid bacteria. *Clin Diagn Lab Immunol*. 2003;10(4):696-701.
18. van Minnen LP, Timmerman HM, Lutgendorff F, et al. Modification of intestinal flora with multispecies probiotics reduces bacterial translocation and improves clinical course in a rat model of acute pancreatitis. *Surgery*. 2007;141(4):470-480.
19. Clark JM, Brancati FL, Diehl AM. Nonalcoholic fatty liver disease. *Gastroenterology*. 2002;122(6):1649-1657.
20. Angulo P. Nonalcoholic fatty liver disease. *N Engl J Med*. 2002;346(16):1221-1231.
21. Joseph AE, Saverymuttu SH, al-Sam S, Cook MG, Maxwell JD. Comparison of liver histology with ultrasonography in assessing diffuse parenchymal liver disease. *Clin Radiol*. 1991;43(1):26-31.

22. Saadeh S, Younossi ZM, Remer EM, et al. The utility of radiological imaging in nonalcoholic fatty liver disease. *Gastroenterology.* 2002;123(3):745-750.
23. Marrero JA, Fontana RJ, Su GL, Conjeevaram HS, Emick DM, Lok AS. NAFLD may be a common underlying liver disease in patients with hepatocellular carcinoma in the United States. *Hepatology.* 2002;36(6):1349-1354.
24. Vuppalanchi R, Chalasani N. Nonalcoholic fatty liver disease and nonalcoholic steatohepatitis: selected practical issues in their evaluation and management. *Hepatology.* 2009;49(1):306-317.
25. Nanji AA, Khettry U, Sadrzadeh SM. *Lactobacillus* feeding reduces endotoxemia and severity of experimental alcoholic liver (disease). *Proc Soc Exp Biol Med.* 1994;205(3):243-247.
26. Diehl AM. Nonalcoholic steatosis and steatohepatitis IV. Nonalcoholic fatty liver disease abnormalities in macrophage function and cytokines. *Am J Physiol Gastrointest Liver Physiol.* 2002;282(1):G1-G5.
27. Li Z, Yang S, Lin H, et al. Probiotics and antibodies to TNF inhibit inflammatory activity and improve nonalcoholic fatty liver disease. *Hepatology.* 2003;37(2):343-350.
28. Pappo I, Bercovier H, Berry E, Gallilly R, Feigin E, Freund HR. Antitumor necrosis factor antibodies reduce hepatic steatosis during total parenteral nutrition and bowel rest in the rat. *JPEN J Parenter Enteral Nutr.* 1995;19(1):80-82.
29. Velayudham A, Dolganiuc A, Ellis M, et al. VSL#3 probiotic treatment attenuates fibrosis without changes in steatohepatitis in a diet-induced nonalcoholic steatohepatitis model in mice. *Hepatology.* 2009;49(3):989-997.
30. Li Z, Yang S, Lin H, et al. Probiotics and antibodies to TNF inhibit inflammatory activity and improve nonalcoholic fatty liver disease. *Hepatology.* 2003;37(2):343-350.
31. Segawa S, Wakita Y, Hirata H, Watari J. Oral administration of heat-killed *Lactobacillus brevis* SBC8803 ameliorates alcoholic liver disease in ethanol-containing diet-fed C57BL/6N mice. *Int J Food Microbiol.* 2008;128(2):371-377.
32. Ma X, Hua J, Li Z. Probiotics improve high fat diet-induced hepatic steatosis and insulin resistance by increasing hepatic NKT cells. *J Hepatol.* 2008;49(5):821-830.
33. Solga SF, Buckley G, Clark JM, Horska A, Diehl AM. The effect of a probiotic on hepatic steatosis. *J Clin Gastroenterol.* 2008;42(10):1117-1119.
34. Loguercio C, De Simone T, Federico A, et al. Gut-liver axis: a new point of attack to treat chronic liver damage? *Am J Gastroenterol.* 2002;97(8):2144-2146.
35. Loguercio C, Federico A, Tuccillo C, et al. Beneficial effects of a probiotic VSL#3 on parameters of liver dysfunction in chronic liver diseases. *J Clin Gastroenterol.* 2005;39(6):540-543.
36. Lirussi F, Mastropasqua E, Orando S, Orlando R. Probiotics for non-alcoholic fatty liver disease and/or steatohepatitis. *Cochrane Database Syst Rev.* 2007;(1):CD005165.
37. Planas R, Ballesté B, Álvarez MA, et al. Natural history of decompensated hepatitis C virus-related cirrhosis. A study of 200 patients. *J Hepatol.* 2004;40(5):823-830.
38. Strauss E, Gomes de Sá Ribeiro MF. Bacterial infections associated with hepatic encephalopathy: prevalence and outcome. *Ann Hepatol.* 2003;2(1):41-45.
39. Yoneyama K, Miyagishi K, Kiuchi Y, Shibata M, Mitamura K. Risk factors for infections in cirrhotic patients with and without hepatocellular carcinoma. *J Gastroenterol.* 2002;37(12):1028-1034.
40. Fernandez J, Navasa M, Gomez J, et al. Bacterial infections in cirrhosis: epidemiological changes with invasive procedures and norfloxacin prophylaxis. *Hepatology.* 2002;35(1):140-148.
41. Borzio M, Salerno F, Piantoni L, et al. Bacterial infection in patients with advanced cirrhosis: a multicentre prospective study. *Dig Liver Dis.* 2001;33(1):41-48.
42. Thulstrup AM, Sorensen HT, Schonheyder HC, Moller JK, Tage-Jensen U. Population-based study of the risk and short-term prognosis for bacteremia in patients with liver cirrhosis. *Clin Infect Dis.* 2000;31(6):1357-1361.
43. Yoshida H, Hamada T, Inuzuka S, Ueno T, Sata M, Tanikawa K. Bacterial infection in cirrhosis, with and without hepatocellular carcinoma. *Am J Gastroenterol.* 1993;88(12):2067-2071.
44. Caly WR, Strauss E. A prospective study of bacterial infections in patients with cirrhosis. *J Hepatol.* 1993;18(3):353-358.
45. Zhao C, Chen SB, Zhou JP, et al. Prognosis of hepatic cirrhosis patients with esophageal or gastric variceal hemorrhage: multivariate analysis. *Hepatobiliary Pancreatic Dis Int.* 2002;1(3):416-419.
46. Deschênes M, Villeneuve JP. Risk factors for the development of bacterial infections in hospitalized patients with cirrhosis. *Am J Gastroenterol.* 1999;94(8):2193-2197.
47. Bernard B, Cadranel JF, Valla D, Escolano S, Jarlier V, Opolon P. Prognostic significance of bacterial infection in bleeding cirrhotic patients: a prospective study. *Gastroenterology.* 1995;108(6):1828-1834.
48. Riordan SM, Williams R. The intestinal flora and bacterial infection in cirrhosis. *J Hepatol.* 2006;45(5):744-757.
49. Rajkovic IA, Williams R. Abnormalities of neutrophil phagocytosis, intracellular killing and metabolic activity in alcoholic cirrhosis and hepatitis. *Hepatology.* 1986;6(2):252-262.

50. Ewaschuk J, Endersby R, Thiel D, et al. Probiotic bacteria prevent hepatic damage and maintain colonic barrier function in a mouse model of sepsis. *Hepatology.* 2007;46(3):841-850.
51. Chiva M, Soriano G, Rochat I, et al. Effect of *Lactobacillus johnsonii* La1 and antioxidants on intestinal flora and bacterial translocation in rats with experimental cirrhosis. *J Hepatol.* 2002;37(4):456-462.
52. Bauer TM, Fernandez J, Navasa M, Vila J, Rodes J. Failure of *Lactobacillus* spp. to prevent bacterial translocation in a rat model of experimental cirrhosis. *J Hepatol.* 2002;36(4):501-506.
53. Liu Q, Duan ZP, Ha DK, Bengmark S, Kurtovic J, Riordan SM. Synbiotic modulation of gut flora: effect on minimal hepatic encephalopathy in patients with cirrhosis. *Hepatology.* 2004;39(5):1441-1449.
54. Lata J, Novotny I, Pribramska V, et al. The effect of probiotics on gut flora, level of endotoxin and Child-Pugh score in cirrhotic patients: results of a double-blind randomized study. *Eur J Gastroenterol Hepatol.* 2007;19(12):1111-1113.
55. Shigeta H, Nagino M, Kamiya J, et al. Bacteremia after hepatectomy: an analysis of a single-center, 10-year experience with 407 patients. *Langenbecks Arch Surg.* 2002;387(3-4):117-124.
56. Bengmark S. Aggressive peri- and intraoperative enteral nutrition—strategy for the future. In: Shikora SA, Martindale RG, Schwaitzberg SD, eds. *Nutritional Considerations in the Intensive Care Unit—Science, Rationale and Practice.* Dubuque, IA: Kendall Hunt Publishing; 2002:365-380.
57. Bolton JS, Fuhrman GM. Survival after resection of multiple bilobar hepatic metastases from colorectal carcinoma. *Ann Surg.* 2000;231(5):743-751.
58. Seehofer D, Rayes N, Schiller R, et al. Probiotics partly reverse increased bacterial translocation after simultaneous liver resection and colonic anastomosis in rats. *J Surg Res.* 2004;117(2):262-271.
59. Stadlbauer V, Mookerjee RP, Hodges S, Wright GA, Davies NA, Jalan R. Effect of probiotic treatment on deranged neutrophil function and cytokine responses in patients with compensated alcoholic cirrhosis. *J Hepatol.* 2008;48(6):945-951.
60. Rayes N, Seehofer D, Hansen S, et al. Early enteral supply of *Lactobacillus* and fiber versus selective bowel decontamination: a controlled trial in liver transplant recipients. *Transplantation.* 2002;74(1):123-127.
61. Rayes N, Seehofer D, Theruvath T, et al. Supply of pre- and probiotics reduces bacterial infection rates after liver transplantation: a randomized, double-blind trial. *Am J Transplant.* 2005;5(1):125-130.
62. Gurusamy KS, Kumar Y, Davidson BR. Methods of preventing bacterial sepsis and wound complications for liver transplantation. *Cochrane Database Syst Rev.* 2008;(4)(4):CD006660.
63. Besselink MG, van Santvoort HC, Buskens E, et al. Probiotic prophylaxis in predicted severe acute pancreatitis: a randomised, double-blind, placebo-controlled trial. *Lancet.* 2008;371(9613):651-659.
64. Munoz SJ. Hepatic encephalopathy. *Med Clin North Am.* 2008;92(4):795-812, viii.
65. Kalaitzakis E, Olsson R, Henfridsson P, et al. Malnutrition and diabetes mellitus are related to hepatic encephalopathy in patients with liver cirrhosis. *Liver Int.* 2007;27(9):1194-1201.
66. Das A, Dhiman RK, Saraswat VA, Verma M, Naik SR. Prevalence and natural history of subclinical hepatic encephalopathy in cirrhosis. *J Gastroenterol Hepatol.* 2001;16(5):531-535.
67. Nicaise C, Prozzi D, Viaene E, et al. Control of acute, chronic, and constitutive hyperammonemia by wild-type and genetically engineered *Lactobacillus plantarum* in rodents. *Hepatology.* 2008;48(4):1184-1192.
68. Jia L, Zhang MH. Comparison of probiotics and lactulose in the treatment of minimal hepatic encephalopathy in rats. *World J Gastroenterol.* 2005;11(6):908-911.
69. Bajaj JS, Saeian K, Christensen KM, et al. Probiotic yogurt for the treatment of minimal hepatic encephalopathy. *Am J Gastroenterol.* 2008;103(7):1707-1715.
70. Zhao HY, Wang HJ, Lu Z, Xu SZ. Intestinal microflora in patients with liver cirrhosis. *Chin J Dig Dis.* 2004;5(2):64-67.
71. Malaguarnera M, Greco F, Barone G, Gargante MP, Malaguarnera M, Toscano MA. *Bifidobacterium longum* with fructo-oligosaccharide (FOS) treatment in minimal hepatic encephalopathy: a randomized, double-blind, placebo-controlled study. *Dig Dis Sci.* 2007;52(11):3259-3265.
72. Osman N, Adawi D, Ahrne S, Jeppsson B, Molin G. Endotoxin- and D-galactosamine-induced liver injury improved by the administration of *Lactobacillus, Bifidobacterium* and blueberry. *Dig Liver Dis.* 2007;39(9):849-856.
73. Adawi D, Ahrne S, Molin G. Effects of different probiotic strains of *Lactobacillus* and *Bifidobacterium* on bacterial translocation and liver injury in an acute liver injury model. *Int J Food Microbiol.* 2001;70(3):213-220.
74. Marotta F, Barreto R, Wu CC, et al. Experimental acute alcohol pancreatitis-related liver damage and endotoxemia: synbiotics but not metronidazole have a protective effect. *Chin J Dig Dis.* 2005;6(4):193-197.
75. Kirpich IA, Solovieva NV, Leikhter SN, et al. Probiotics restore bowel flora and improve liver enzymes in human alcohol-induced liver injury: a pilot study. *Alcohol.* 2008;42(8):675-682.

76. Vleggaar FP, Monkelbaan JF, van Erpecum KJ. Probiotics in primary sclerosing cholangitis: a randomized placebo-controlled crossover pilot study. *Eur J Gastroenterol Hepatol.* 2008;20(7):688-692.

77. El-Nezami HS, Polychronaki NN, Ma J, et al. Probiotic supplementation reduces a biomarker for increased risk of liver cancer in young men from Southern China. *Am J Clin Nutr.* 2006;83(5):1199-1203.

78. el-Nezami H, Kankaanpaa P, Salminen S, Ahokas J. Physicochemical alterations enhance the ability of dairy strains of lactic acid bacteria to remove aflatoxin from contaminated media. *J Food Prot.* 1998;61(4):466-468.

79. Pierides M, El-Nezami H, Peltonen K, Salminen S, Ahokas J. Ability of dairy strains of lactic acid bacteria to bind aflatoxin M1 in a food model. *J Food Prot.* 2000;63(5):645-650.

80. Qian GS, Ross RK, Yu MC, et al. A follow-up study of urinary markers of aflatoxin exposure and liver cancer risk in Shanghai, People's Republic of China. *Cancer Epidemiol Biomarkers Prev.* 1994;3(1):3-10.

81. Roebuck BD, Liu YL, Rogers AE, Groopman JD, Kensler TW. Protection against aflatoxin B1-induced hepatocarcinogenesis in F344 rats by 5-(2-pyrazinyl)-4-methyl-1,2-dithiole-3-thione (oltipraz): predictive role for short-term molecular dosimetry. *Cancer Res.* 1991;51(20):5501-5506.

24

Probiotics Use in Bacterial Vaginosis and Vulvovaginal Candidiasis

Paola Mastromarino, PhD; Beatrice Vitali, PhD; and Luciana Mosca, PhD

The female lower genital tract, consisting of vagina and ectocervix, is an ecological niche where several aerobe and anaerobe microorganisms coexist in a dynamic balance. The homeostasis of the vaginal ecosystem results from complex interactions and synergies among the host and different microorganisms that colonize the vaginal mucosa.[1,2] This ecosystem is dynamic with changes in structure and composition being influenced by age, menarche, time in menstrual cycle, pregnancy, infections, methods of birth control, sexual activity, use of medication, and hygiene.[3]

In healthy women, the vaginal ecosystem is dominated by *Lactobacillus* spp., but a diverse array of other bacteria can be present in much lower numbers. *L. iners*, *L. acidophilus*, *L. gasseri*, *L. crispatus*, and *L. vaginalis* are the predominant vaginal *Lactobacillus* species.[4,5] Mainly, frequent undesirable organisms are yeasts (*Candida albicans*, *C. tropicalis*, *C. krusei*), anaerobic bacteria responsible for vaginosis (*Gardnerella vaginalis*, *Atopobium vaginae*, *Prevotella*, *Veillonella*), uropathogens (*E. coli*, *Proteus*, *Klebsiella*, *Serratia*), and sexually transmitted viruses (HIV, Herpes virus).[5] Lactobacilli are involved in maintaining the normal vaginal microflora by preventing overgrowth of pathogenic and opportunistic organisms.[6] The principal mechanisms by which lactobacilli exert their protective functions are (1) stimulation of the immune system, (2) competition with other microorganisms for the nutrients and for adherence to the vaginal epithelium, (3) reduction of the vaginal pH by the production of organic acids, especially lactic acid, and (4) production of antimicrobial substances, such as bacteriocins, and hydrogen peroxide.[7] This latter microbial metabolite represents one of the most effective protective agents against pathogens. It has been observed that 70% to 95% of lactobacilli present in the vaginal flora of healthy women produce hydrogen peroxide. This percentage drops to 5% in women affected by vaginal infections.[8]

Floch MH, Kim AS, eds.
Probiotics: A Clinical Guide (pp 321-334)
© 2010 Taylor & Francis Group

BACTERIAL VAGINOSIS

Bacterial vaginosis (BV) represents the most common vaginal syndrome affecting fertile, premenopausal, and pregnant women, with an incidence rate ranging from 5% to 50%.[2] BV is a complex, polymicrobial disorder characterized by an overgrowth of strict or facultative anaerobic bacteria (*G. vaginalis*, *Prevotella*, *Mobiluncus*, *Mycoplasma hominis*) and a reduction in lactobacilli, particularly those producing hydrogen peroxide.[9,10] Women with BV typically complain of vaginal discomfort and homogeneous malodorous vaginal discharge, which is more noticeable after unprotected intercourse, although a substantial fraction of women are asymptomatic.[11] The overgrowth of vaginal anaerobes determines an increased production of amines (putrescine, cadaverine, and trimethylamine) that become volatile at alkaline pH, that is, after sexual intercourse and during menstrual cycle, and contribute to the typical malodor of the vaginal discharge.[12] BV is frequently underestimated because the symptoms are often insignificant; however, the clinical consequences could be important. In fact, the alterations in the vaginal microbiology have been associated with ascending infections and obstetrical complications,[13] as well as with urinary tract infections.[14] Increasing data also indicate that BV facilitates the acquisition of sexually transmitted diseases such as *Neisseria gonorrhoeae*, *Chlamydia trachomatis*, HIV, and Herpes simplex virus type-2 infection (HSV-2).[15-17] Moreover, genital tract shedding of HSV-2[18] and cytomegalovirus[19] is significantly higher in women affected by BV than in BV-free women, and female genital tract HIV load correlates inversely with *Lactobacillus* count.[20] Therefore, vaginal lactobacilli exert in vivo an important role in sexually transmitted infections both in relation to the protection of female health or by reducing the risk of virus transmission from an infected woman to a healthy man.

Two methods are used for BV diagnosis: the first was described by Amsel et al,[21] which implies the presence of at least 3 of the following criteria: (1) thin, homogeneous vaginal discharge; (2) vaginal pH higher than 4.5; (3) "fishy" odor of vaginal fluid after addition of 10% KOH (whiff test); and (4) presence of clue cells on microscopic evaluation of saline wet preparations. The second method, the Gram stain score of vaginal smears according to Nugent et al,[22] involves the microscopic quantitation of bacterial morphotypes yielding a score between 0 and 10. A Gram stain score ≥ 7 is considered indicative of BV.

In recent years, culture-independent techniques based on the analysis of rRNA gene sequences have been developed, providing powerful tools to reveal the phylogenetic diversity of the microorganisms found within the vaginal ecosystem and to understand community dynamics.[9,23-25] These molecular studies indicate that the vaginal bacterial communities are dramatically different between women with and without BV. BV is associated with increased taxonomic richness and diversity. The microbiota composition is highly variable among subjects at a fine taxonomic scale (species or genus level), but, at the phylum level, actinobacteria and bacteroidetes are strongly associated with BV, while higher proportions of firmicutes are found in healthy subjects. Several vaginal bacteria have been indicated as excellent markers of BV, either alone or in combination, including *Megasphaera*, 3 novel bacteria in the order *Clostridiales*, *Leptotrichia/Sneathia*, *A. vaginae*, and an *Eggerthella*-like bacterium.

Therapy of BV involves oral or local administration of metronidazole or intravaginal clindamycin and varies in efficacy (48% to 85% for absence of infection 4 or more weeks after treatment).[13] The long-term cure rate is low; BV recurs in up to 40% of women within 3 months after initiation of antibiotic therapy and in up to 50% of women after 6 months.[26] There are several unpleasant side effects and disadvantages associated with these therapies, including superinfections by pathogenic microorganisms[27] and susceptibility of lactobacilli to clindamycin.[28] Moreover, vaginal pathogens, particularly *G. vaginalis* and anaerobic bacteria, are showing increasing drug resistance.[29,30] The high recurrence rates resulting in repeated exposure to antibiotics and the emergence of drug-resistant strains suggest a need for alternative therapeutic tools.

VULVOVAGINAL CANDIDIASIS

Vaginitis is a common gynecological condition that may significantly affect the patient's quality of life and is one of the most common reasons for a gynecologic consultation. It is characterized by abnormal or increased discharge, itching, burning, irritation, and sometimes even painful urination or vaginal bleeding. The most common causative agents of vaginitis in adults are *Candida* spp. and *Trichomonas vaginalis*.[2]

Vulvovaginal candidiasis (VVC) accounts for the majority of vaginitis cases. There are tens of different species of *Candida*, and the most common causative agent for vaginitis is *C. albicans*.[2] It has been estimated that 75% of women can be affected by VVC at least once during their lifetime. Between 40% and 50% of these women are affected by recurrent VVC, and 5% to 8% experience chronic *Candida* infections, which may indicate underlying immunodeficiency or diabetes.[2,31] Topical and systemic drugs are available for the treatment of VVC. Antifungal imidazoles, such as fluconazole, clotrimazole, miconazole, terconazole, or tioconazole, with dosing schedules ranging from 1 to 7 days depending on the particular product and on the route of administration, usually achieve cure rates between 75% and 90%. Despite treatment, however, symptoms may persist or recur, with recurrent VVC defined as 4 or more confirmed candidal infections in 1 year.[31] The pathogenesis of VVC remains elusive; however, it seems that a microflora imbalance may facilitate *Candida* overgrowth.

RATIONALE FOR USING PROBIOTICS IN GENITOURINARY INFECTIONS

Probiotics have been defined as "live microorganisms which, when administered in adequate amounts, confer a health benefit on the host."[32] The rationale for the use of probiotics in women is based on the genitourinary regulatory role played by the vaginal health microbiota and the need for restoration of this microbial ecosystem after insult. Lactobacilli are the organisms commonly used as probiotics. The use of lactobacilli to reestablish a physiological microbial flora of the female urogenital tract dates back to early 1900s (reviewed by Sieber and Dietz).[33] From the beginning of the 1990s, there has been a renewed interest in the use of probiotic products in the treatment and prevention of BV and vaginitis. Because antimicrobial treatment of urogenital infections is not always effective, and problems remain due to bacterial and yeast resistance, recurrent infections, as well as side effects, it is not surprising that alternative remedies are of interest to patients and their caregivers.

This chapter reviews the most relevant current literature and investigations on probiotics' potential to prevent and treat BV and VVC.

CLINICAL TRIALS

Clinical Trials of Lactobacilli in the Treatment or Prevention of Bacterial Vaginosis

Two types of experimental approaches have been used in clinical trials using probiotics for treatment of BV. In the first, BV therapy was carried out using only probiotics. In the second, probiotics were administered following a conventional antibiotic therapy. The more relevant trials using the first type of approach on women affected by BV are reported in Table 24-1. Only 2 studies employing different species of lactobacilli have been performed using well-characterized and well-selected strains specific for treatment of genitourinary infections.[34,35] In both studies, a combination of different species of lactobacilli with different biological properties has been used on fertile, nonpregnant women. *L. rhamnosus* GR-1 and *L. fermentum* RC-14 were the strains used in the first study.[34] *L. rhamnosus* GR-1 adheres strongly to uroepithelial cells and inhibits adhesion and growth of uropathogens.[36] *L. fermentum* RC-14 produces significant amounts of hydrogen peroxide, adheres to uroepithelial cells, and inhibits pathogen binding.[37] These strains can be recovered from the vagina after oral administration.[38] In the second, study a product called Florisia containing a combination of 3 strains of lactobacilli (*L. brevis* CD2, *L. salivarius* FV2, and *L. plantarum* FV9) has been used. *L. salivarius* FV2 and *L. plantarum* FV9 produce anti-infective agents, including hydrogen peroxide, and are able to coaggregate efficiently with vaginal pathogens.[39] *L. plantarum* FV9 and *L. brevis* CD2 strains are able to adhere at high levels to human epithelial cells, displacing vaginal pathogens.[39] All the strains were able to temporarily colonize the human vagina after 5 days of treatment.[40] A single-blind comparison of intravaginal probiotics (*L. rhamnosus* GR-1 and *L. fermentum* RC-14) and metronidazole gel for the treatment of BV was carried out on a group of Nigerian women.[34] Cure of BV was based on a Nugent score ≤ 3 at 30 days. A BV cure rate of 55% was achieved after probiotic treatment compared to 33% of the metronidazole therapy (P = NS). In the double-blind, placebo-controlled trial,[35] both the Amsel criteria and Nugent scores were utilized to assess BV cure, as recommended by FDA.[41] In the intravaginal probiotic-treated group (*L. brevis* CD2, *L. salivarius* FV2, and *L. plantarum* FV9), a BV cure rate of 50% was obtained compared to 6% of placebo-treated group with the combined test methods, whereas 67% vs 12% cure rate was obtained when considering only the Amsel criteria. The other clinical studies were performed using different strains of *L. acidophilus*. In pregnant women, a high BV cure rate according to the Amsel criteria was reported in the probiotic group (87%) treated with a commercial yogurt douche, containing *L. acidophilus* of unknown designation, compared to 15% cure rate in untreated control group.[42] A similar BV cure rate (88%) was observed in a placebo-controlled study using a pharmaceutical product called Gynoflor (containing a H_2O_2-producing *L. acidophilus* strain plus estriol) that included both pregnant and nonpregnant women.[43] However, the results reported in this trial may have been invalidated by the enrollment criteria in which only 2 of the 4 Amsel criteria needed to be positive. In 2 trials, *Lactobacillus* treatment of BV assessed according to Amsel criteria turned out to be ineffective.[44,45] In the first study,[44] a commercially available yogurt was used, whereas in the second,[45] a product called Vivag, made up of H_2O_2-producing freeze-dried *L. acidophilus*, was utilized. It is difficult to evaluate the real efficacy of the product tested in the last study because 50% of the patients in the active group and 86% of the placebo group did not complete the trial.

TABLE 24-1

CLINICAL TRIALS ON PROBIOTICS USE FOR TREATMENT OF BACTERIAL VAGINOSIS

REFERENCES	SIZE/N° OF ARMS	TYPE OF STUDY/ DURATION	INTERVENTION	RESULTS
Anukam et al[34]	40; 2	R, AC; 30 days	Daily vaginal capsule containing *L. rhamnosus* GR-1 (10^9 CFU) and *L. reuteri* RC-14 (10^9 CFU) or 0.75% metronidazole gel bid for 5 days	BV cure rate: 55% compared to 33% metronidazole ($P = .056$)
Mastromarino et al[35]	34; 2	R, DB, PC; 3 weeks	Daily vaginal tablet containing $\geq 10^9$ CFU of *L. brevis* CD2, *L. salivarius* FV2, and *L. plantarum* FV9 for 7 days	BV cure rate: 50% compared to 6% control ($P = .017$)
Neri et al[42]	84; 3	R, OL; 60 days	Intravaginal yogurt containing *L. acidophilus* $>10^9$ CFU, bid for 7 days, repeated 1 week later	BV cure rate: 87% probiotic group compared to 37% acetic acid tampon-treated group ($P = .04$) or 5% untreated control group ($P < .0005$)
Parent et al[43]	32; 2	R, PC; 4 weeks	1 to 2 daily vaginal tablets containing *L. acidophilus* $\geq 10^7$ CFU and 0.03 mg estriol for 6 days	BV cure rate: 88% compared to 22% control ($P < .05$)
Fredricsson et al[44]	61; 4	R, OL, AC; 4 weeks	Intravaginal fermented milk containing *L. acidophilus* (2.5×10^9 to 1×10^{10} CFU), or 500 mg metronidazole tablet, bid, for 7 days	BV cure rate: 7% probiotic compared to 93% metronidazole, 18% acetic acid jelly, 6% estrogen cream
Hallén et al[45]	57; 2	R, DB, PC; 20 to 40 days	Vaginal suppository containing *L. acidophilus* 10^{8-9} CFU or placebo bid for 6 days	BV cure rate: 21% compared to 0% control ($P = NS$)

R = randomized; DB = double-blind; PC = placebo-controlled; AC = active-controlled; OL = open-label; CFU = colony-forming units.

TABLE 24-2

CLINICAL TRIALS ON PROBIOTICS USE FOLLOWING ANTIBIOTIC TREATMENT FOR BACTERIAL VAGINOSIS

AUTHORS	SIZE	TYPE OF STUDY/ DURATION	INTERVENTION	RESULTS
Anukam et al[46]	125	R, DB, PC; 30 days	Oral metronidazole 500 mg bid for 7 days and oral capsules containing *L. rhamnosus* GR-1 (10^9 CFU) and *L. reuteri* RC-14 (10^9 CFU) or placebo bid for 30 days starting on day 1 of metronidazole treatment	BV cure rate: 88% probiotic compared to 40% control ($P < .001$)
Petricevic and Witt[47]	190	R, OB, PC; 4 weeks	Oral clindamycin 300 mg bid for 7 days, then vaginal capsules containing 10^9 CFU of *L. casei rhamnosus* for 7 days	BV cure rate: 83% probiotic compared to 35% control ($P < .001$)
Larsson et al[48]	100	R, DB, PC; 6 menstrual periods	Vaginal 2% clindamycin cream directly followed by vaginal capsules containing *L. gasseri* Lba EB01-DSM 14869 (10^{8-9} CFU) and *L. rhamnosus* Lbp PB01-DSM 14870 (10^{8-9} CFU) for 10 days, probiotic treatment repeated for 10 days after each menstruation during 3 menstrual cycles	BV cure rate: 65% probiotic compared to 46% control ($P = .042$)
Eriksson et al[49]	187	R, DB, PC; 2 menstrual periods	Vaginal 100 mg clindamycin ovules for 3 days, then tampons containing 10^8 CFU of *L. gasseri, L. casei rhamnosus, L. fermentum,* or placebo tampons during the next menstrual period	BV cure rate: 56% compared to 62% control ($P = NS$)

R = randomized; DB = double-blind; PC = placebo-controlled; OB = observe-blind; CFU = colony-forming units.

In 4 randomized controlled trials, lactobacilli were used following conventional antibiotic treatment (Table 24-2).[46-49] A trial in Nigeria evaluated augmentation of antimicrobial metronidazole therapy of BV by a 30-day oral probiotic treatment (*L. rhamnosus* GR-1 and *L. fermentum* RC-14) compared to placebo-treated control.[46] At the end of treatment, a significantly greater number of women in the probiotic group were BV-free compared to the placebo group (Nugent score ≤ 3). In the other trials, *Lactobacillus* treatment was performed after clindamycin therapy. In the first study, a product called Gynophilus containing *L. casei rhamnosus* (Lcr35) was used in the intervention group, whereas women in the control group did not receive Lcr35.[47] BV cure rate was evaluated by Nugent method 4 weeks after the last administration of medication in both groups. A significantly higher cure rate was obtained in the intervention group. The efficacy of *Lactobacillus* supplementation after clindamycin treatment on the recurrence rate of BV was evaluated.[48] A 10-day repeated treatment with EcoVag (*L. gasseri* Lba EB01-DSM 14869 and *L. rhamnosus* Lbp PB01-DSM 14870) during 3 menstrual cycles was compared with a placebo treatment on BV-affected women enrolled according to Amsel criteria. The cure was evaluated by the Hay/Ison score.[50] Lactobacilli did not improve the efficacy of BV therapy during the first month of treatment, but it significantly reduced the recurrence rate of BV at 6 months from initiation of treatment. Administration of tampons impregnated with *L. gasseri*, *L. casei* subsp. *rhamnosus*, and *L. fermentum* or placebo tampons during the menstrual period following clindamycin treatment was exploited.[49] Cure rates assessed by Amsel criteria after the second menstrual period did not show a significant difference between the 2 groups. Possible explanations for the lack of effects could be the low amount of lactobacilli in tampons at the end of the study (10^6CFU) or the unfavorable period of administration, ie, during the menstrual flow.

Clinical Trials of Lactobacilli in the Treatment or Prevention of Recurrence of Candida Vaginitis

Candida treatment with lactobacilli has been recently extensively reviewed by Jeavons and Falagas et al.[31,51] This chapter will focus only on the most relevant clinical reports (Tables 24-3 and 24-4).

Trials were designed to prevent the recurrence of candidiasis in women affected by recurrent VVC[52-54] or to treat *Candida* infection.[55,56] Two trials evaluated the effectiveness of 2 different yogurt preparations containing viable *L. acidophilus* strains of unknown designation on the recurrence rate of VVC in women who reported a history of recurrent candidiasis. In the first study,[52] which had a crossover design, 8 ounces of a commercial yogurt preparation containing >10^8 CFU/mL were ingested daily for 6 months, followed by 6 months in which the patient was instructed not to eat yogurt, and vice versa in the second arm. The mean number of candidiasis episodes was 2.54 ± 1.66 in the control arm and 0.38 ± 0.51 in the treatment arm ($P = .001$). Yogurt treatment was also effective in hindering *Candida* colonization regardless of clinical evidence of infection ($P < .001$). The second study[53] evaluated the effect of a daily dose of 150 mL of another yogurt preparation containing viable *L. acidophilus* (>10^8 CFU/mL) compared to a pasteurized yogurt. Though the vaginal colonization by *L. acidophilus* was greater in treated women, there was no significant difference in *Candida* vaginitis or *Candida* colonization between the 2 arms. Both of these studies had some flaws. The attrition rate was very high, with only a small percentage of women completing the study protocol as originally designed (13/33 for the Hilton study[52] and 7/46 for the Shalev study[53]). In the Hilton study,[52] randomization was inappropriate, as women did not want to change treatment and switch to control when first assuming yogurt; hence, 8 months into the study, the authors decided to change the protocol so that all the patients started the treatment in the control arm. The original design of the Shalev[53] trial was also a crossover design. However, due to the high attrition rate, the study only reports data from the first 4-month period.

A third study[54] evaluated the incidence of VVC in HIV-positive women who were using 2 self-care approaches as prophylaxis—ie, weekly intravaginal application of

TABLE 24-3

CLINICAL TRIALS ON PROBIOTICS USE FOR TREATMENT OR PREVENTION OF RECURRENCE OF VULVOVAGINAL CANDIDIASIS

REFERENCES	SIZE/N OF ARMS	TYPE OF STUDY/ DURATION	INTERVENTION	RESULTS
Hilton et al[52]	33; 2	R, OL, CO; 12 months	Crossover study. Ingested yogurt containing *L. acidophilus* >2.4 × 10^{10} CFU for 6 months and then 6 months with no yogurt. Vice versa in the other group	Mean number of Candida infections lower during the 6 months of consuming yogurt ($P = .001$)
Shalev et al[53]	46; 2	R, OL, CO; 4 months	Ingested yogurt containing *L. acidophilus* >1.5 × 10^{10} CFU for 2 months vs pasteurized yogurt, then 2 months of washout. Vice versa in the other group	No significant difference in Candida cultures or candidiasis in the 2 groups ($P = .67$)
Williams et al[54]	164; 3	R, DB, PC; 21 months	Intravaginal *L. acidophilus* or vaginal clotrimazole (100 mg) once a week vs placebo	Relative risk vs placebo: 0.5 for *Lactobacillus*-treated group (not significant) and 0.4 for clotrimazole-treated group (significant)

R = randomized; DB = double-blind; PC = placebo-controlled; OL = open-label; CO = crossover; CFU = colony-forming units.

clotrimazole tablets or intravaginal application of *L. acidophilus* of unknown definition and unknown amount. The trial was a randomized, double-blind, placebo-controlled study, in which women underwent a complete medical evaluation every 6 months for a median period of 21 months. The primary study outcome was the relative risk of experiencing an episode of VVC while on treatment. The rate of VVC in each of the treatment groups was approximately half of that in the placebo group, with a relative risk of 0.4 for clotrimazole and 0.5 for *L. acidophilus*, respectively. However, in comparison with the placebo arm, the reduction risk was statistically significant only for clotrimazole. This is a well-designed trial with a large number of enrolled subjects, but it applied very restrictive case definition for VVC, which required visualization of spores or hyphae on microscopic examination. This could have negatively affected the results, leading to a result not statistically significant for *L. acidophilus* treatment.

TABLE 24-4

CLINICAL TRIALS ON PROBIOTICS USE IN TREATMENT/PREVENTION OF VULVOVAGINAL CANDIDIASIS AFTER ANTIBIOTIC TREATMENT

REFERENCES	SIZE/N OF ARMS	TYPE OF STUDY/ DURATION	INTERVENTION	RESULTS
Martinez et al[55]	55; 2	R, DB, PC; 4 weeks	Single dose of fluconazole (150 mg) followed by a 4-week treatment of daily oral *L. rhamnosus* GR-1 and *L. reuteri* RC-14 (4 × 10⁹ CFU) or placebo	Probiotic group showed a lower yeast colonization (P = .014)
Witt[56]	150; 3	R, OL; 12 months	One group was treated with itraconazole (200 mg bid) twice a week for the first month, then once a month for the following 5 months. A second group was treated with itraconazole as in the first group, plus intravaginal *L. gasseri* (2 × 10⁸·⁹ CFU) for 6 consecutive days/ month during maintenance period. A third group was treated only with classic homeopathy	Lactobacilli do not confer an added benefit to monthly cycles of itraconazole

R = randomized; DB = double-blind; PC = placebo-controlled; OL = open-label; CFU = colony-forming units.

A less restrictive case definition might have resulted in a greater number of cases and stronger treatment effect.

Two recently published trials evaluated the efficacy of probiotic products in the treatment of women affected by active VVC.[55,56] The first study[55] evaluated the effectiveness of a combination of single-dose fluconazole plus *L. rhamnosus* GR-1 and *L. reuteri* RC-14. Women were treated with fluconazole and then with the probiotic strains or a placebo for 4 weeks. At the end of treatment, women in the active group showed a lower presence of yeast detected by culture (10.3% vs 38.5%, *P* = .014) and less vaginal discharge. The second study[56] evaluated the efficacy of a combination of itraconazole plus probiotic vs itraconazole alone in women affected by recurrent VVC who presented at the clinic with active symptoms. After an initial treatment with a single dose of itraconazole for all the patients, they were randomized to the 2 different groups for the maintenance regimen. At the end of the 5-month maintenance period, 61% of women treated with itraconazole alone and 67% of women treated with itraconazole plus probiotic were free of *Candida*, while at the end of the study period (12 months), 76% of women treated with itraconazole alone and 78% of women treated with the combination were free of *Candida*. These data indicate that lactobacilli association with itraconazole does not seem to confer an additional benefit to the patients. This study was well designed and involved a large number of subjects; however, attrition rate was very high (only 71/150 women completed the trial).

DISCUSSION

In the past years, several studies have evaluated the effect of probiotic treatment in vaginal infections. The studies using lactobacilli to treat BV, albeit small in size, showed the potential of probiotics to cure BV. Although the species used in the various trials were different, 4 out of the 6 studies reported a significant cure rate.[34,35,42,43] When probiotics were used following antibiotic treatment, BV cure rate was increased and recurrence rates were reduced.[46-48] On the contrary, the effectiveness of lactobacilli treatment in *Candida* vaginitis is controversial. Though some studies have shown that some *Lactobacillus* strains are able to inhibit the growth of *C. albicans* in vitro and/or its adherence to the vaginal epithelium, in vivo studies are not always positive. However, there is a lack of well-designed, properly powered studies. A major drawback of all the trials reported is that a very high attrition rate was observed and the analysis of the data was performed only as per protocol and not as intention to treat, thus introducing a potential bias in the interpretation of the results.

The preferred route of delivery for probiotic lactobacilli was intravaginal. However, some authors delivered lactobacilli orally to repopulate the vagina, on the basis of the observation that pathogens can pass from the gut into the urogenital system and that orally administered *Lactobacillus* strains have been recovered from the vagina. It is noteworthy that the capability of the lactobacilli to colonize the vagina after oral ingestion is strictly dependent on their viability and on their potential to survive gastric acid and bile salts. Furthermore, the fact that lactobacilli can reach the vagina is not to be taken for granted as the gut microbiota and the vaginal microbiota are greatly different, which excludes a direct passage of all the species and strains present in the gut. It is also to be pointed out that because none of the trials on oral use of lactobacilli in BV or VVC evaluated the vaginal colonization by the administered strains, it cannot be excluded that the bacteria may have exerted a systemic immunomodulating effect, thus conferring an improvement of the clinical conditions. Obviously, the timing of vaginal colonization after oral administration is longer compared to direct administration at the vaginal level. Also, the load of lactobacilli that can be delivered orally to the vagina is clearly lower than direct vaginal administration.

CONCLUSION

In conclusion, lactobacilli use in VVC is at present not sufficiently supported by scientific results, while positive results have been obtained for the treatment of BV. However, lack of large and properly designed studies does not confer a high level of recommendation for the use of probiotics in vaginal infections. Also, it has to be pointed out that there were differences in the species and in the strains used, in the dosage regimen, in the route of administration, in the duration of treatment, and in the population under study in the trials conducted with probiotics. All these differences could act as confounding factors, hindering a real comparison among the trials, and also may account for the different effectiveness of the treatments in a given clinical condition.

According to the trials conducted to date, only a Level C evidence can be attributed to probiotic use in BV and VVC.[57]

REFERENCES

1. Mårdh PA. The vaginal ecosystem. *Am J Obstet Gynecol.* 1991;165:1163-1168.
2. Sobel JD. Vaginitis. *N Engl J Med.* 1997;337:1896-1903.
3. Srinivasan S, Fredricks DN. The human vaginal bacterial biota and bacterial vaginosis. *Interdiscip Perspect Infect Dis.* 2008;2008:750479.
4. Antonio MA, Hawes SE, Hillier SL. The identification of vaginal *Lactobacillus* species and the demographic and microbiologic characteristics of women colonized by these species. *J Infect Dis.* 1999;180:1950-1956.
5. Larsen B, Monif GR. Understanding the bacterial flora of the female genital tract. *Clin Infect Dis.* 2001;32: e69-e77.
6. Rönnqvist PD, Forsgren-Brusk UB, Grahn-Håkansson EE. Lactobacilli in the female genital tract in relation to other genital microbes and vaginal pH. *Acta Obstet Gynecol Scand.* 2006;85:726-735.
7. Aroutcheva A, Gariti D, Simon M, et al. Defense factors of vaginal lactobacilli. *Am J Obstet Gynecol.* 2001;185:375-379.
8. Eschenbach DA, Davick PR, Williams BL, et al. Prevalence of hydrogen peroxide-producing *Lactobacillus* species in normal women and women with bacterial vaginosis. *J Clin Microbiol.* 1989;27:251-256.
9. Fredricks DN, Fiedler TL, Marrazzo JM. Molecular identification of bacteria associated with bacterial vaginosis. *N Engl J Med.* 2005;353:1899-1911.
10. Eschenbach DA. History and review of bacterial vaginosis. *Am J Obstet Gynecol.* 1993;169:441-445.
11. Klebanoff MA, Schwebke JR, Zhang J, Nansel TR, Yu KF, Andrews WW. Vulvovaginal symptoms in women with bacterial vaginosis. *Obstet Gynecol.* 2004;104:267-272.
12. Chen KC, Forsyth PS, Buchanan TM, Holmes KK. Amine content of vaginal fluid from untreated and treated patients with nonspecific vaginitis. *J Clin Invest.* 1979;63:828-835.
13. Koumans EM, Markowitz LE, Hogan V. Indications for therapy and treatment recommendations for bacterial vaginosis in non-pregnant and pregnant women: a synthesis of data. *Clin infect Dis.* 2002;35(suppl 2): S152-S172.
14. Harmanli OH, Cheng GY, Nyirjesy P, Chatwani A, Gaughan JP. Urinary tract infections in women with bacterial vaginosis. *Obstet Gynecol.* 2000;95:710-712.
15. Martin HL, Richardson BA, Nyange PM, et al. Vaginal lactobacilli, microbial flora, and risk of human immunodeficiency virus type 1 and sexually transmitted disease acquisition. *J Infect Dis.* 1999;180: 1863-1868.
16. Cherpes TL, Meyn LA, Krohn MA, Lurie JG, Hillier SL. Association between acquisition of herpes simplex virus type 2 in women and bacterial vaginosis. *Clin Infect Dis.* 2003;37:319-325.
17. Wiesenfeld H, Hillier S, Krohn MA, Landers D, Sweet R. Bacterial vaginosis is a strong predictor of *Neisseria gonorrhoeae* and *Chlamydia trachomatis* infection. *Clin Infect Dis.* 2003;36:663-668.
18. Cherpes TL, Melan MA, Kant JA, Cosentino LA, Meyn LA, Hillier SL. Genital tract shedding of Herpes simplex virus type 2 in women: effects of hormonal contraception, bacterial vaginosis and vaginal group B *Streptococcus* colonization. *Clin Infect Dis.* 2005;40:1422-1428.
19. Ross SA, Novak Z, Ashrith G, et al. Association between genital tract cytomegalovirus infection and bacterial vaginosis. *J Infect Dis.* 2005;192:1727-1730.
20. Sha BE, Zariffard MR, Wang QJ, et al. Female genital-tract HIV load correlates inversely with *Lactobacillus* species but positively with bacterial vaginosis and *Mycoplasma hominis. J Infect Dis.* 2005;191:25-32.
21. Amsel R, Totten PA, Spiegel CA, Chen KCS, Eschenbach D, Holmes KK. Non specific vaginitis: diagnostic criteria and microbial and epidemiologic associations. *Am J Med.* 1983;74:14-22.
22. Nugent RP, Krohn MA, Hillier SL. Reliability of diagnosing bacterial vaginosis is improved by a standardized method of Gram stain interpretation. *J Clin Microbiol.* 1991;29:297-301.
23. Biagi E, Vitali B, Pugliese C, Candela M, Donders GG, Brigidi P. Quantitative variations in the vaginal bacterial population associated with asymptomatic infections: a real-time polymerase chain reaction study. *Eur J Clin Microbiol Infect Dis.* 2009;28:281-285.
24. Oakley BB, Fiedler TL, Marrazzo JM, Fredricks DN. Diversity of human vaginal bacterial communities and associations with clinically defined bacterial vaginosis. *Appl Environ Microbiol.* 2008;15: 4898-4909.
25. Vitali B, Pugliese C, Biagi E, et al. Dynamics of vaginal bacterial communities in women developing bacterial vaginosis, candidiasis, or no infection, analyzed by PCR-denaturing gradient gel electrophoresis and real-time PCR. *Appl Environ Microbiol.* 2007;73:5731-5741.

26. Bradshaw CS, Morton AN, Hocking J, et al. High recurrence rates of bacterial vaginosis over the course of 12 months after oral metronidazole therapy and factors associated with recurrence. *J Infect Dis.* 2006;193:1478-1486.

27. Sobel JD, Ferris D, Schwebke J, et al. Suppressive antibacterial therapy with 0.75% metronidazole vaginal gel to prevent recurrent bacterial vaginosis. *Am J Obstet Gynecol.* 2006;194:1283-1289.

28. Bayer AS, Chow AW, Concepcion N, Guze LB. Susceptibility of 40 lactobacilli to six antimicrobial agents with broad gram-positive anaerobic spectra. *Antimicrob Agents Chemother.* 1978;14:720-722.

29. McLean NW, McGroarty JA. Growth inhibition of metronidazole-susceptible and metronidazole-resistant strains of *Gardnerella vaginalis* by lactobacilli in vitro. *Appl Environ Microbiol.* 1996;62: 1089-1092.

30. Beigi RH, Austin MN, Meyn LA, Krohn MA, Hillier SL. Antimicrobial resistance associated with the treatment of bacterial vaginosis. *Am J Obstet Gynecol.* 2004;191:1124-1129.

31. Jeavons HS. Prevention and treatment of vulvovaginal candidiasis using exogenous *Lactobacillus*. *J Obstet Gynecol Neonatal Nurs.* 2003;32:287-296.

32. Joint FAO/WHO Working Group Report on Drafting Guidelines for the Evaluation of Probiotics in Food. London, Ontario, Canada, April 30 and May 1, 2002. http://www.who.int/foodsafety/fs_management/en/probiotic_guidelines.pdf. Accessed July 2, 2009

33. Sieber R, Dietz UT. *Lactobacillus acidophilus* and yogurt in the prevention and therapy of bacterial vaginosis. *Int Dairy J.* 1998;8:599-607.

34. Anukam KC, Osazuwa E, Osemene GI, Ehigiagbe F, Bruce AW, Reid G. Clinical study comparing probiotic *Lactobacillus GR-1* and RC-14 with metronidazole vaginal gel to treat symptomatic bacterial vaginosis. *Microbes Infect.* 2006;8:2772-2776.

35. Mastromarino P, Macchia S, Meggiorini L, et al. Effectiveness of *Lactobacillus*-containing vaginal tablets in the treatment of symptomatic bacterial vaginosis. *Clin Microbiol Infect.* 2009;15:67-74.

36. Reid G, Cook RL, Bruce AW. Examination of strains of lactobacilli for properties that may influence bacterial interference in the urinary tract. *J Urol.* 1987;138:330-335.

37. Reid G, Bruce AW. Selection of *Lactobacillus* strains for urogenital probiotic applications. *J Infect Dis.* 2001;183(suppl 1):S77-S80.

38. Reid G, Bruce AW, Fraser N, Heinemann C, Owen J, Henning B. Oral probiotics can resolve urogenital infections. *FEMS Immunol Med Microbiol.* 2001;30:49-52.

39. Mastromarino P, Brigidi P, Macchia S, et al. Characterization and selection of vaginal *Lactobacillus* strains for the preparation of vaginal tablets. *J Appl Microbiol.* 2002;93:884-893.

40. Massi M, Vitali B, Federici F, Matteuzzi D, Brigidi P. Identification method based on PCR combined with automated ribotyping for tracking probiotic *Lactobacillus* strains colonizing the human gut and vagina. *J Appl Microbiol.* 2004;96:777-786.

41. US Dept of Health and Human Services, Food and Drug Administration, Center for Drug Evaluation and Research. Guidance for industry: Bacterial vaginosis—developing antimicrobial drugs for treatment. http://www.fda.gov/downloads/Drugs/GuidanceComplianceRegulatoryInformation/Guidances/ucm070969.pdf. Accessed February 12, 2010.

42. Neri A, Sabah G, Samra Z. Bacterial vaginosis in pregnancy treated with yoghurt. *Acta Obstet Gynecol Scand.* 1993;72:17-19.

43. Parent D, Bossens M, Bayot D, et al. Therapy of bacterial vaginosis using exogenously-applied lactobacilli acidophili and a low dose of estriol: a placebo-controlled multicentric clinical trial. *Arzneimittelforschung.* 1996;46:68-73.

44. Fredricsson B, Englund K, Weintraub L, Olund A, Nord CE. Bacterial vaginosis is not a simple ecological disorder. *Gynecol Obstet Invest.* 1989;28:156-160.

45. Hallén A, Jarstrand C, Påhlson C. Treatment of bacterial vaginosis with lactobacilli. *Sex Transm Dis.* 1992;19:146-148.

46. Anukam K, Osazuwa E, Ahonkhai I, et al. Augmentation of antimicrobial metronidazole therapy of bacterial vaginosis with oral probiotic *Lactobacillus rhamnosus* GR-1 and *Lactobacillus reuteri* RC-14: randomized, double-blind, placebo-controlled trial. *Microbes Infect.* 2006;8:1450-1454.

47. Petricevic L, Witt A. The role of *Lactobacillus casei rhamnosus* Lcr35 in restoring the normal vaginal flora after antibiotic treatment of bacterial vaginosis. *BJOG.* 2008;115:1369-1374.

48. Larsson PG, Stray-Pedersen B, Ryttig KR, Larsen S. Human lactobacilli as supplementation of clindamycin to patients with bacterial vaginosis reduce the recurrence rate; a 6-month, double-blind, randomized, placebo-controlled study. *BMC Women's Health.* 2008;8:3.

49. Eriksson K, Carlsson B, Forsum U, Larsson PG. A double-blind treatment study of bacterial vaginosis with normal vaginal lactobacilli after an open treatment with vaginal clindamycin ovules. *Acta Derm Venereol.* 2005;85:42-46.

50. Ison CA, Hay PE. Validation of a simplified grading of Gram stained vaginal smears for use in genitourinary medicine clinics. *Sex Transm Infect.* 2002;78:413-415.

51. Falagas ME, Betsi GI, Athanasiou S. Probiotics for prevention of recurrent vulvovaginal candidiasis: a review. *J Antimicrob Chemother.* 2006;58:266-272.
52. Hilton E, Isenberg HD, Alperstein P, France K, Borenstein MT. Ingestion of yogurt containing *Lactobacillus acidophilus* as prophylaxis for candidal vaginitis. *Ann Intern Med.* 1992;116:353-357.
53. Shalev E, Battino S, Weiner E, Colodner R, Keness Y. Ingestion of yogurt containing *Lactobacillus acidophilus* compared with pasteurized yogurt as prophylaxis for recurrent candidal vaginitis and bacterial vaginosis. *Arch Fam Med.* 1996;5:593-596.
54. Williams AB, Yu C, Tashima K, Burgess J, Danvers K. Evaluation of two self-care treatments for prevention of vaginal candidiasis in women with HIV. *J Assoc Nurses AIDS Care.* 2001;12:51-57.
55. Martinez RC, Franceschini SA, Patta MC, et al. Improved treatment of vulvovaginal candidiasis with fluconazole plus probiotic *Lactobacillus rhamnosus* GR-1 and *Lactobacillus reuteri* RC-14. *Lett Appl Microbiol.* 2009;48:269-274.
56. Witt A, Kaufmann U, Bitschnau M, et al. Monthly itraconazole versus classic homeopathy for the treatment of recurrent vulvovaginal candidiasis: a randomised trial. *BJOG.* 2009;116(11):1499-1505.
57. Floch MH, Walker WA, Guandalini S, et al. Recommendations for probiotic use—2008. *J Clin Gastroenterol.* 2008;42(suppl 2):S104-S108.

FINANCIAL DISCLOSURES

Katie L. Blackett, BSc, PhD has no financial or proprietary interest in the materials presented herein.

Ian M. Carroll, PhD has not disclosed any relevant financial relationships.

Erika C. Claud, MD has no financial or proprietary interest in the materials presented herein.

Anne M. Dattilo, PhD, RD, CDE is a nutrition consultant to Nestle Nutrition, North America.

Levinus A. Dieleman, MD, PhD is supported by the Crohn's and Colitis Foundation of Canada (CCFC) and Canadian Institutes of Health Research (CIHR).

Shira Doron, MD has not disclosed any relevant financial relationships.

Sylvia H. Duncan, BSc, PhD has no financial or proprietary interest in the materials presented herein.

Giuseppe Famularo, MD, PhD has no financial or proprietary interest in the materials presented herein.

Richard N. Fedorak, MD, FRCP(C) has no financial or proprietary interest in the materials presented herein.

Harry J. Flint, BSc, PhD is a member of the Scientific Advisory Board of Syral.

Miguel Freitas, PhD is a full-time employee of The Dannon Company Inc.

Pramod Gopal, PhD is employed by Fonterra Co-operative Group.

Sherwood L. Gorbach, MD has not disclosed any relevant financial relationships.

Stefano Guandalini, MD has not disclosed any relevant financial relationships.

Mario Guslandi, MD, FACG has not disclosed any relevant financial relationships.

Ailsa Hart, PhD has no financial or proprietary interest in the materials presented herein.

Laurel H. Hartwell, MD has no financial or proprietary interest in the materials presented herein.

Erika Isolauri, MD, PhD has not disclosed any relevant financial relationships.

Karen Kroeker, MD, FRCP(C) has not disclosed any relevant financial relationships.

Kirsi Laitinen, PhD has not disclosed any relevant financial relationships.

George T. Macfarlane, BSc, PhD has not disclosed any relevant financial relationships.

Sandra Macfarlane, BSc, PhD has no financial or proprietary interest in the materials presented herein.

Karen L. Madsen, PhD has not disclosed any relevant financial relationships.

Paola Mastromarino, PhD has no financial or proprietary interest in the materials presented herein.

Daniel Merenstein, MD currently serves as an expert witness for General Mills.

Giovanni Minisola, MD has no financial or proprietary interest in the materials presented herein.

Luciana Mosca, PhD has no financial or proprietary interest in the materials presented herein.

Peter Neuhaus, PhD has not disclosed any relevant financial relationships.

Siew C. Ng, PhD has no financial or proprietary interest in the materials presented herein.

Eamonn M. M. Quigley, MD, FRCP, FACP, FACG, FRCPI is the Director of Alimentary Health, University College, Cork, Ireland.

Samuli Rautava, MD, PhD has not disclosed any relevant financial relationships.

Nada Rayes, MD has no financial or proprietary interest in the materials presented herein.

Yehuda Ringel, MD has not disclosed any relevant financial relationships.

Tamar Ringel-Kulka, MD, MPH has not disclosed any relevant financial relationships.

Jose M. Saavedra, MD, FAAP is the Medical and Scientific Director, Nestle Nutrition, North America.

Seppo Salminen, PhD has not disclosed any relevant financial relationships.

Mary Ellen Sanders, PhD has not disclosed any relevant financial relationships.

Daniel Seehofer, MD has not disclosed any relevant financial relationships.

Anish Sheth, MD has no financial or proprietary interest in the materials presented herein.

Christina M. Surawicz, MD, MACG has not disclosed any relevant financial relationships.

Gerald W. Tannock, PhD has no financial or proprietary interest in the materials presented herein.

Vito Trinchieri, MD has no financial or proprietary interest in the materials presented herein.

Beatrice Vitali, PhD has no financial or proprietary interest in the materials presented herein.

W. Allan Walker, MD has not disclosed any relevant financial relationships.

Index

BV (bacterial vaginosis), 123, 322-323, 324-327, 330-331

carbohydrate assimilation, regulatory mechanisms of, 85-87
carbohydrates. *See* dietary fiber and nondigestible carbohydrates; prebiotics
carbon availability, effect on fermentation product formation, 87, 88
catabolite regulatory processes, 85-87
children. *See* pediatrics
cholesterol levels, 7, 10, 76, 101, 103-104
claudins, 22
clinical studies, quality and results of, 125-126, 131, 135-136
clinical trials, charts of
  probiotic benefits in pediatric populations
    emerging areas of research, 166-168
    immune effects and acute illness, 152-155
    management of acute diarrhea, 155-160
    prevention and management of allergic conditions, 162-165
    prevention of acute diarrhea, 160-161
    prevention of antibiotic-associated diarrhea, 162
  probiotic maintenance of remission in ulcerative colitis, 249
  probiotic use following antibiotic treatment for bacterial vaginosis, 326
  probiotic use following antibiotic treatment for vulvovaginal candidiasis, 329
  probiotic use in induction/maintenance of remission in Crohn's disease, 258-260
  probiotic use in the induction of remission in ulcerative colitis, 246
  probiotic use in treatment of bacterial vaginosis, 325
  probiotic use in vulvovaginal candidiasis, 328
  yogurt, effect on diarrhea, 98-100
  yogurt, effect on fecal microbiota and biochemistry, 110-112
  yogurt, effect on *Helicobacter pylori*, 102
  yogurt, effect on lactose digestion, 106-107
  yogurt, effect on nutritional status, 108
  yogurt, effect on serum lipids, 103-104
  yogurt, effect on various immune endpoints, 115-116
Clostridium difficile infection (CDI)
  AAD, related to, 207, 211-212
  children and infants, 143, 149, 150, 198, 199
  mechanisms of action, 208
  prevention, 57, 149, 198, 199, 207, 208, 210, 212, 214
  probiotic products, 122, 123
  recurrent, 57, 212, 213-214
  treatment, 207, 212-214
colic, 122, 150-151, 167, 168

colonic transit rates, 76, 83, 85, 113
commercial probiotic products and companies, 122-123, 146-147
community-acquired diarrhea, 99, 197, 203
constipation
  prebiotics, 9, 76
  probiotics, 122, 166, 168, 275, 276, 277
Crohn's disease (CD), 253-265
  pathogenesis, 15, 16, 254-255
  prebiotics, 75, 256, 257, 259, 262
  probiotics, 126, 150, 167, 253-254, 255, 256-263
cross-feeding interactions, 75, 77, 84, 91-92, 170
culture techniques, 9, 56-58, 65, 66, 72, 113, 133-134
cystic fibrosis, 166
cytokine products, functions of, 15
cytoprotective molecules, 25

dairy products, 9
  allergic disease, 96, 97, 105, 106-107, 108, 110, 112, 114, 115, 162, 165, 237, 238
  development of, 131-138
    clinical studies, features of, 131, 135-136
    consumer appeal, 114, 134, 135
    preclinical screening of strains, 133-134
    production techniques, 96, 109, 134, 134-135
    quality control, 136-137
    safety, 136, 151
    strain specificity, 96, 109, 113, 132-133
  diarrhea, 97-101, 108, 196, 197, 198, 201-202, 208, 209
  DNA-based detection, 61, 109, 110, 111, 112, 113
  Helicobacter pylori, 296, 298-300, 301, 302
  immune system function, 113-114, 115-116
  lipid profiles, 101, 103-104
  liver disease, 309, 314, 317
  microbiological effects of, 109-113
  nutritional status, 105, 108, 114, 155
  pouchitis, 269, 270, 271
  probiotic products, 146
  ulcerative colitis, 247
  vaginal infections, 101, 105, 324, 325, 327, 328
daycare-acquired diarrhea, 197-198, 202, 203
defensins, structure and functions of, 5-6, 14, 17-18, 24
denaturing gradient gel electrophoresis (DGGE), 61, 62, 65, 66, 73
dendritic cells, functions of, 17-18, 22, 30, 31-32
DGGE (denaturing gradient gel electrophoresis), 61, 62, 65, 66, 73
diabetes, 6, 76, 313
diarrhea
  acute diarrhea
    community-acquired diarrhea, 99, 197, 197-198, 202, 203
    Helicobacter pylori, 97, 101, 102, 210

Printed in the United States
by Baker & Taylor Publisher Services

Printed in the United States
by Baker & Taylor Publisher Services